D0846928

Straight A's *in* Nursing Pharmacology

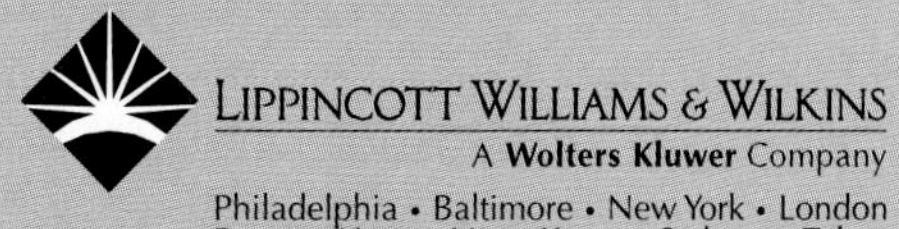
LIPPINCOTT WILLIAMS & WILKINS
A **Wolters Kluwer** Company
Philadelphia • Baltimore • New York • London
Buenos Aires • Hong Kong • Sydney • Tokyo

STAFF

Executive Publisher
Judith A. Schilling McCann, RN, MSN

Senior Acquisitions Editor
Elizabeth Nieginski

Editorial Director
David Moreau

Clinical Director
Joan M. Robinson, RN, MSN

Senior Art Director
Arlene Putterman

Clinical Project Manager
Minh N. Luu, RN, BSN, JD

Drug Information Editor
Melissa M. Devlin, PharmD

Editor
Karen C. Comerford

Copy Editors
Kimberly Bilotta (supervisor),
Doris Weinstock, Pamela Wingrod

Designers
Lynn Foulk, Debra Moloshok

Digital Composition Services
Diane Paluba (manager),
Joyce Rossi Biletz, Donna S. Morris

Manufacturing
Patricia K. Dorshaw (director),
Beth Janae Orr

Editorial Assistants
Megan L. Aldinger,
Tara L. Carter-Bell, Linda K. Ruhf

Indexer
Karen C. Comerford

The clinical treatments described and recommended in this publication are based on research and consultation with nursing, medical, and legal authorities. To the best of our knowledge, these procedures reflect currently accepted practice. Nevertheless, they can't be considered absolute and universal recommendations. For individual applications, all recommendations must be considered in light of the patient's clinical condition and, before administration of new or infrequently used drugs, in light of the latest package-insert information. The authors and publisher disclaim any responsibility for any adverse effects resulting from the suggested procedures, from any undetected errors, or from the reader's misunderstanding of the text.

© 2004 by Lippincott Williams & Wilkins. All rights reserved. This book is protected by copyright. No part of it may be reproduced, stored in a retrieval system, or transmitted, in any form or by any means — electronic, mechanical, photocopy, recording, or otherwise — without prior written permission of the publisher, except for brief quotations embodied in critical articles and reviews and testing and evaluation materials provided by publisher to instructors whose schools have adopted its accompanying textbook. Printed in the United States of America. For information, write Lippincott Williams & Wilkins, 323 Norristown Road, Suite 200, Ambler, PA 19002-2758.

STRPHM — D N O S A J
05 04 10 9 8 7 6 5 4 3 2

Library of Congress Cataloging-in-Publication Data

Straight A's in Nursing Pharmacology
p. ; cm.
Includes bibliographical references and index.
1. Pharmacology—Examinations, questions, etc.
2. Nursing—Examinations, questions, etc.
[DNLM: 1. Pharmaceutical Preparations—Examination Questions. 2. Pharmaceutical Preparations—Nurses' Instruction. 3. Pharmacology, Clinical—Examination Questions. 4. Pharmacology, Clinical—Nurses' Instruction. QV 18.2 S896 2004]
I. Lippincott Williams & Wilkins.
RM301.14.S75 2004
615'.1'076--dc22
ISBN 1-58255-286-X (pbk., hardcover : alk. paper)
2003018316

Contents

Advisory board

Ivy Alexander, PhD, CANP
Assistant Professor, Yale University, New Haven, Conn.

Susan E. Appling, RN, MS, CRNP
Assistant Professor, Johns Hopkins University School of Nursing, Baltimore

Paul M. Arnstein, PhD, APRN-BC, FNP-C
Assistant Professor, Boston College

Bobbie Berkowitz, PhD, CNAA, FAAN
Chair and Professor, Psychosocial and Community Healt, University of Washington, Seattle

Michael A. Carter, BSN, MNSc, DNSc, FAAN, APRN-BC
University Distinguished Professor, University of Tennessee, Memphis

Karla Jones, RN, MSN
Nursing Faculty; Treasure Valley Community College; Ontario, Ore.

Manon Lemonde, RN, PhD
Associate Professor, University of Ontario (Oshawa) Institute of Technology

Sheila Sparks Ralph, DNSc, RN, FAAN
Director and Professor; Division of Nursing and Respiratory Care; Shenandoah University; Winchester, Va.

Kristine Anne Scordo, PhD, RN, CS, ACNP
Director; Acute Care Nurse Practitioner Program; Wright State University, Dayton, Ohio

Contributors and consultants

Ruth Ann Benfield, RNCS, MSN, MEd, APRN, CRNP
Professor of Nursing; Montgomery County Community College; Blue Bell, Pa.

Diane S. Benson, RN, EdD(c)
Assistant Professor of Nursing; Humboldt State University; Arcata, Calif.

Daphne B. Bernard, PharmD
Assistant Professor/Clinical Pharmacist; Howard University School of Pharmacy; Washington, D.C.

Kathleen Bode, RN, MS
Chair; Division of Health & Human Services; Flint Hills Technical College; Emporia, Kan.

Lisa M. Bonsall, RN, MSN, CRNP
Independent Clinical Consultant; West Chester, Pa.

Cheryl L. Brady, RN, MSN
Adjunct Faculty; Kent State University; East Liverpool, Ohio

Sandra H. Clark, RN, MSN
Assistant Professor; Armstrong Atlantic State University; Savannah, Ga.

Valerie Daily, RN, BSN
Cardiovascular Clinical Nurse, Cardiovascular Center, Hospital of the University of Pennsylvania, Philadelphia

Teresa S. Dunsworth, PharmD, BCPS
Clinical Associate Professor of Clinical Pharmacy, West Virginia University, Morgantown

JoAnne Christa Fante, RN, BSN
Staff Nurse, Hospital of the University of Pennsylvania, Philadelphia

Susan Sard, PharmD
Clinical Pharmacist; Anne Arundel Medical Center; Annapolis, Md.

Michele F. Shepherd, PharmD, MS, BCPS, FASHP
Clinical Specialist, Abbott Northwestern Hospital, Minneapolis

Joseph F. Steiner, PharmD, RPh
Dean and Professor, College of Pharmacy, Idaho State University, Pocatello

Barbara S. Wiggins, PharmD
Clinical Pharmacy Specialist – Cardiology, University of Virginia Health System, Charlottesville

How to use this book

Straight A's is a multivolume study guide series developed especially for nursing students. Each volume provides essential course material in a unique two-column design. The easy-to-read interior outline format offers a succinct review of key facts as presented in leading textbooks on the subject. The bulleted exterior columns provide only the most crucial information, allowing for quick, efficient review right before an important quiz or test.

Special features appear in every chapter to make information accessible and easy to remember. **Learning objectives** encourage the student to evaluate knowledge before and after study. **Chapter overview** highlights the chapter's major concepts. Within the outlined text, color is used to highlight critical information and key points. Key points may include cardinal signs and symptoms, current theories, important steps in a nursing procedure, critical assessment findings, crucial nursing interventions, or successful therapies and treatments. **NCLEX checks** at the end of each chapter offer additional opportunities to review material and assess knowledge gained before moving on to new information.

Other features appear throughout the book to facilitate learning. **Time-out for teaching** highlights key areas to address when teaching patients. **Go with the flow** charts promote critical thinking. Finally, a brand-new Windows-based software program (see CD-ROM on inside back cover) poses more than 250 multiple-choice and alternate-format NCLEX-style questions in random or sequential order to assess your knowledge.

The *Straight A's* volumes are designed as learning tools, not as primary information sources. When read conscientiously as a supplement to class attendance and textbook reading, *Straight A's* can enhance understanding and help improve test scores and final grades.

Foreword

Nurses face many challenges in today's complex health care environment. More advanced technology, shrinking staffing patterns, and increased patient acuity all interact to make the nurse's work more demanding than ever. In addition, new drugs hit the market daily. Current standards of practice require that the nurse know about each medication administered. To be a safe practitioner, the nurse must dispense drugs skillfully and observe the patient for untoward effects.

Indeed, the public's concern over safe medication practices looms large. In a recent survey, nearly 25% of Americans said that they or a family member were given the wrong medication by a health care professional, and a recent headline claimed that more than 7,000 people die each year from medication errors. In fact, two preventable adverse drug events occur for every 100 admissions to U.S. hospitals. Many more incidents may not be reported. Adverse events drove up hospital costs an estimated $2.8 million annually for a 700-bed hospital. In the face of these statistics, consumers demand a safe health care environment for themselves and their families.

Responding to consumer concerns over safety, the Joint Commission on Accreditation of Healthcare Organizations recently announced six national patient safety goals for health care institutions. Three of these goals relate directly to medication administration. The National Coordinating Council for Medicine Error Reporting and Prevention recommends that nurses know the indications, precautions, and adverse reactions related to each medication given. The Council also recommends that drug information for quick reference be readily available in the direct vicinity where drugs are being prepared for administration. Implementing these guidelines is helpful in reducing the number of errors made, but no strategies are foolproof. In an attempt to further ensure patient safety, some hospitals have implemented Bar Code Systems which require scanning of the patient arm band and medication to ensure delivery of the correct medicine to the correct patient at the correct time. But errors can still be made. No matter how sophisticated the electronic equipment, the nurse remains the last line of defense against medication errors. There is no substitute for the knowledgeable nurse who can skillfully administer and carefully observe for adverse effects of drugs the patient receives.

A necessary tool in the safe administration of medicines is a reference book that can be easily and quickly checked for important facts. This text is a valuable resource for meeting the demands of current knowledge and ease of use. The format of *Straight A's in Nursing Pharmacology* provides quick accessibility to the core knowledge of each class of drugs. It is a valuable reference for student nurses who must learn an ever-increasing body of knowledge and endless bits of data which can be forgotten. Nursing students often ask, "How can I learn about thousands of different drugs?" The answer, of course, is that they can't. They can, however, learn about broad groups of drugs and indications and side effects of each group. Once that is mastered, additional information specific to individual drugs can be accessed to supplement core knowledge. This text is organized to provide quick reference to the most important facts about each drug category. The chapters begin with objectives that highlight the most critical points to master in that chapter. Drugs are organized into broad groups and then discussed as a group, including the pharmacodynamics, pharmacokinetics, indications, contraindications, and adverse reactions. Important nursing considerations conclude the discussion of each group. At the end of each chapter are several NCLEX-type questions and answers with rationales for student practice.

Straight A's in Nursing Pharmacology will be helpful to both practicing nurses and nursing students. Armed with core knowledge of broad groups of drugs, and supplemented by information from this book, the nurse can become safe and skillful in the administration of medications and an astute observer of the effects of drugs on the patient.

Hannah R. DeToma, PhD, RN, FNP-C
Assistant Professor of Nursing
Medical University of South Carolina
Charleston

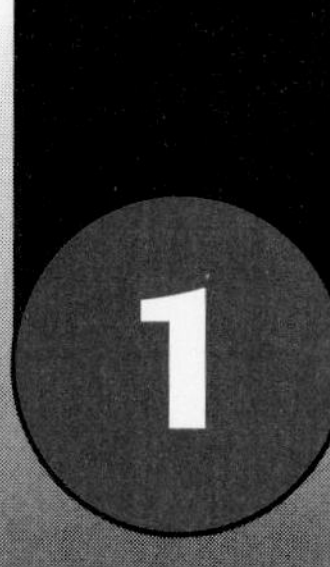

Fundamentals of nursing pharmacology

LEARNING OBJECTIVES

After studying this chapter, you should be able to:

- Identify the pharmacodynamic and pharmacokinetic phases of drug action.
- Identify those patients at risk for drug toxicities.
- Discuss use of the nursing process with patients and families when administering medications.
- Discuss measures to avoid or reduce the risk of medication errors.
- Describe techniques for administering intramuscular, subcutaneous, and intradermal medications.
- Describe special drug considerations in pregnant women, children, and elderly patients.

CHAPTER OVERVIEW

This chapter begins by exploring two major concepts in pharmacology: pharmacodynamics — the mechanism by which drugs produce chemical and physiologic changes in the body — and pharmacokinetics — the movement of drugs into systemic circulation. The chapter also provides guidelines for using the nursing process as a framework for administering medications, teaching patients and families about their drug therapy, and evaluating pharmacologic effects. In order to safely administer medications, the nurse also must understand key drug concepts: therapeutic effects, adverse reactions, drug interactions, and toxic effects of each drug. Finally, the nurse needs to be aware of federal legislation and regulations governing the manufacture and sale of drugs and laws governing administration of controlled substances.

What is pharmacodynamics?

- Mechanisms by which specific drugs produce biochemical and physiologic changes in the body

PHARMACODYNAMICS

Definition

- The mechanisms by which specific drugs produce biochemical and physiologic changes in the body

Pharmacodynamic events

- A given drug interacts with specific receptor sites: agonist drugs stimulate receptors; antagonist drugs inhibit receptors
- It causes a general interaction with cell metabolism
- The cellular environment and function are altered to produce the desired response

What is pharmacokinetics?

- Movement of drugs across body membranes to reach the target organ

4 ways drugs move through the body

- Absorption: movement of a drug from its administration site through or across tissue into the systemic circulation
- Distribution: movement of a drug from the systemic circulation into the tissues
- Metabolism: alteration of a drug to a more active or less active form, usually in the liver
- Excretion: elimination of a drug from the circulation

PHARMACOKINETICS

General information

- Refers to the movement of drugs across body membranes to reach the target organ
- The movement of drugs may be categorized in four components: absorption, distribution, metabolism, and excretion
- Pharmacokinetics of a drug influences the determination of proper dosing schedules
- Pharmacokinetic profiles also describe the drug's onset of activity, peak level, duration, and bioavailability

Absorption

- Refers to movement of a drug from its administration site through or across tissue into the systemic circulation
- The percentage of drug absorbed into the systemic circulation for activity is known as bioavailability; drugs injected intravenously (I.V.) have 100% bioavailability
- The degree and rate of drug absorption depend on the administration route, the patient's age and physical condition, the lipid or water solubility of the drug, and any potential drug interactions with other drugs or food
- The degree and rate of absorption also depend on the drug's mechanism of absorption, such as passive transport (including diffusion, passive diffusion, and carrier-mediated diffusion), active transport, or pinocytosis

Distribution

- Refers to movement of a drug from the systemic circulation into the tissues
- Distribution may be affected by several physiologic factors, including the blood-brain barrier, cardiac output, body composition (amount of adipose

tissue), blood supply to target tissues, the degree of vessel constriction or dilation, and the degree to which the drug binds to plasma proteins such as albumin

- Blood-brain barrier refers to limited distribution of drugs into the central nervous system (CNS); only highly lipid-soluble drugs can pass through tightly packed glial cells

Metabolism

- Refers to the alteration of a drug to a more active or less active form, usually in the liver
- Metabolism may be affected by genetic factors, the patient's age and physical condition, and the drug itself (for example, the suitability of the metabolites for drug activity or the drug's lipid solubility)
- Orally administered drugs pass through the liver and are partially metabolized before entering the systemic circulation. This first pass effect usually requires higher doses. Some drugs have almost complete first pass metabolism and are ineffective when given orally

Excretion

- Refers to elimination of a drug from the circulation
- A drug may be excreted in various ways:
  - Most drugs are excreted by the kidney via the urine; by the liver via the bile, then into the feces; by the lungs via exhaled air; or into breast milk
  - Minor excretion routes include saliva, tears, and sweat

Dosing schedules

- Dosing schedules are determined by the drug's pharmacokinetic properties
- The following factors are considered when establishing dosing schedules:
  - Route of administration: the area of the body where the drug's absorption will take place — bioavailability may change when the route of administration is changed
  - Onset of action: the time when a drug's effects first become noticeable
  - Peak concentration level: the maximum blood concentration level achieved through absorption: at this level most of the drug reaches the site of action and provides the therapeutic response
  - Duration of action: the length of time a drug acts on the body
  - Half-life: the time required for a drug's plasma concentration to decrease by 50%

PHARMACOTHERAPEUTICS

General information

- Refers to the use of drugs to treat a specific disease or produce a desired effect

Metabolism highlights

- Alteration of a drug to a more active or less active form
- Usually occurs in the liver
- May be affected by genetic factors, age, physical condition and the drug
- Orally administered drugs pass through the liver and are partially metabolized before entering the systemic circulation; effect usually requires higher doses (first pass)

Excretion highlights

- Elimination of drug from circulation
- Excretion occurs:
  - by the kidneys via urine
  - by the liver via bile and into feces
  - by the lungs via exhaled air
  - into breast milk
  - through saliva, tears, and sweat

Dosing schedule highlights

- Determined by the drug's pharmacokinetic properties
- Routing factors are considered when establishing dosing schedules
- Route of administration: area where drug absorption occurs
- Onset of action: time when drug effects are noticeable
- Peak concentration level: maximum blood concentration level achieved through absorption
- Duration of action: time a drug acts on the body
- Half-life: time required for a drug's plasma concentration to decrease by 50%

- Types of drug therapy include acute, empiric, supportive, palliative, maintenance, supplemental, and replacement
- Therapeutic steps include assessing the nature and extent of the patient's health problem, assessing the options, selecting the type of therapy, implementing the therapy, monitoring effectiveness of the therapy, and reassessing the problem
- Factors affecting response to a drug include the disease or disorder, the route of administration, the patient's body size, weight, sex, and past medical condition, psychological and emotional factors, and tolerance and dependence
- A loading dose refers to administration of one or more doses at the onset of therapy to quickly reach the therapeutic blood level and thereby hasten a therapeutic effect; commonly, the loading dose is larger than the maintenance dose
- Drug efficacy refers to a drug's maximal effectiveness
- Measures of drug efficacy include vital signs, body weight, and easing of symptoms that the drug is expected to relieve; the nurse can document efficacy using these parameters
- Therapeutic drug levels may be monitored to individualize drug dosage, to evaluate toxicity, and to monitor compliance

Types of drug therapy

- Acute
- Empiric
- Supportive
- Palliative
- Maintenance
- Supplemental
- Replacement

ADVERSE REACTIONS

Definition

- Refers to unwanted or potentially harmful effects of a drug; all drugs have one or more adverse reactions in addition to having the desired effect

Key facts about adverse reactions

- Unwanted or potentially harmful effects of a drug
- Range from mild responses to debilitating, chronic or life-threatening problems
- Can be dose-related or sensitivity-related

Types of adverse reactions

- May range from mild responses that resolve spontaneously or that disappear upon discontinuing the drug to debilitating, potentially chronic or life-threatening problems
- Adverse reactions may be dose-related; careful prescription and administration may prevent such reactions
- Some adverse reactions are inseparable from the drug's intended effect
- Adverse reactions may be related to patient sensitivity; such reactions may be unpredictable

Classifying adverse reactions

- Dose-related reactions: reactions to the drug's primary or secondary effect
- Sensitivity-related: reaction due to hypersensitivity or allergy
- Toxicity: reaction when drug levels exceed therapeutic range
- Idiosyncrasy: reaction that's unexpected or peculiar

Classifications of adverse reactions

- Dose-related reactions may be reactions to the drug's primary effect, such as bleeding from anticoagulants, or a secondary effect, such as drowsiness after taking antihistamines
- Sensitivity-related reactions occur when a patient is hypersensitive or allergic to a drug or one of its components
  - In hypersensitivity or allergic reactions, a sensitized patient is exposed to a drug that elicits an antigen-antibody reaction
  - Reactions may be immediate, resulting in anaphylaxis or urticaria or delayed, as in serum sickness

- Toxicity occurs when drug levels exceed the therapeutic range and may cause additional adverse effects
  - Toxicity may develop due to overdosage caused by failure to consider hepatic impairment, renal function, or the patient's age; toxicity may also result from patient's or family member's failure to understand drug dosing or administration
  - Dosage modification may be necessary if toxic effects occur
  - For many drugs, established therapeutic blood levels help to monitor for therapeutic effect and prevent toxicity
- Idiosyncrasy refers to an unexpected or peculiar response to a drug—for example, diphenhydramine (Benadryl) may cause hyperexcitability in children
- Other adverse reactions
  - A patient may develop blood dyscrasias, nephrotoxicity, or hepatic toxicity
  - Carcinogenicity, teratogenicity, photosensitivity, and disease-related effects also should be considered

Other adverse reactions

- Blood dyscrasias
- Nephrotoxicity
- Hepatic toxicity
- Carcinogenicity
- Teratogenicity
- Photosensitivity
- Disease-related effects

INTERACTIONS

General information

- Interactions can alter the pharmacokinetic, pharmacodynamic, or pharmacotherapeutic characteristics of the drugs involved, thereby affecting the overall therapeutic effect of a drug
- A drug's therapeutic effect may be altered by other drugs, foods, herbs, or the environment; for example, taking monoamine oxidase (MAO) inhibitors with tyramine-containing foods, such as aged cheese or beer, may lead to hypertensive crisis
- Contraindications and precautions warn against drug use or advise caution in patients with specific medical conditions, patients in a specific age-group, or patients who are taking another, potentially incompatible or interacting drug
- Some drug interactions are used for their therapeutic benefits; for example, one drug may block the elimination of another drug, thus keeping the drug in systemic circulation longer
- Interactions may affect and alter laboratory test values
- Categories of interactions include incompatibilities, pharmacokinetic interactions, and pharmacodynamic interactions

Interactions

- Can alter the pharmacokinetic, pharmacodynamic, or pharmacotherapeutic drug characteristics
- Contraindications and precautions: warn against drug use or advise caution in patients with specific medical conditions, patients in a specific age-group, or patients who are taking another, potentially incompatible or interacting drug

Three types of interactions

1. Incompatibilities
2. Pharmacokinetic interactions
3. Pharmacodynamic interactions

Incompatibilities

- Incompatibilities are chemical or physical reactions between two or more drugs
- Incompatibilities may occur when preparing I.V. admixtures, administering medications in I.V. bolus or piggyback, or mixing medications in a syringe

Pharmacokinetic interactions

- Absorption may be affected by stomach pH changes and the presence of food or other drugs
- Administration of some drugs may cause induction or inhibition of hepatic metabolism or excretion

Additive effect

- Combining two or more drugs to cause an effect equal to the sum of their separate effects

Synergistic effect

- Combining two or more drugs to cause an effect greater than the sum of their separate effects

Antagonistic effects

- Combining two or more drugs to produce an effect less than the sum of their separate effects

U.S. drug legislation

- Began in 1906; create uniform drug standards, ensure quality and regulation, and promote safety
- FFDCA empowers federal government to enforce U.S. USP and National Formulary standards

Pharmacokinetic interactions

- Absorption may be affected by changes in stomach pH, presence or absence of food in the GI tract, and the presence of other drugs or herbs in the stomach
- Many drugs bound to plasma protein may compete for binding sites; as drugs displace one another from binding sites, more of the displaced drug circulates and toxicity may occur
- Administration of some drugs may cause induction or inhibition of hepatic metabolism, possibly causing an increase or decrease in some hepatically metabolized drugs
- Administration of drugs may be coordinated to enhance or inhibit excretion; for example, probenecid may be administered with penicillin to delay renal excretion and prolong the antibiotic's effect

Pharmacodynamic interactions

- Additive effect: combining two or more drugs to cause an effect equal to the sum of their separate effects; for example, aspirin and codeine may be combined to relieve pain
- Synergism: combining two or more drugs to cause an effect greater than the sum of their separate effects
- Potentiation, a type of synergism, occurs when one of two or more drugs are combined and one of the drugs exerts an action greater than if it was given alone
- Antagonistic effect: combining two or more drugs to produce an effect less than the sum of their separate effects; for example, a drug antidote works by an antagonistic effect

DRUG LEGISLATION IN THE UNITED STATES

General information

- Legislative drug control in the United States began in 1906
- Since 1906, many acts have been passed to create uniform drug standards to ensure the quality and regulation of drugs and the pharmaceutical industries and to promote patient safety

Federal Food, Drug, and Cosmetic Act (FFDCA) of 1906

- Empowers the federal government to enforce standards set by the United States Pharmacopeia (USP) and the National Formulary
- Requires drugs meet standards of strength and purity
- Requires the type and amount of narcotic be listed on the label of opiate mixtures
- The Sherley Amendment to the FFDCA (1912) increases federal involvement in drug control by prohibiting drug companies from using fraudulent therapeutic claims

- **Food, Drug, and Cosmetic Act — Amendment of 1938**
  - Requires all drugs and drug products be tested for harmful effects in four stages of clinical trials involving animal and human subjects before Food and Drug Administration (FDA) approval of a new drug for sale
  - Requires that drug labels and literature be complete and accurate and state the dose, manufacturer's name and address, names and amounts of potentially harmful ingredients, a warning if the drug might be habit-forming, directions for use, and contraindications
  - States that medical devices must be safe and effective and that cosmetics must be safe
- **Food, Drug, and Cosmetic Act — Durham-Humphrey Amendment of 1952**
  - Distinguishes between prescription and over-the-counter medications
  - States that a prescription for narcotics, hypnotics, habit-forming drugs, and potentially harmful drugs can be refilled only with a new prescription and requires that the label state this fact
- **Food, Drug, and Cosmetic Act — Kefauver-Harris Amendment of 1962**
  - Gives the FDA additional control over drug safety
  - Allows the FDA to evaluate the testing methods of drug manufacturers
  - Requires manufacturers to prove that a drug is effective, not just nontoxic
- **Controlled Substances Act or Comprehensive Drug Abuse Prevention Act of 1970**
  - Groups controlled substances (such as narcotics, tranquilizers, barbiturates, and amphetamines) into five categories (schedules) based on a drug's potential for abuse and medical effectiveness
  - Limits the number of prescription refills for controlled substances
- **Drug Price Competition and Patent Time Restoration Act of 1984**
  - Makes it possible for generic versions of bioequivalent equals to be marketed without duplicating clinical trials
  - Grants longer patent protection to companies introducing new drugs

CONTROLLED SUBSTANCES

- **General information**
  - Controlled substances are drugs that have potential for abuse or physical and psychological dependence
  - Proper handling of controlled substances is essential; any violations by a nurse may result in suspension of your nursing license
  - There are five groups or schedules of controlled substances (see *Schedule of Controlled Substances,* page 8)

FDA regulations

- All drugs need testing for harmful effects in four stages of clinical trials
- Drug labels need to be accurate
- Medical devices and cosmetics must be safe
- Durham-Humphrey Amendment: distinguishes between prescription and OTC drugs
- Controlled Substances Act: groups controlled substances; limits the number of refills
- Drug Price Competition and Patent Time Restoration Act: generic version equivalents don't need to duplicate trials; longer patent protection granted

Key facts about controlled substances

- Drugs with potential for abuse or physical and psychological dependence
- Proper handling of controlled substances is essential; any violations by a nurse may result in suspension of your nursing license
- Five groups or schedules of controlled substances

Schedules

- Schedule I: highest risk for abuse
- Schedule II: high potential for abuse; may lead to physical and psychological dependence
- Schedule III: lesser abuse potential
- Schedule IV: low abuse potential; psychological dependence more common than physical
- Schedule V: least abuse potential

Schedule of Controlled Substances

SCHEDULE I

1. Schedule I drugs carry the highest risk for abuse.

These drugs, which include cannabinols, such as marijuana, and hallucinogens, such as LSD, heroin, and mescaline, are not acceptable for prescription use; they may be available for investigational use.

SCHEDULE II

1. Schedule II drugs carry high potential for abuse and may lead to physical and psychological dependence.
2. This group includes certain barbiturates, narcotics, opiates, and stimulants.

SCHEDULE III

1. Schedule III drugs carry a lesser abuse potential than schedules I and II.
2. This group includes barbiturates such as butabarbital, narcotics in combination with other drugs, stimulants, androgens, anabolic steroids, and paregoric.

SCHEDULE IV

1. Schedule IV drugs carry a low abuse potential, with psychological dependence more common than physical dependence.
2. This group includes benzodiazepines, propoxyphene (Darvon), and chlordiazepoxide (Librium).

SCHEDULE V

1. Schedule V drugs carry the least abuse potential.
2. Most drugs in this class have a small amount of narcotic combined with an antitussive or antidiarrheal.

NURSING PROCESS IN DRUG ADMINISTRATION

Assessment

- Determine whether the patient has food or drug allergies; document clearly on patient's chart all food and drug allergies
- Find out which prescription and nonprescription medications the patient currently takes, the frequency, the purpose of each medication for this patient, and whether adverse effects have occurred
- Obtain a history of patient's medical conditions, socioeconomic status, and psychosocial support
- Perform a physical examination; pay particular attention to body systems that may be affected by current or newly prescribed medications or to where the patient has complaints or concerns

Assessment for drug administration

- Determine food or drug allergies
- Obtain a drug history
- Obtain a medical history
- Perform a physical examination

Nursing diagnosis

- Develop a nursing diagnosis consisting of the patient's disease process and its etiology

- Begin by addressing problems that pose immediate threats to the patient's health
- Common nursing diagnoses include
  - Deficient knowledge
  - Risk for injury
  - Ineffective management of therapeutic regimen
  - Noncompliance

Planning

- Develop outcomes using the nursing diagnosis; if possible, obtain input from the patient and family
- Use these goals as outcome criteria for evaluation

Implementation — Avoiding Medication Errors

- Follow the six rights of drug administration at all times
  - Verify the medication order for the RIGHT DRUG
    - Ensure that the medication order is properly composed and includes the patient's full name, drug name, dosage form, dose amount, administration route, time schedule, prescriber's signature, and date and time of order
    - Check the medication order against the drug label three times
    - Know why the patient is receiving this specific drug at this time
  - Check the order and medication supplied to ensure the RIGHT ROUTE
    - Drugs can be administered orally (by mouth or through a gastric tube), parenterally (by intradermal, subcutaneous, intramuscular, or intravenous injection), topically, otically, ophthalmically, or via the mucous membranes (by sublingual, buccal, vaginal, rectal, intranasal, transdermal, or inhaled methods)
    - Be aware of the routes available for the specified drug ordered; if a patient cannot swallow the pill form of a drug, suggest to the prescriber an alternative route, such as I.M. or I.V.
    - Be aware that drugs forms or types are not always interchangeable
  - Perform dosage calculation to ensure the RIGHT DOSE
    - Use a ratio and proportion to arrive at the ordered dose; for example: A nurse must administer Demerol 75 mg I.M. taken from a 1-cc prefilled syringe containing 100 mg of Demerol; the ratio reads 75 mg is to X cc as 100 mg is to 1 cc; the equation reads as follows:
      $$\frac{75\text{ mg}}{X\text{ cc}} :: \frac{100\text{ mg}}{1\text{ cc}}$$
      Solve for X
      X = 75/100 or X = 0. 75 cc
    - Alternatively, the nurse may use the desired/on hand × cc's method (for example, 75/100 × 1 cc = 0.75 cc).
  - Verify the frequency of dosage with the medication order to ensure the RIGHT TIME
  - Confirm the patient's identity by checking the patient's armband before administering each drug to ensure the RIGHT PATIENT

Nursing diagnosis and planning

- Begin by addressing immediate threat to patient's health.
- Include deficient knowledge, injury risk, ineffective mangement of therapeutic regimen, noncompliance.
- Develop manageable outcomes using the nursing diagnosis.

6 rights to drug administration

- Right drug
- Right route
- Right dose
- Right time
- Right patient
- Right documentation

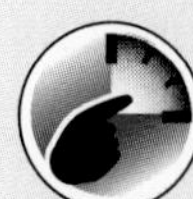

TIME-OUT FOR TEACHING

Patient teaching and medication therapy

Make sure to include the following topics in your teaching plan for the patient receiving medication therapy.

- Name of medication
- Purpose of medication
- How and when to take medication; what to do about missed doses
- How to monitor medication's effectiveness (for example, monitoring blood glucose level when taking a hypoglycemic)
- Drugs that may interact with the prescribed medication (include over-the-counter and herbal medications)
- Any required dietary changes, including use of alcohol
- Possible adverse effects and what to do if these occur
- Signs and symptoms to bring to the doctor's attention
- Required follow-up procedures
- Storing and handling medication

Topics for patient discussion

- Medication name and purpose
- Monitoring medication's effectiveness
- Drugs that could interact with the prescribed medication
- Possible adverse effects

Key ways to avoid medication errors

- Never give a drug poured or prepared by someone else.
- Never allow the medication cart or tray out of your sight once you have prepared a dose.
- Never leave a drug at a patient's bedside; rather, watch the patient swallow the drug.
- Never return unwrapped or prepared drugs to the stock supply; instead, dispose of the medication and notify the pharmacist.
- Keep the medication cart locked at all times.
- Medication errors can easily be caused by similar sounding drug names, unclear orders, wrong route of administration, and miscalculation of dosages; take extra care to avoid these errors.

  - Make sure the physician's order is clear and complete to ensure the RIGHT DOCUMENTATION
    - Compare the original physician's order with the medication label to ensure accuracy
    - Record the medication in the patient's chart immediately after administering it
- Administer medication as prescribed and according to the manufacturer's instructions. If there is any concern or question regarding the look, consistency, dosage, or proper administration technique for a drug, consult the pharmacist and document the consultation. Whenever administering a drug, follow these safety procedures:
- **Never give a drug poured or prepared by someone else**
- **Never allow the medication cart or tray out of your sight once you have prepared a dose**
- **Never leave a drug at a patient's bedside; rather, watch the patient swallow the drug**
- **Never return unwrapped or prepared drugs to the stock supply; instead, dispose of the medication and notify the pharmacist**
- **Keep the medication cart locked at all times**
- Follow standard precautions, as appropriate
- Monitor the patient for therapeutic effects; regularly evaluate the serum drug level and the results of relevant laboratory tests
- Evaluate the patient for adverse reactions; notify the physician if adverse reactions occur and intervene, as necessary
- Provide patient teaching essential to proper medication administration; include family members in patient teaching (for specific teaching tips, see *Patient teaching and medication therapy*)
- Consider legal aspects associated with drug therapy

  - Make sure that there is a complete medication order
  - Question any order when handwriting is difficult to read, the drug's use in the patient's condition is questionable, or dosages are unclear, or if drug incompatibilities or interactions may occur
- Consider ethical principles when dealing with medication errors, medications during pregnancy, and investigational protocols
- Medication errors can easily be caused by similar sounding drug names, unclear orders, wrong route of administration, and miscalculation of dosages; take extra care to avoid these errors

Evaluation

- Appropriate evaluation statements include
  - The patient obtains expected effects of the prescribed medication
  - The patient avoids adverse effects or interactions with other drugs, foods, or alcohol
  - The patient demonstrates an understanding of information taught
  - The patient complies with the therapeutic regimen (if the patient does not comply, determine reasons for noncompliance)
  - Therapeutic drug levels are maintained
- Based on patient evaluation, modify outcomes and interventions, as needed

DRUG ADMINISTRATION TECHNIQUES

Oral (P.O.) administration

- Most medications are administered via oral route because it is safe, convenient and least expensive
- Some oral drugs are prescribed at higher doses than their parenteral equivalent because of first pass metabolism or poor bioavailability
- Oral formulations include tablets, enteric-coated tablets, capsules, syrups, elixirs, oils, liquids, suspensions, powders, and granules
- Some drugs require special preparation before administration such as mixing with juice to improve palatability
- Many drugs can be mixed with juice or foods if patients have difficulty taking medications; make sure that the drug is able to be crushed or mixed with foods because some drugs are sustained-release formulations
- Oral administration via the nasogastric (NG) route
  - Useful in patients with NG tubes in place who are unable to swallow or take drugs by mouth
  - Some tablets should not be crushed and some capsules should not be opened; if there is any question, consult the pharmacist
  - Some drugs may interact with tube feedings, causing decreased drug absorption; in these situations, tube feeding should be held for at least 1 hour before and 2 hours after drug administration
  - If the NG tube is hooked to suction, the suction should be held for 20 to 30 minutes after drug administration

When to question a medication order

- When handwriting is difficult to read
- When the drug's use in the patient's condition is questionable
- When dosages are unclear
- When drug incompatibilities or interactions may occur

Evaluation

- Determine if outcome goals were met; if not, modify outcome goals and interventions, as needed

Oral drug highlights

- Most medications delivered orally; safe, convenient, and least expensive
- Oral forms include tablets, enteric-coated tablets, capsules, syrups, elixirs, oils, liquids, suspensions, powders, and granules
- Remember that many drugs can be mixed with juice or foods
- Make sure that the drug is able to be crushed or mixed with foods because some drugs are sustained-release formulations

Buccal and sublingual administration

- Buccally administered medications are placed between the cheek and the teeth
- Sublingually administered medications are placed under the tongue
- These drugs bypass the digestive tract and are immediately absorbed into systemic circulation

4 methods of parenteral administration

- Intravenous: deposits drug directly into the systemic circulation
- Intramuscular: deposits drug into the muscle
- Subcutaneous: deposits drug directly into fatty tissue
- Intradermal: deposits drug into corium of skin

Topical drugs

- Applied directly to the skin
- Include lotions, creams, ointments, drops, and transdermal patches
- When applying, never place a heating pad over the application site; never place a defibrillator paddle over a transdermal patch

- Buccal and sublingual (S.L.) administration
  - Buccally administered medications are placed between the cheek and the teeth
  - Sublingually administered medications are placed under the tongue
  - Buccally and sublingually administered drugs bypass the digestive tract and are immediately absorbed into systemic circulation
  - Administration via these routes requires either concentrated liquid formulations or specially formulated disintegrating tablets
  - Make sure patient doesn't swallow drug because this will involve the digestive tract in the absorption and eliminate immediate absorption

Parenteral administration

- Many medications that can't be delivered orally can be administered parenterally
- Medications can be administered via injection directly into the vein (I.V.), into the muscle (I.M.), into the subcutaneous tissue (S.C.), or intradermally (I.D.)
  - I.V. administration
    - Provides direct delivery of drugs into the systemic circulation; direct intravenous push (I.V.P.), I.V. administration by bolus infusions, and I.V. administration by continuous infusion are all different methods of I.V. delivery
    - Effects are immediate
    - Bypasses absorption process and enters directly in the systemic circulation
    - Bioavailability of the drug is 100% when given I.V.
  - I.M. administration
    - Deposits the drug into the muscle; the medication is then absorbed into the systemic circulation from the muscle
    - When injecting I.M., avoid areas that look inflamed, edematous, or irritated and areas that contain moles, birthmarks, scars, or other lesions
    - The dorsogluteal and ventrogluteal muscles are the most commonly used muscle groups
    - The deltoid muscle can be used for injections of 2 cc or less
    - The vastus lateralis muscle is used most often in children
    - The rectus formus may be used in infants
  - S.C. administration
    - S.C. administration involves injection into fatty tissue
    - It allows for a slower, more sustained administration than I.M. injection
  - I.D. administration
    - I.D. administration involves an injection into the corium, a skin layer consisting of dense vascular tissue

Topical administration

- Topical drugs are applied directly to the skin and include lotions, creams, ointments, and transdermal patches

- Lotions, creams, and ointments are typically used for their local effects
- Transdermal delivery systems (which include some ointments and patches) are designed to allow delivery of the drug into systemic circulation after absorption through the skin
- Topically administered drugs must be applied to areas of skin that are intact (unless the drug is prescribed to treat a skin lesion), clean and dry; application of the drug to callused or scarred areas may result in impaired absorption

Ophthalmic administration

- Ophthalmic drugs are used for their local effects within the eye
- They're absorbed into the mucus membrane
- These drugs are available as either ointments or drops
- When administering eyedrops or ointment
  - Have the patient lie in supine position and tilt his head back and toward the affected eye; this will direct flow of the drug away from the tear duct and minimize the risk of systemic absorption through the nasal mucosa
  - Gently pull down the lower lid of the affected eye and instill the drops into the conjunctival sac
  - **Never instill the drug directly onto the eyeball**
  - **Never touch the eye or lid with the applicator tip**

Otic administration

- Drugs are administered into the ear to treat local infection and inflammation, to soften cerumen, and to provide local anesthesia
- When administering eardrops, have the patient lie on the side opposite the affected ear; straighten the patient's ear canal—for adults, gently pull the auricle up and back; for an infant or child younger than age 3, gently pull the auricle down and back
- Gently massage the anterior area of the ear and have the patient remain lying on his side for 5 minutes after drug administration
- If ordered, insert a cotton ball into the external ear and observe for reactions

Inhalation administration

- Inhaled medications are topical medications delivered into the respiratory tract for local and systemic effects
- The mucosal lining of the lung absorbs the drug almost immediately
- Drugs can be administered into the respiratory tract by an inhaler or nebulizer

Vaginal administration

- Vaginally administered drugs are used as topical treatments for vaginal infections and inflammation
- Suppositories and creams are used to deliver drugs vaginally

Rectal administration

- Rectal administration of drugs is used when other routes of administration aren't available

Ophthalmic administration

- Ointments or drops used for local effects within the eye
- Absorbed into mucus membrane
- When administering, never instill the drug directly onto the eyeball; never touch the eye or lid with applicator tip

Otic administration

- Administered to the ear to treat local infection and inflammation, soften cerumen, and provide local anesthesia
- When administering, straighten the patient's ear canal; in adults, gently pull the auricle up and back; in infants or children younger than age 3, gently pull the auricle down and back

Inhalation administration

- Topical medications delivered into the respiratory tract by inhaler or nebulizer
- Lung's mucosal lining aborbs the drug almost immediately

Vaginal administration

- Used as topical treatments for vaginal infections and inflammation
- Suppositories or creams

- Medications administered rectally include drugs that treat constipation, nausea and vomiting, hemorrhoids, colitis, and pain
  - Drugs administered rectally are absorbed into the large intestine; the degree of absorption depends on the patient's ability to retain the suppository or enema
  - Administer these drugs while the patient is in the Sim's position; urge him to remain in this position for 30 minutes, if possible

Rectal administration

- Used when other routes are not available
- Include drugs that treat constipation, nausea and vomiting, hemorrhoids, colitis, and pain
- Absorbed into the large intestine

SPECIAL POPULATIONS

Pregnant or breast-feeding women

- The FDA has established six pregnancy risk categories for pregnant patients or patients considering pregnancy (see *Pregnancy risk categories*).
- Teratogenic effects may occur in the fetus secondary to drug exposure, including topically administered drugs
- **Caution the pregnant woman to avoid all drugs except those that are approved by her health care provider and instruct her to check with her health care provider before taking any drugs, including herbal and over-the-counter drugs**
- Drugs may appear in breast milk, producing a pharmacologic effect in the infant; this may warrant discontinuing the drug or avoiding breast-feeding
- Weigh the potential fetal and neonatal risks and potential benefits to the mother when administering medications

Drug considerations in pregnant and breast-feeding women

- Six pregnancy risk categories
- Teratogenic effects may occur in the fetus secondary to drug exposure
- Drugs may appear in breast milk, producing a pharmacologic effect in the infant; this may warrant discontinuing the drug or avoiding breast-feeding

Children

- Usually, pediatric dosing is based on milligram of drug per kilogram of body weight (mg/kg) or body surface area expressed as milligrams per square meter (mg/m^2)
- Pharmacokinetics in children
  - Absorption: may vary between neonates and infants; thin epidermis in children causes increased absorption of topical drugs
  - Distribution: may be altered because neonates have a larger percentage of body water, less protein levels, and less fat than adults, which may result in reduced plasma levels of water-soluble drugs and less storage
  - Metabolism: immaturity of the liver may delay metabolism in infants; some drugs may be metabolized more rapidly in children than in adults
  - Excretion: immaturity of the kidneys may delay excretion in infants

Drug considerations in children

- Pediatric dosing is based on mg of drug/kg of body weight or mg/m^2
- Immaturity of liver may delay metabolism; some drugs may be metabolized more rapidly in children than adults
- Immaturity of the kidneys may delay excretion in infants

Elderly patients

- Elderly patients absorb, distribute, and eliminate drugs less efficiently
- These patients usually require a decrease in dosage
- Elderly patients usually have an increased likelihood of having multiple disorders, such as cardiac disease, renal disease, hepatic disturbances, or diabetes, which may alter drug action and excretion, thereby placing them at an increased risk for adverse reactions and drug toxicities

Pregnancy risk categories

Category A: controlled studies failed to demonstrate a risk to the fetus
Category B: animal studies showed no risk to the fetus or there were no studies performed on pregnant women.
Category C: either animal studies showed adverse effects to the fetus or no studies in women or animals are available.
Category D: fetal risk exists.
Category X: fetal risk has been shown in animals and in women. Drug is contraindicated in women who are or who may become pregnant.
Category NR: no rating is available.

- Be alert for adverse reactions and toxicities, especially from the following drugs: antiarrhythmics, diuretics, antihypertensives, corticosteroids, anticoagulants, benzodiazepines, and narcotics
- Poor compliance (because of lack of family support, fixed income, and decreased access to transportation or resources, for example) is a factor in the elderly population
- Patient teaching may be difficult because of sensory deficits, such as hearing impairment and poor eyesight, and cognitive deficits, such as poor memory

NCLEX CHECKS

It's never too soon to begin your NCLEX preparation. Now that you've reviewed this chapter, carefully read each of the following questions and choose the best answer. Then compare your responses to the correct answers.

1. A 65-year-old patient carefully follows a diabetic diet and exercise program prescribed by her physician. Because her blood glucose level remains elevated, her physician prescribes glipizide (Glucotrol) daily. The nurse wants to learn more about this drug's absorption, distribution, metabolism, and excretion. Which of the following branches of pharmacology provides this information?

☐ **A.** Pharmacognosy
☐ **B.** Pharmacokinetics
☐ **C.** Pharmacodynamics
☐ **D.** Pharmacotherapeutics

2. While giving scheduled drugs at 9:00 a.m., you realize that your patient is in the bathroom. Through the door, the patient tells you to leave the pills by his bed and he'll take them when he comes out. Which of the following actions is the most appropriate for you to take?

Categories for pregnancy risk

- Category A: studies failed to demonstrate a risk to fetus
- Category B: animal studies showed no risk to fetus; no studies on pregnant women
- Category C: animal studies showed adverse effects to fetus or no studies available
- Category D: fetal risk exists
- Category X: fetal risk shown in animals and women; drug is contraindicated in pregnant women or those who may become pregnant
- Category NR: no rating available

Drug considerations in elderly patients

- Absorb, distribute, and eliminate drugs less efficiently
- Usually require a decrease in dosage
- Increased likelihood of having multiple disorders
- Adverse reactions and toxicities may occur

☐ **A.** Take the drugs away, but return in 10 minutes to give them.
☐ **B.** Return the drugs to the patient's drug drawer and chart "drugs refused."
☐ **C.** Go into the bathroom and give them to the patient to take with you standing there.
☐ **D.** Leave the drugs at the bedside with a note for the patient to take them as soon as possible.

3. In 1938, Congress passed an amendment to the Federal Food, Drug, and Cosmetic Act. As a result of this amendment, drug labels must consist of:
☐ **A.** only the name of the distributor.
☐ **B.** a warning if the drug comes from a foreign source.
☐ **C.** the name of the scientist who discovered the drug.
☐ **D.** a statement describing the contents of the package, including manufacturer, ingredients, a warning if the drug is habit-forming, contraindications, and directions for use.

4. A new drug order is written for your patient. After reviewing the order, you think that the dosage is unusually high. How should you proceed?
☐ **A.** Ignore the drug order.
☐ **B.** Give the drug exactly as prescribed.
☐ **C.** Question the physician about the dosage.
☐ **D.** Have another nurse double-check the order.

5. You are preparing to give cortisone to your patient. Which item must you always check before giving a drug?
☐ **A.** Family history
☐ **B.** Blood pressure
☐ **C.** Respiratory rate
☐ **D.** Identification bracelet

6. You are teaching a patient about a newly prescribed drug. What could cause an elderly patient to have difficulty learning about prescribed medications?
☐ **A.** Decreased drug excretion
☐ **B.** Sensory deficits
☐ **C.** Lack of family support
☐ **D.** Fixed income

7. During an acute infection, a patient with diabetes develops severe hyperglycemia and requires insulin therapy. Which administration route provides an immediate systemic response?
☐ **A.** Intramuscular (I.M.)
☐ **B.** Intradermal
☐ **C.** Intravenous (I.V.)
☐ **D.** Subcutaneous (S.C.)

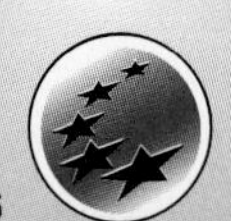

TOP 6

Items to study for your next test on fundamentals of nursing pharmacology

1. Pharmacodynamic and pharmacokinetic phases of drug action
2. Patients at risk for drug toxicities
3. Use of the nursing process with patients and families when administering medications
4. Measures to avoid or reduce the risk of medication errors
5. Techniques for administering intramuscular, subcutaneous, and intradermal medications
6. Special drug considerations in pregnant women, children, and elderly patients

8. The cardiologist prescribes digoxin (Lanoxin) 125 µg by mouth every morning for a client diagnosed with heart failure. The pharmacy dispenses tablets that contain 0.25 mg each. How many tablets should the nurse administer in each dose?

____

ANSWERS AND RATIONALES

1. CORRECT ANSWER: B
Look for a word that refers to movement. Pharmacokinetics refers to the absorption, distribution, metabolism, and excretion of the drug in a living organism. Pharmacognosy deals with natural drug resources. Pharmacodynamics is the study of the biochemical and physical effects of drugs and the mechanism of drug actions in living organisms. Pharmacotherapeutics, also known as clinical pharmacology, is a general term covering the use of drugs to prevent and treat diseases.

2. CORRECT ANSWER: A
Legally, you must witness the patient taking the drugs. Thus, coming back with the drugs in 10 minutes would be the best action to make sure the patient takes his drugs. The patient didn't refuse to take the drugs, so it wouldn't be appropriate to chart this. Going into the bathroom wouldn't be the best option because you wouldn't be respecting the patient's privacy. Drugs should never be left at the bedside.

3. CORRECT ANSWER: D
Drug labels must be clear and contain a warning if a drug is habit-forming. The manufacturer, packager, and distributor also must be listed.

4. CORRECT ANSWER: C
As the nurse, you are obliged to act as the patient's advocate and legally are required to question an order that doesn't seem safe or correct. To ignore the drug order or give an unusually high dose can harm the patient. Because the physician ordered the dosage, you should question him, not another nurse.

5. CORRECT ANSWER: D
Remember the six "rights" of drug administration — right drug, right dose, right patient, right time, right route, and right documentation. Always check the patient's identification bracelet before giving a drug. Checking the patient's history (not the family history) is also important before giving a drug. Checking blood pressure and respiratory rate is needed only when the drug to be given affects these factors.

6. CORRECT ANSWER: B
Sensory deficits could cause a geriatric patient to have difficulty retaining knowledge about prescribed medications. Decreased drug excretion doesn't alter the patient's knowledge about a drug. A lack of family support or limited finances may affect compliance, but not knowledge retention.

7. CORRECT ANSWER: C

The I.V. route bypasses the body's absorption barriers and provides an immediate systemic response. Drugs given intradermally, I.M., or S.C. all require absorption.

8. CORRECT ANSWER: 1/2

The nurse should begin by converting 125 µg to milligrams:

125 µg/1,000 = 0.125 mg

The following formula is used to calculate drug dosages:

Dose on hand/Quantity on hand = Dose desired/X

The nurse should use the following equations:

0.25 mg/1 = 0.125mg/1 tablet

0.25X = 0.125

X = 0.5 tablet

2

Drugs and the autonomic nervous system

LEARNING OBJECTIVES

After studying this chapter, you should be able to:

- Correlate the mechanisms of action of cholinergics and adrenergics to the receptor stimulated or blocked.
- Identify indications for the various types of drugs.
- Describe nursing responsibilities related to each class of cholinergic and adrenergic.
- Understand the indications and mechanism of action for neuromuscular blockades.

CHAPTER OVERVIEW

Cholinergics include parasympathomimetics, which mimic the effects of the parasympathetic nervous system, and parasympatholytics, which oppose or block the effects of the parasympathetic system. Parasympathomimetics include cholinergic agonists and acetylcholinesterase inhibitors. Parasympatholytics include anticholinergics or cholinergic blockers.

Adrenergics include sympathomimetics (also known as adrenergic agonists), which mimic the effects of the sympathetic system, and sympatholytics (also known as adrenergic blockers), which antagonize or inhibit the adrenergic activity.

A&P highlights

- The autonomic nervous system (ANS) consists of the sympathetic nervous system, the parasympathetic nervous system, and the enteric nervous system.
- ANS pathways consist of two neurons, which transmit information to the effector organs: preganglionic neuron and postganglionic neuron.
- The ANS controls involuntary body functions, glands, and organs.
- The sympathetic system helps the body cope with external stimuli and functions during stress (triggers "fight or flight" response).
- The parasympathetic system works to save energy, aids in digestion, and supports restorative, resting body functions.

Key facts about ANS neurotransmitters

- Help neurons transmit impulses in the CNS
- Acetylcholine
  - Is released in response to a stressful event
  - Stimulates postganglionic neurons, causing epinephrine and norepinephrine release
  - Activates effector organs by combining with cholinergic receptors
  - Is inactivated by cholinesterase
- Norepinephrine
  - Causes sympathetic stimulation by triggering release of epinephrine and more norepinephrine
  - Combines with adrenergic receptors on effector organs

ANATOMY AND PHYSIOLOGY

Anatomy

- The autonomic nervous system (ANS) consists of the sympathetic nervous system (adrenergic system), parasympathetic nervous system (cholinergic system), and the enteric nervous system (which is not often discussed)
- ANS pathways consist of two neurons, which transmit information to the effector organs
  - Preganglionic neuron — extends from the central nervous system (CNS) to a ganglion
  - Postganglionic neuron — extends from the ganglion to the effector organ or gland

Function

- The ANS controls involuntary (or automatic) body functions, glands, and organs, such as the activity of the cardiac muscle and smooth muscle of the blood vessels, eye, stomach, and intestines
- The sympathetic system helps the body cope with external stimuli and functions during stress. It triggers the "fight or flight" response (vasoconstriction, increased heart and respiratory rate; cold, sweaty palms; and pupil dilation)
- The parasympathetic system works to save energy, activates the GI system (aids in digestion), and supports restorative, resting body functions (decreased heart rate, increased GI tract tone and peristalsis, urinary sphincter relaxation, and vasodilation)

ANS neurotransmitters

- The ANS neurotransmitters acetylcholine and norepinephrine help neurons transmit impulses in the CNS
- Acetylcholine
  - Released in response to a stressful event
  - Released from the axons of preganglionic neurons
  - Stimulates the postganglionic neurons, causing the release of epinephrine and norepinephrine
  - Activates effector organs by combining with cholinergic receptors on the effector organs
  - Inactivated by cholinesterase
- Norepinephrine
  - Released from postganglionic neurons and causes sympathetic stimulation by triggering release of epinephrine and more norepinephrine
  - Norepinephrine produces its effects by combining with adrenergic receptors found on the effector organs
    - Adrenergic receptors are divided into alpha and beta receptors; most effector organs contain both alpha and beta receptors
    - Alpha receptors contain two subgroups, $alpha_1$ and $alpha_2$
      - Stimulation of $alpha_1$ receptors produces contractions (vasoconstriction) of smooth-muscle walls of blood vessels

Adrenergic receptor uses and effects

RECEPTOR ACTIVATED	THERAPEUTIC USES	ADVERSE EFFECTS
$Alpha_1$	• Control topical superficial bleeding • Treat nasal decongestion • Elevate blood pressure • Delay absorption of local anesthetics • Decrease intraocular pressure	• Hypertension • Necrosis with extravasation • Bradycardia
$Alpha_2$	• Treat glaucoma	• Burning sensation • Ptosis • Redness and swelling of eyelid
$Beta_1$	• Treat heart failure, cardiac arrest, and shock	• Tachycardia • Arrhythmias • Angina
$Beta_2$	• Produce bronchodilation • Delay preterm labor	• Hyperglycemia • Tremors
Dopamine	• Increase renal blood flow • Increase cardiac output • Elevate blood pressure	• Ectopy • Nausea and vomiting • Tachycardia • Palpitations

  - Stimulation of $alpha_2$ receptors produces the opposite effect by inhibiting norepinephrine release from sympathetic nerve endings
- Beta receptors contain two subgroups, $beta_1$ and $beta_2$
  - Stimulation of $beta_1$ receptors (which are mostly found in the heart) causes the heart to beat faster and more forcefully
  - Stimulation of $beta_2$ receptors (which are found mostly in the smooth muscles of the bronchial walls and blood vessels) dilate bronchi and relaxes blood vessels
  - For more information, see *Adrenergic receptor uses and effects*
- After its release, some norepinephrine is inactivated by reuptake (when some of it is taken back into the synaptic vesicles in the axon terminals) or by the enzymes catechol O-methyl-transferase or monoamine oxidase

Key facts about cholinergic agonists

- Directly stimulate cholinergic receptors
- Mimic action of acetylcholine
- Metabolized by cholinesterases at the muscarinic and nicotinic receptor sites, in the plasma, and in the liver
- Excreted in urine

CHOLINERGIC DRUGS

PARASYMPATHOMIMETICS: CHOLINERGIC AGONISTS

Mechanism of action

- Directly stimulate cholinergic receptors, mimicking the action of acetylcholine

When to use cholinergic agonists

- Glaucoma
- Bladder and intestinal function stimulation
- Nonobstructive urine retention
- Neurogenic bladder

When NOT to use cholinergic agonists

- Prostate enlargement
- Possible urinary or GI obstruction
- Hyperthyroidism
- Bradycardia or atrioventricular (AV) conduction defects
- Asthma
- Pregnancy

Adverse reactions to watch for

- Hypotension, headache, flushing, sweating, increased salivation, abdominal cramps, nausea, vomiting, diarrhea, blurred vision, bronchial constriction

Key nursing actions

- For bethanechol chloride
  - Base patient evaluation on increased bladder tone and function.
  - Assess urinary status.
  - Administer by mouth or S.C.
  - Observe patient for 20 to 60 minutes after S.C. administration.
  - Monitor for toxicity.
- For pilocarpine
  - Base patient evaluation on decreased intraocular pressure.
  - Teach patient how to instill eyedrops.

Pharmacokinetics

- Absorption: Varies widely; rarely administered intramuscularly (I.M.) or intravenously (I.V.) because they would be subject to immediate breakdown by cholinesterases; usually given orally or subcutaneously (S.C.)
- Distribution: Widely distributed, binding primarily to muscarinic receptors
- Metabolism: Metabolized by cholinesterases at the muscarinic and nicotinic receptor sites, in the plasma, and in the liver
- Excretion: Excreted in the urine

Drug examples

- bethanechol chloride (Duvoid, Myotonachol), pilocarpine (Isopto Carpine, Pilocar)

Indications

- Cholinergic agonists are used to treat glaucoma and to stimulate bladder and intestinal function
- Bethanechol is used to treat nonobstructive urine retention and neurogenic bladder
- Pilocarpine is used to treat glaucoma

Contraindications and precautions

- Prostate enlargement, possible urinary or GI obstruction, hyperthyroidism, bradycardia or atrioventricular (AV) conduction defects, asthma, and pregnancy

Adverse reactions

- Hypotension, headache, flushing, sweating, increased salivation, abdominal cramps, nausea, vomiting, diarrhea, blurred vision, bronchial constriction

Interactions

- Inhibits parasympathomimetic action when used with atropine-like drugs (antimuscarinics) and sympathomimetics.
- Acetylcholinesterase inhibitors and cholinergic agonists potentiate each other
- Causes additive effects when parasympatholytics are used with other anticholinergic
- Quinidine and procainamide may antagonize effects of bethanechol chloride

Nursing responsibilities

- When administering bethanechol chloride:
  - Base patient evaluation on increased bladder tone and function
  - Assess the patient's urinary status
  - **Never give bethanechol chloride I.V. or I.M. (only give by mouth [P.O.] or S.C.)**
  - Observe the patient for 20 to 60 minutes after S.C. administration
  - Monitor the patient for signs and symptoms of drug toxicity, such as urinary urgency, excessive secretions, respiratory depression or spasm, bradycardia, abdominal cramping, and involuntary defecation
  - **Administer atropine as the antidote for toxicity, as prescribed**

- When administering pilocarpine:
  - Base patient evaluation on decreased intraocular pressure
  - Teach the patient how to instill the eyedrops

PARASYMPATHOMIMETICS: ACETYLCHOLINESTERASE INHIBITORS

Mechanism of action

- Inhibit acetylcholinesterase, the enzyme that inactivates acetylcholine, thereby stimulating cholinergic receptors and producing prolonged activation of the parasympathetic nervous system

Pharmacokinetics

- Absorption: Absorbed readily in the GI tract, subcutaneous tissues, and mucous membranes, except for neostigmine, which is absorbed poorly if given orally
- Distribution: Only physostigmine readily penetrates the blood-brain barrier
- Metabolism: Most are metabolized by the plasma esterases
- Excretion: Excreted in the urine; half-life (of neostigmine) — oral, 40 to 60 minutes; injection, 50 to 90 minutes

Drug examples

- ambenonium (Mytelase), edrophonium (Enlon, Reversol, Tensilon), neostigmine (Prostigmin), physostigmine (Antilirium), pyridostigmine (Mestinon, Regonol)

Indications

- Acetylcholinesterase inhibitors are used to treat myasthenia gravis and glaucoma and to prevent or treat postoperative paralytic ileus
- Edrophonium and neostigmine are used to diagnose myasthenia gravis
- Ambenonium, neostigmine, and pyridostigmine promote muscle contraction and are used to treat myasthenia gravis
- Neostigmine is used to prevent or treat postoperative ileus, prevent or treat postoperative distention, and treat nonobstructive urine retention
- Physostigmine is used to treat anticholinergic poisoning (including tricyclic antidepressant overdose)
- Edrophonium, neostigmine, and pyridostigmine are used to reverse the effects of nondepolarizing neuromuscular blockers

Contraindications and precautions

- Possible urinary or GI obstruction

Adverse reactions

- Parasympathomimetic or muscarinic adverse effects are common and include nausea, vomiting, diarrhea, increased salivation, bradycardia, hypotension, dyspnea, diaphoresis, blurred vision, and miosis
- Nicotinic adverse effects include muscle cramps, fatigue, weakness, paralysis, hypertension, and respiratory depression

Key facts about acetylcholinesterase inhibitors

- Inhibit acetylcholinesterase, the enzyme that inactivates acetylcholine, thereby stimulating cholinergic receptors and producing prolonged activation of the parasympathetic nervous system
- Metabolized by plasma esterases
- Excreted in urine

When to use acetylcholinesterase inhibitors

- Myasthenia gravis
- Glaucoma
- Postoperative paralytic ileus or distention
- Nonobstructive urine retention
- Anticholinergic poisoning

When NOT to use acetylcholinesterase inhibitors

- Possible urinary or GI obstruction

Adverse reactions to watch for

- Nausea, vomiting, diarrhea, increased salivation, bradycardia, hypotension, dyspnea, diaphoresis, blurred vision, miosis, muscle cramps, fatigue, weakness, paralysis, hypertension, and respiratory depression

Key nursing actions

- Assess the patient's neuromuscular status before and during drug therapy.
- Monitor for drug toxicity.
- Monitor vital signs and breath sounds every 4 hours.
- Take seizure precautions.

Key facts about parasympatholytics

- Block the action of acetylcholine at muscarinic receptors in the parasympathetic nervous system
- Metabolized in the liver or the GI tract
- Excreted in feces and urine

When to use parasympatholytics

- Salivation and gastric secretion reduction
- Heart block
- Mydriasis
- Parkinson's disease
- GI spasms
- Motion sickness
- Enuresis

Interactions

- Use of edrophonium, neostigmine, and pyridostigmine with nondepolarizing neuromuscular blockers (for example, tubocurarine) antagonizes the effect of the neuromuscular blocker, decreasing the drug's therapeutic effectiveness
- Neostigmine and pyridostigmine potentiate depolarizing muscle relaxants (for example, succinylcholine), prolonging muscle paralysis
- Use with cholinergic agonists (such as pilocarpine, bethanechol, and carbachol) will increase the effect of acetylcholine
- Use with anticholinergics (such as atropine and scopolamine) decreases the effect of the anticholinesterase and could mask signs of a cholinergic crisis

Nursing responsibilities

- Assess the patient's neuromuscular status, including gait, muscle strength, reflexes, and heart rate, before and during drug therapy
- **Monitor the patient for signs and symptoms of toxicity, such as generalized weakness, dysphagia, and respiratory weakness; administer atropine as the antidote for toxicity, as prescribed**
- **Monitor the patient's vital signs and auscultate for breath sounds at least once every 4 hours**
- **Take seizure precautions**

PARASYMPATHOLYTICS: CHOLINERGIC BLOCKERS (ANTICHOLINERGICS)

Mechanism of action

- Block the action of acetylcholine at muscarinic receptors in the parasympathetic nervous system

Pharmacokinetics

- Absorption: Absorbed in the GI tract, mucous membranes, skin, and eyes
- Distribution: Belladonna alkaloids are distributed widely and readily cross the blood-brain barrier; the other drugs aren't.
- Metabolism: Alkaloids are metabolized in the liver; the other drugs are hydrolyzed in the GI tract and the liver
- Excretion: Excreted in the feces and the urine

Drug examples

- atropine, belladonna, benztropine (Cogentin), glycopyrrolate (Robinul), propantheline (Pro-Banthine), scopolamine (Scop, Transderm Scop), trihexyphenidyl hydrochloride (Artane)

Indications

- Parasympatholytics are used to reduce salivation and gastric secretions, to reverse heart block, to induce mydriasis, and to treat Parkinson's disease, GI spasms, motion sickness, and enuresis
- Atropine and glycopyrrolate are used to treat bradyarrhythmias, arrhythmias, and sinus arrest

- Benztropine and trihexyphenidyl are used to treat dyskinesia, extrapyramidal reactions, and parkinsonism
- Propantheline and glycopyrrolate are used to treat peptic ulcer and bowel spasms
- Scopolamine is used to prevent nausea and vomiting resulting from motion sickness
- Atropine also is used to induce mydriasis
- Atropine, scopolamine, and glycopyrrolate are used to decrease saliva and bronchial secretions before surgery

Contraindications and precautions

- Contraindicated in angle-closure glaucoma, uncontrolled tachycardia, urinary or GI tract obstruction, hypersensitivity, severe ulcerative colitis, myasthenia gravis, tachycardia caused by cardiac insufficiency or thyrotoxicosis, acute or severe hemorrhage, or unstable cardiovascular status
- Also contraindicated in children and breast-feeding women

Adverse reactions

- Ophthalmic adverse effects with topical application of atropine include blurred vision, conjunctivitis, and photophobia
- Systemic adverse effects include tachycardia, constipation, dry mouth, and urinary hesitancy or urine retention

Interactions

- Use with various drugs (such as tricyclic antidepressants) may increase anticholinergic adverse effects
- Antacids decrease absorption of parasympatholytics

Nursing responsibilities

- Assess the patient for relief of symptoms
- Monitor the patient for adverse reactions
- Teach the patient to reduce dry mouth by using ice chips, hard candy, or gum and to reduce constipation by exercising and increasing fiber and fluid intake
- Instruct the patient to consult a physician or pharmacist before taking nonprescription drugs to prevent adverse drug interactions
- Administer a cholinergic blocker 30 minutes before meals and at bedtime when used to reduce GI motility
- Monitor the patient's intake and output, and watch for signs and symptoms of urine retention, such as urinary frequency with voiding of minimal amounts

ADRENERGIC AGONISTS (SYMPATHOMIMETICS)

Mechanism of action

- Mimic sympathetic activity by activating or inhibiting alpha and beta receptors that normally are activated by the neurotransmitter norepinephrine, or dopamine receptors activated by dopamine

When NOT to use parasympatholytics

- Angle-closure glaucoma
- Uncontrolled tachycardia
- Urinary or GI tract obstruction
- Hypersensitivity
- Severe ulcerative colitis
- Myasthenia gravis
- Tachycardia caused by cardiac insufficiency or thyrotoxicosis
- Acute or severe hemorrhage
- Unstable cardiovascular status
- Children
- Breast-feeding

Adverse reactions to watch for

- Blurred vision, conjunctivitis, photophobia, tachycardia, constipation, dry mouth, urinary hesitancy, urine retention

Key nursing actions

- Monitor for adverse reactions.
- Administer 30 minutes before meals and at bedtime when used to reduce GI motility.
- Monitor intake and output, and watch for signs and symptoms of urine retention.

Key facts about adrenergic agonists

- Mimic sympathetic activity by activating or inhibiting alpha, beta, and dopamine receptors
- Metabolism and excretion vary by drug

Pharmacokinetics

- Absorption: Varies widely with each drug
- Distribution: Varies widely with each drug
- Metabolism: Varies widely with each drug
- Excretion: Varies widely with each drug

Drug examples

- albuterol (Proventil, Ventolin), dobutamine (Dobutrex), dopamine (Intropin), epinephrine (Adrenalin, Susphrine), isoproterenol (Isuprel), metaproterenol sulfate (Alupent), norepinephrine (Levophed), phenylephrine (Neosynephrine), pseudoephedrine (Novafed, Sudafed), terbutaline (Brethine, Bricanyl)

Indications

- Alpha-adrenergic agonists, which increase blood pressure, are used to treat hypotension
- $Beta_1$-adrenergic agonists, which increase cardiac output, myocardial contractility, and heart rate and accelerate AV conduction, are used to treat heart failure
- $Beta_2$-adrenergic agonists, which cause peripheral vasodilation and bronchodilation, are used to treat asthma and allergy
- Dopamine agonists, which dilate renal arteries in low doses, are used to treat mild renal failure caused by decreased cardiac output
- Epinephrine is used for bronchodilation in asthma or allergic reactions, cardiac stimulation in cardiac arrest, and mydriasis; it's also used to stimulate alpha, $beta_1$, and $beta_2$ receptors and, when combined with local anesthetics, to produce local vasoconstriction, thereby decreasing blood flow to the site and prolonging anesthetic action
- Isoproterenol is used for cardiac stimulation and bronchodilation through stimulation of $beta_1$ and $beta_2$ receptors
- Norepinephrine is used to stimulate the heart in cardiac arrest and to increase blood pressure through vasoconstriction in acute hypotension and shock
- Dopamine is used in higher doses for increased blood pressure and cardiac output through positive inotropic action and in lower doses for increased renal and mesenteric blood flow through its action on alpha-adrenergic and $beta_1$-adrenergic receptors
- Dobutamine is used for increased myocardial force and cardiac output through stimulation of $beta_1$-adrenergic receptors for patients with acute congestive heart failure and those undergoing cardiopulmonary bypass
- Albuterol and metaproterenol are used for bronchodilation
- Terbutaline is used for bronchodilation and to delay delivery in preterm labor
- Pseudoephedrine and phenylephrine are used for nasal decongestion
- Phenylephrine is given I.V. to treat severe hypotension or shock

Contraindications and precautions

- Epinephrine is contraindicated in angle-closure glaucoma

When to use adrenergic agonists

- Hypotension
- Heart failure
- Asthma and allergy
- Mild renal failure
- Cardiac arrest
- Mydriasis
- Shock
- Preterm labor
- Nasal congestion

When NOT to use adrenergic agonists

- Angle-closure glaucoma
- Tachyarrhythmias

- Dopamine and isoproterenol are contraindicated in patients with tachyarrhythmias

Adverse reactions

- Arrhythmias, tachycardia, angina, restlessness, urinary urgency or incontinence; overuse of nasal decongestants may result in rebound stuffiness

Interactions

- Antagonize the effects of beta blockers (epinephrine, isoproterenol, and norepinephrine)

Nursing responsibilities

- Explain to the patient the purpose of the drug
- Assess the patient's vital signs, breath sounds, and urine output to prevent the adverse effects listed above
- Monitor the electrocardiogram and hemodynamic parameters for undesirable changes
- Correct hypovolemia before infusing dopamine or norepinephrine to ensure the drug's effectiveness
- **Administer drugs through a large vein to prevent extravasation; if extravasation occurs during infusion of dopamine or norepinephrine, infiltrate the skin with phentolamine (Regitine) and normal saline solution, as ordered**
- Teach the patient how to administer the prescribed inhalation drug, as appropriate
- Base patient evaluation on improved vital signs, urine output, and hemodynamics or on relief of bronchospasms without serious adverse effects

ADRENERGIC BLOCKERS (SYMPATHOLYTICS)

ALPHA-ADRENERGIC BLOCKERS

Mechanism of action

- Inhibit sympathetic activity by activating or inhibiting alpha- and beta-receptors that normally are activated by norepinephrine, or dopamine receptors that are activated by dopamine

Pharmacokinetics

- Absorption: Absorption is erratic when administered orally; more rapidly and completely absorbed when administered sublingually
- Distribution: Unknown
- Metabolism: Metabolized by the liver
- Excretion: Excreted in the feces with only traces in the urine

Drug examples

- doxazosin mesylate (Cardura), ergotamine tartrate (Ergostat), ergotamine tartrate with caffeine (Cafergot), phenoxybenzamine (Dibenzyline), phentolamine (Regitine)

Indications

– As smooth-muscle relaxants and vasodilators; used to treat peripheral

Adverse reactions to watch for

- Arrhythmias, tachycardia, angina, restlessness, urinary urgency or incontinence, rebound stuffiness

Key nursing actions

- Explain purpose of drug to patient.
- Assess vital signs, breath sounds, and urine output.
- Monitor the electrocardiogram and hemodynamic parameters.
- Correct hypovolemia before infusing dopamine or norepinephrine.
- Administer drugs through a large vein to prevent extravasation.

Key facts about alpha-adrenergic blockers

- Inhibit sympathetic activity by activating or inhibiting alpha-, beta-, or dopamine receptors
- Metabolized by the liver
- Excreted in feces

When to use alpha-adrenergic blockers

- Peripheral vascular disorders
- Raynaud's disease
- Vascular headaches
- Adrenergic excess
- Hypertension secondary to pheochromocytoma
- Extravasation of vasopressors

When NOT to use alpha-adrenergic blockers

- Myocardial infarction
- Coronary insufficiency
- Evidence of coronary artery disease
- Pregnancy

Adverse reactions to watch for

- Nasal congestion, orthostatic hypotension, tachycardia, dizziness, GI irritation, arrhythmias, miosis, ergotism (characterized by numbness, tingling of fingers and toes, weakness, and blindness)

Key nursing actions

- Monitor blood pressure for signs of orthostatic hypotension, as appropriate.
- Instruct patient to change positions slowly to minimize orthostatic hypotension.
- Administer drug with milk or food.
- If patient experiences a shocklike state, place in Trendelenburg position, notify prescriber, and begin emergency resuscitation, as appropriate.

vascular disorders, Raynaud's disease, vascular headaches, and adrenergic excess (for example, pheochromocytoma)

- Phenoxybenzamine is used to treat Raynaud's disease
- Phentolamine is used to diagnose and treat hypertension secondary to pheochromocytoma and to treat extravasation of vasopressors
- Ergotamine is used to treat vascular headache

Contraindications and precautions

- Patients who have had a myocardial infarction (MI), coronary insufficiency, or other evidence of coronary artery disease; pregnant women

Adverse reactions

- Phenoxybenzamine and phentolamine may cause nasal congestion, orthostatic hypotension, tachycardia, dizziness, GI irritation, arrhythmias, and miosis
- Ergotamine may cause ergotism (chronic poisoning from excessive ergot use), characterized by numbness, tingling of fingers and toes, weakness, and blindness

Interactions

- Use with antihypertensives (phenoxybenzamine) potentiates hypotensive effects
- Use of adrenergic agonists with other adrenergics causes additive effects
- Use of adrenergic blockers with other sympatholytics increases effects
- Use with epinephrine or ephedrine will antagonize their vasoconstricting and hypertensive effects
- Use of ergotamine tartrate and caffeine suppository with potent CYP3A4 inhibitors (such as macrolides and protease inhibitors) can cause ergot toxicity (vasospasms, ischemic extremities, and cerebral ischemia)

Nursing responsibilities

- **When administering phenoxybenzamine or phentolamine, monitor blood pressure for signs of orthostatic hypotension**
- If a phentolamine test is scheduled, withhold all antihypertensives, as ordered, and explain the test to the patient
- Instruct the patient to change positions slowly to minimize orthostatic hypotension.
- Inform the patient that the intended effects of phenoxybenzamine may take 1 week to appear
- Instruct the patient with vascular headache to take ergotamine at onset of the headache and then lie down in a dark, quiet room
- **Monitor the patient receiving ergotamine for signs and symptoms of vascular insufficiency due to ergotism, such as numbness, tingling, or weakness in extremities**
- Administer with milk or food to minimize gastric irritation
- **If the patient experiences a shocklike state, place the patient in a Trendelenburg position, notify the prescriber, and begin emergency resuscitation, as appropriate**

BETA-ADRENERGIC BLOCKERS

Mechanism of action

- Reduce or block myocardial stimulation and cause vasodilation, reducing glycogenolysis and bronchodilator effects
- Selective beta blockers block $beta_1$ receptors found predominantly in the heart
- Nonselective beta blockers block both $beta_1$ and $beta_2$ receptors, which may result in bronchospasm in individuals with asthma or obstructive lung disease

Pharmacokinetics

- Absorption: Usually absorbed rapidly and well from the GI tract and some drugs are absorbed more completely than others; food may enhance absorption
- Distribution: Somewhat protein-bound; distributed widely in the body tissues, with highest concentrations in the heart, liver, lungs, and saliva
- Metabolism: Except for nadolol and atenolol, usually metabolized in the liver
- Excretion: Excreted in feces, urine, and breast milk

Drug examples

- acebutolol (Sectral), atenolol (Tenormin), betaxolol (Betoptic, Kerlone), carteolol (Cartrol), carvedilol (Coreg), esmolol (Brevibloc), labetalol (Normodyne, Trandate), levobunolol (Betagan), metipranolol (OptiPranolol), metoprolol (Lopressor), nadolol (Corgard), penbutolol (Levatol), pindolol (Visken), propranolol (Inderal), sotalol (Betapace), timolol (Blocadren)

Indications

- Beta blockers are used to treat hypertension, angina, and tachyarrhythmias and to prevent migraine headache, MI, glaucoma, and acute anxiety reaction
- Acebutolol, atenolol, betaxolol, carteolol, carvedilol, labetalol, metoprolol, nadolol, penbutolol, pindolol, propranolol, and timolol are used to treat hypertension
- Atenolol, metoprolol, nadolol, and propranolol are used to treat angina
- Acebutolol, esmolol, sotalol and propranolol are used to treat tachyarrhythmias
- Carvedilol is used to treat mild to severe heart failure and left ventricular dysfunction after MI
- Metoprolol, propranolol, and timolol are used to prevent MI
- Propranolol is used to prevent vascular headache
- Betaxolol, levobunolol, metipranolol, and timolol are used to treat glaucoma

Contraindications and precautions

- Bradyarrhythmias, bronchospasm, heart block

Adverse reactions

- Arrhythmias, bradycardia, bronchospasm, nausea, vomiting, diarrhea, increased sensitivity to cold

Key facts about beta-adrenergic blockers

- Reduce or block myocardial stimulation
- Cause vasodilation
- Usually metabolized in the liver
- Excreted in feces, urine, and breast milk

When to use beta-adrenergic blockers

- Hypertension
- Angina
- Tachyarrhythmias
- Migraines
- MI
- Glaucoma
- Acute anxiety reaction
- Mild to severe heart failure
- Left ventricular dysfunction after MI
- Vascular headache

When NOT to use beta-adrenergic blockers

- Bradyarrhythmias
- Bronchospasm
- Heart block

Adverse reactions to watch for

- Arrhythmias, bradycardia, bronchospasm, nausea, vomiting, diarrhea, increased sensitivity to cold

Topics for patient discussion

- Medication regimen, including proper administration
- Methods to assess pulse and blood pressure
- Signs and symptoms of adverse reactions
- Avoidance of over-the-counter drugs
- Importance of carrying identification about his disease and drug regimen
- Follow-up care

Key nursing actions

- Assess pulse rate; withhold drug and notify physician if rate is below 50 beats/minute (or according to hospital policy).
- After administering eyedrops, apply pressure to inner canthus for 1 minute.
- Encourage the patient to comply with other recommended antihypertensive interventions.

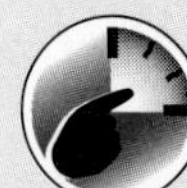

TIME-OUT FOR TEACHING

Teaching about beta-adrenergic blockers

Make sure to include the following topics in your teaching plan for the patient receiving a beta-adrenergic blocker.

- Medication prescribed, including name, dose, frequency, action, and adverse effects
- Proper technique for administration
- Methods to assess pulse and blood pressure
- Signs and symptoms of adverse reactions
- Avoidance of over-the-counter products
- Follow-up care

Interactions

- Use with drugs having similar effects (such as antiarrhythmics and calcium channel blockers) may cause additive myocardial depression and bradycardia
- Use with insulin or hypoglycemics increases the risk of hypoglycemia, may alter insulin requirements, and may mask signs and symptoms of hypoglycemia (such as tachycardia and sweating)

Nursing responsibilities

- **Assess the patient's pulse rate; withhold the drug and notify the physician if the rate is below 50 beats/minute (or according to hospital policy)**
- After administering eyedrops, apply pressure to the inner canthus of the eye for 1 minute to minimize systemic absorption
- Teach the patient to monitor pulse and blood pressure for adverse changes (for specific teaching tips, see *Teaching about beta-adrenergic blockers*)
- If appropriate, encourage the patient to comply with other recommended antihypertensive interventions (such as weight reduction, smoking cessation, dietary sodium restriction, moderation of alcohol consumption, regular exercise, and stress management)
- Instruct the patient to carry identification describing the disease and drug regimen
- **Advise the patient who is receiving long-term therapy not to discontinue the drug suddenly because this may precipitate an MI or arrhythmias**

NEUROMUSCULAR BLOCKERS

NONDEPOLARIZING DRUGS (COMPETITIVE OR STABILIZING DRUGS)

Mechanism of action
- Compete with acetylcholine at the cholinergic receptor sites of the skeletal muscle membrane, thereby blocking acetylcholine transmitter action and preventing muscle membranes from depolarizing

Pharmacokinetics
- Absorption: Absorbed parenterally because they are poorly absorbed after oral administration
- Distribution: Distributed rapidly throughout the body but don't cross blood-brain barrier; therefore, they don't alter consciousness or pain perception
- Metabolism: Partially metabolized in the liver
- Excretion: Most are excreted unchanged in the urine

Drug examples
- atracurium besylate (Tacrium), cisatracurium besylate (Nimbex), doxacurium chloride (Nuromax), pancuronium bromide, vecuronium bromide (Norcuron)

Indications
- For prolonged or intermediate muscle relaxation during surgery or facilitation of endotracheal (ET) intubation
- For paralysis in patients who are insufficiently ventilated or who fight with the ET tube or ventilator

Contraindications and precautions
- Contraindicated in patients hypersensitive to drug and in neonates because these drugs contain benzyl alcohol
- Use cautiously in pregnant and breast-feeding women

Adverse reactions
- Apnea, hypotension, skin reactions, bronchospasms, excessive bronchial or salivary excretions

Interactions
- Most drugs, such as antibiotics and anesthetics, that interact with a nondepolarizing blocker will have an additive effect
- **Anticholinesterases (neostigmine, pyridostigmine, and edrophonium) are antagonistic and are used as antidotes to nondepolarizing blockers**

Nursing responsibilities
- Monitor the patient for any adverse reactions, especially apnea or bronchospasm, during drug therapy
- **Have oxygen and ET and suction equipment available at all times in case respiratory support is needed**

Key facts about nondepolarizing drugs
- Compete with acetylcholine at cholinergic receptor sites of skeletal muscle membrane, thereby blocking acetylcholine transmitter action and preventing muscle membranes from depolarizing
- Partially metabolized in the liver
- Excreted in urine

When to use nondepolarizing drugs
- Prolonged or intermediate muscle relaxation for surgery or ET intubation

When NOT to use nondepolarizing drugs
- Hypersensitivity
- Neonates
- Pregnancy
- Breast-feeding

Adverse effects to watch for
- Apnea, hypotension, skin reactions, bronchospasms, excessive bronchial or salivary excretions

Key nursing actions
- Monitor for adverse reactions.
- Have oxygen and ET and suction equipment available.
- Monitor respirations frequently until the patient is fully recovered.
- Suction the patient as needed.
- Frequently check the mechanical ventilator settings and functions to ensure proper functioning.

Key facts about depolarizing drugs

- Compete with acetylcholine at cholinergic receptors of the skeletal muscle membrane and depolarize that postsynaptic membrane of the muscle
- Cause persistent depolarization followed by muscle fasciculations and paralysis or flaccidity
- Metabolized in the liver and plasma
- Excreted in urine

When to use depolarizing drugs

- Endotracheal intubation
- Skeletal muscle relaxation for surgery or mechanical ventilation

When NOT to use depolarizing drugs

- Hypersensitivity
- Genetic disorder of plasma pseudocholinesterase
- History of malignant hyperthermia
- Myopathies associated with elevated creatine phosphokinase levels
- Acute angle-closure glaucoma
- Penetrating eye injuries

Adverse effects to watch for

- Prolonged apnea and cardiovascular effects, muscle pain, increased intraocular pressure

- **Monitor respirations frequently until the patient is fully recovered from the neuromuscular blockade, as evidenced by increased muscle strength (peripheral nerve stimulation, hand grip, head lift, and ability to cough)**
- Keep drugs refrigerated to maintain their potency
- Suction the patient as needed because the drug will suppress the cough reflex and increase respiratory secretions
- **Frequently check the mechanical ventilator settings and functions to ensure that that it's working properly; never turn off the ventilator alarm**

DEPOLARIZING DRUGS

Mechanism of action

- Produce a biphasic effect at the skeletal muscle
  - First phase: These drugs compete with acetylcholine at the cholinergic receptors of the skeletal muscle membrane and depolarize that postsynaptic membrane of the muscle; NOT counteracted by anticholinesterase causing persistent depolarization followed by muscle fasciculations and paralysis or flaccidity
  - The second phase is seen only in high doses

Pharmacokinetics

- Absorption: Absorbed poorly in the GI tract; I.V. administration is the preferred route
- Distribution: Unknown
- Metabolism: Hydrolyzed in the liver and plasma by pseudocholinesterase
- Excretion: Excreted in the urine; about 10% is excreted unchanged

Drug examples

- succinylcholine chloride (Anectine, Quelicin)

Indications

- For short-term muscle relaxation as an adjunct to general anesthesia to facilitate ET intubation
- To induce skeletal muscle relaxation during surgery or mechanical ventilation

Contraindications and precautions

- Contraindicated in patients with a known hypersensitivity to the drug or its components, a genetic disorder of plasma pseudocholinesterase, personal or family history of malignant hyperthermia, myopathies associated with elevated creatine phosphokinase levels, acute angle-closure glaucoma, or penetrating eye injuries
- Use cautiously in pregnant or breast-feeding women, children, and patients with cardiovascular, hepatic, pulmonary, metabolic, or renal disorders

- **Adverse reactions**
  - Prolonged apnea and cardiovascular effects, possible muscle pain and increased intraocular pressure
- **Interactions**
  - Anticholinesterases increase succinylcholine blockade
  - Many antibiotics and anesthetics increase action of succinylcholine
- **Nursing responsibilities**
  - **Maintain a patent airway for the patient at all times.**
  - **Check the patient's respiratory rate and pattern every 5 minutes during drug infusion**
  - Monitor the patient closely until recovery from the neuromuscular blockade is complete; signs of recovery include a renewed ability to cough, and a return of previous levels of muscle strength on hand-grip and head-lift tests

NCLEX CHECKS

It's never too soon to begin your NCLEX preparation. Now that you've reviewed this chapter, carefully read each of the following questions and choose the best answer. Then compare your responses to the correct answers.

1. A patient with Parkinson's disease asks why he is taking trihexyphenidyl hydrochloride. You should respond by explaining that the drug:

☐ **A.** helps patients relax so they can sleep.
☐ **B.** counteracts the adverse reactions of levodopa.
☐ **C.** prevents patients from developing depression.
☐ **D.** controls the symptoms of drooling and muscle rigidity.

2. A 73-year-old patient is scheduled for a cholecystectomy. The physician prescribes preoperative sedation with meperidine (Demerol), 75 mg I.M., and the cholinergic blocker atropine, 0.4 mg I.M. Which of the following statements describes the purpose of atropine as a preanesthetic agent?

☐ **A.** Atropine reduces hyperreflexia during surgery.
☐ **B.** Atropine minimizes the risk of postoperative ileus.
☐ **C.** Atropine prevents respiratory depression during surgery.
☐ **D.** Atropine reduces excess salivation and gastric secretions.

3. A patient with an endotracheal (ET) tube receiving mechanical ventilation becomes more conscious and begins to fight both the ET tube and the ventilator. Pancuronium bromide, 0.1 mg/kg of body weight, is ordered. This drug exerts its therapeutic effect by:

☐ **A.** stimulating muscarinic receptors at effector organs.
☐ **B.** inhibiting the action of cholinesterase at the motor end plate.
☐ **C.** enhancing the muscle's ability to respond to the neurotransmitter acetylcholine.
☐ **D.** competing with acetylcholine at cholinergic receptor sites in the skeletal muscle.

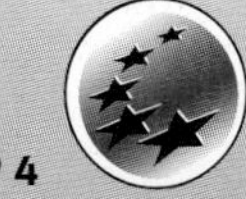

TOP 4

Items to study before your next test on drugs and the autonomic nervous system

1. Mechanisms of action of cholinergics and adrenergics
2. Indications for various autonomic nervous system drugs
3. Nursing responsibilities related to each class of cholinergic and adrenergic
4. Indications and mechanisms of action for neuromuscular blockades

4. A patient with a history of asthma occasionally gets bronchospasm attacks. You review the patient's drug history, questioning the use of which drug?

☐ **A.** Ergotamine tartrate (Ergomar)
☐ **B.** Metoprolol tartrate (Lopressor)
☐ **C.** Phenoxybenzamine hydrochloride (Dibenzyline)
☐ **D.** Phentolamine mesylate (Regitine)

5. Essential hypertension, Raynaud's disease, and pheochromocytoma respond effectively to which class of drugs?

☐ **A.** Alpha-adrenergic blockers
☐ **B.** Beta-adrenergic blockers
☐ **C.** Central nervous system (CNS) stimulants
☐ **D.** Cholinergic blockers

6. A patient taking an anticholinergic for 1 month arrives at an outpatient clinic with complaints of constipation, dry mouth, and decreased sweating. You realize that these complaints are:

☐ **A.** rare.
☐ **B.** normal.
☐ **C.** dose-related adverse reactions.
☐ **D.** symptoms of anaphylactic reaction.

7. The nurse is caring for a patient with a T5 complete spinal cord injury. On assessment, the nurse notes flushed skin, diaphoresis above T5, and a blood pressure of 162/96 mm Hg. The patient reports a severe, pounding headache. Which of the following nursing interventions would be appropriate for this patient?

Select all that apply:

☐ **A.** Elevate the head of the bed 90 degrees.
☐ **B.** Loosen constrictive clothing.
☐ **C.** Use a fan to reduce diaphoresis.
☐ **D.** Assess for bladder distention and bowel impaction.
☐ **E.** Administer antihypertensive medication.
☐ **F.** Place the patient in a supine position with legs elevated.

ANSWERS AND RATIONALES

1. CORRECT ANSWER: D

Anticholinergics antagonize functions controlled by the parasympathetic nervous system. Trihexyphenidyl hydrochloride is an anticholinergic and is used to control the symptoms of drooling and muscle rigidity. It isn't used for the other reasons listed.

2. CORRECT ANSWER: D

The ultimate goal of giving atropine is to prevent the patient from aspirating. Atropine will reduce the amount of excess salivation and gastric secretions preoperatively. This effect aims to prevent nausea, vomiting, and possible aspiration intraoperatively and postoperatively. Atropine is not used to reduce hyperreflexia, to minimize postoperative ileus, or to prevent respiratory depression during surgery.

3. CORRECT ANSWER: D
Pancuronium is a neuromuscular blocking agent, thereby blocking depolarization. It disrupts nerve impulse transmission at the motor end plate by competing with acetylcholine at receptor sites. This drug does not stimulate muscarinic receptors at effector organs, inhibit cholinesterase, or enhance muscle response to acetylcholine.

4. CORRECT ANSWER: B
Metoprolol is a beta-adrenergic blocker. The most common respiratory adverse reaction is bronchospasm. Caution is advisable when giving beta-adrenergic blockers to patients with bronchial asthma, bronchitis, or emphysema. Ergotamine, phenoxybenzamine, and phentolamine are alpha-adrenergic blockers, which cause smooth muscle relaxation and vasodilation, not bronchospasm.

5. CORRECT ANSWER: A
Alpha-adrenergic blockers increase blood flow by relaxing smooth muscles and causing vasodilation. This mechanism makes them useful in treating essential hypertension, Raynaud's disease, and pheochromocytoma. Beta-adrenergic blockers, cholinergic blockers, and CNS stimulants don't produce this action.

6. CORRECT ANSWER: C
Constipation, dry mouth, and decreased sweating are dose-related adverse reactions to anticholinergics. These usually decrease as treatment continues. These symptoms aren't normal or rare, and some physicians will try to reduce the dose to decrease them. Anticholinergics don't cause anaphylactic reactions, but patient sensitivity reactions, including urticaria and allergic rashes that may lead to exfoliation, may occur.

7. CORRECT ANSWER: A, B, D, E
The patient is exhibiting signs and symptoms of autonomic dysreflexia. The condition is a potentially life-threatening emergency caused by an uninhibited response from the sympathetic nervous system resulting from a lack of control over the autonomic nervous system. The nurse should immediately elevate the head of the bed to 90 degrees and place the extremities in a dependent position to decrease venous return to the heart and increase venous return from the brain. Because tactile stimuli can trigger autonomic dysreflexia, any constrictive clothing should be loosened. The nurse should also assess for distended bladder and bowel impaction — which may trigger autonomic dysreflexia — and correct any problems. Elevated blood pressure is the most life-threatening complication of autonomic dysreflexia because it can cause stroke, myocardial infarction, or seizure activity. If removing the triggering event doesn't reduce the patient's blood pressure, I.V. antihypertensives should be administered. A fan shouldn't be used because drafts of cold may trigger autonomic dysreflexia.

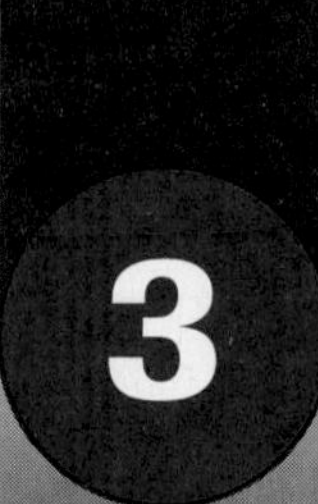

Drugs and the central nervous system

LEARNING OBJECTIVES

After studying this chapter, you should be able to:

- Explain the general mechanism of action of central nervous system (CNS) stimulants, anticonvulsants, antiparkinsonians, and antimyasthenics.
- Name the most common adverse effects of the various CNS stimulants, anticonvulsants, antiparkinsonians, and antimyasthenics.
- Identify nursing responsibilities when administering CNS stimulants, anticonvulsants, antiparkinsonians, and antimyasthenics.
- Discuss appropriate teaching for the patient who is receiving a CNS stimulant, anticonvulsant, antiparkinsonian, or antimyasthenic.
- Compare and contrast dopaminergic and cholinergic blocking drugs.
- Explain the importance of patient compliance with antimyasthenic therapy.

CHAPTER OVERVIEW

Central nervous system (CNS) stimulants (amphetamines, caffeine, analeptics, and anorexiants) increase neurotransmitter levels in the CNS, causing CNS and respiratory stimulation, pupil dilation, increased motor activity, heightened mental alertness, brighter spirits, and a diminished sense of fatigue.

Anticonvulsants are used to reduce or eliminate seizures. The current trend in therapy is maintenance with one drug (monotherapy) to avoid drug interactions.

Antiparkinsonians, drugs used to treat parkinsonism, include dopaminergic agonists and cholinergic blockers. Parkinson's disease results from an imbalance of neurotransmitters, particularly excess acetylcholine and insufficient dopamine, in the CNS. It is a chronic, disabling disorder of motor function characterized by tremors, rigidity, bradykinesia, depression, and dementia. Drug therapy reduces cholinergic activity and enhances dopamine activity.

Antimyasthenics (cholinergics) are used to treat myasthenia gravis, which is an autoimmune disease caused by a deficiency of acetylcholine. It results in muscle weakness exacerbated by physical or emotional stress or infection. Myasthenic crisis and cholinergic crisis are two important complications associated with the administration of antimyasthenics.

Nursing responsibilities for all these drugs focus on monitoring the therapeutic effectiveness of the drug, as evidenced by improvement in the condition and avoidance of overdosage, and patient education about all aspects of the drug therapy, complications and possible adverse effects.

ANATOMY AND PHYSIOLOGY

Anatomy

- The CNS consists of the spinal cord and the brain
  - The spinal cord carries messages from the body to the brain
  - The brain, once it receives the message, analyzes and interprets it and sends a response message from the brain, through the spinal cord, to the rest of the body
- The brain and the spinal cord are protected by bony structures (the skull and the vertebrae), membranous meninges, and cerebrospinal fluid
- Neurons are the basic functional unit of the nervous system

Function

- The CNS is considered the control center of the body; it relays messages, processes information, and compares and analyzes information
- Neurons conduct the impulses across a synapse to and from muscles, glands, and organs and the CNS

CNS neurotransmitters

- The CNS neurotransmitters acetylcholine, norepinephrine, serotonin, dopamine, and gamma-aminobutyric acid (GABA) help neurons transmit impulses in the CNS
- Acetylcholine—inactivated by the enzyme cholinesterase
- Norepinephrine—inactivated by reuptake (when some of it is taken back into the synaptic vesicles in the axon terminals) or by the enzymes catechol O-methyl-transferase (COMT) or monoamine oxidase (MAO)
- Serotonin—inactivated by reuptake and by enzymatic (MAO) breakdown
- Dopamine—inactivated by reuptake or by COMT or MAO
- GABA—inactivated by enzymatic breakdown

A&P highlights

- The CNS consists of the spinal cord and the brain.
- The spinal cord carries messages from the body to the brain.
- The brain analyzes and interprets messages and sends response messages, through the spinal cord, to the rest of the body.
- Neurons are the basic functional unit of the nervous system.
- Neurons conduct impulses across a synapse to and from muscles, glands, and organs and the CNS.

Five CNS neurotransmitters

1. Acetylcholine
2. Norepinephrine
3. Serotonin
4. Dopamine
5. Gamma-aminobutyric acid

CNS STIMULANTS

Key facts about CNS stimulants

- Increase neurotransmitter levels in the CNS
- Metabolized by the liver
- Excreted in urine

When to use CNS stimulants

- Hyperactivity in children
- ADHD
- Narcolepsy

When NOT to use CNS stimulants

- Glaucoma
- Severe cardiovascular disease

Adverse reactions to watch for

- Restlessness, tremor, irritability, insomnia, hypotension, arrhythmias, angina, CV collapse, weight loss, fatigue, depression, growth suppression

Mechanism of action

- Increase neurotransmitter levels in the CNS, either by increasing neuronal discharge or by blocking an inhibitory neurotransmitter, causing CNS and respiratory stimulation, pupil dilation, increased motor activity, heightened mental alertness, brighter spirits, and a diminished sense of fatigue

Pharmacokinetics

- Absorption: Absorbed in the GI tract after oral administration
- Distribution: Varies with each drug
- Metabolism: Usually metabolized by the liver
- Excretion: Excreted in the urine

Drug examples

- dexmethylphenidate hydrochloride (Focalin), dextroamphetamine (Dexedrine), doxapram (Dopram), methylphenidate hydrochloride (Concerta, Metadate, Methylin, Ritalin), pemoline (Cylert, PemADD)

Indications

- To increase mental alertness and respiratory rate
- To treat hyperactivity in children
- Dexmethylphenidate hydrochloride effectively manages symptoms of attention deficit hyperactivity disorder (ADHD) at half the dose of Ritalin
- Dextroamphetamine, methylphenidate, and pemoline are used to treat narcolepsy and ADHD
- Doxapram is used to treat respiratory stimulation after anesthesia

Contraindications and precautions

- Contraindicated in patients with glaucoma and severe cardiovascular (CV) disease
- Use with caution in patients with psychosis and in pregnant and breast-feeding women

Adverse reactions

- Acute adverse effects (toxicity) include restlessness, tremor, irritability, insomnia, hypotension, arrhythmias, angina, and CV collapse
- Chronic adverse effects include marked weight loss, fatigue, irritability, depression, and growth suppression (in children)

Interactions

- Concurrent use with similar-acting drugs causes additive sympathomimetic effects
- Altered urine pH may alter the effectiveness of CNS stimulants
  - Urine acidification enhances renal excretion of the drug
  - Urine alkalinization enhances renal absorption of the drug

Nursing responsibilities

- Assess the patient's behavior to determine drug effectiveness
- Monitor growth in a child who is receiving long-term therapy

- When administering doxapram, assess the patient's respiratory status (including lung sounds and rate and depth of respirations) and arterial blood gas (ABG) measurements for changes
- Keep in mind that most CNS stimulants are controlled substances and that amphetamines may cause dependence and abuse
- Instruct the patient to take the last daily dose at least 6 hours before bedtime to prevent insomnia
- Instruct the patient to avoid beverages containing caffeine to prevent added stimulation
- Base patient evaluation on the reason for using the drug
  - In the patient with narcolepsy, base evaluation on increased activity and alertness, diminished fatigue, and brighter spirits
  - In the patient with ADHD, base evaluation on increased calmness, decreased hyperactivity, and a prolonged attention span (these effects usually appear in 3 to 4 weeks)
  - In the patient receiving doxapram to treat respiratory depression after anesthesia, base evaluation on improved respiratory status and ABG measurements

Key nursing actions

- Assess patient behavior to determine drug effectiveness.
- Monitor growth in a child receiving long-term therapy.
- Instruct patient to take last daily dose 6 hours before bedtime to prevent insomnia.
- Instruct patient to avoid caffeine.

ANTICONVULSANTS

HYDANTOINS

Mechanism of action

- Inhibit seizure activity by promoting sodium outflow from the neurons, thereby depressing abnormal neuronal stimulation and discharge

Pharmacokinetics

- Absorption: Usually slowly absorbed in the small intestines after oral administration; bioavailability varies among products.
- Distribution: Protein-bound; distributed in breast milk
- Metabolism: Metabolized in the liver
- Excretion: Excreted in the urine; half-life varies and is dose-dependent

Drug examples

- ethotoin (Peganone), fosphenytoin sodium (Cerebyx), mephenytoin (Mesantoin), phenytoin (Dilantin, Phenytek)

Indications

- To treat tonic-clonic (grand mal) seizures, status epilepticus (I.V.), and complex partial seizures
- Phenytoin also is used to treat arrhythmias and painful conditions, such as trigeminal neuralgia

Contraindications and precautions

- Contraindicated in patients hypersensitive to drug or its components
- Phenytoin is contraindicated in patients with sinus bradycardia, sinoatrial block, second- and third-degree heart block, or Adam-Stokes syndrome

Key facts about anticonvulsants

- Inhibit seizure activity
- Metabolized in the liver
- Excreted in urine

When to use anticonvulsants

- Tonic-clonic seizures
- Status epilepticus
- Complex partial seizures
- Arrhythmias
- Painful conditions, such as trigeminal neuralgia

When NOT to use anticonvulsants

- Hypersensitivity
- Sinus bradycardia
- Sinoatrial block
- Second- and third-degree heart block
- Adam-Stokes syndrome

Topics for patient discussion

- Medication regimen
- Signs and symptoms to discuss with the physician
- Oral hygiene measures to minimize gingival hyperplasia
- Urine discoloration
- Activity allowances and restriction
- Avoidance of alcohol and over-the-counter drug use
- Compliance with therapy, including adherence to regimen, avoidance of abrupt discontinuation, and consistent use of same drug preparation
- Follow-up care
- Care during and after a seizure
- Community resources for support and information

Adverse reactions to watch for

- Gingival hyperplasia, rare blood dyscrasias, diplopia, nystagmus, ataxia, drowsiness, slurred speech, tremors, nausea, vomiting

Key nursing actions

- Monitor for signs and symptoms of toxicity.
- Monitor therapeutic hydantoin, complete blood count, and liver enzyme levels.
- If GI upset occurs, administer drug with food.

Signs of anticonvulsant toxicity

- Ataxia
- Nystagmus
- Dysarthria
- Hypotension
- Coma
- Unresponsive pupils

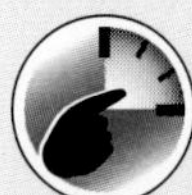

TIME-OUT FOR TEACHING

Teaching about oral hydantoin anticonvulsant therapy

Make sure to include the following topics in your teaching plan for the patient receiving an oral hydantoin anticonvulsant.

- Medication prescribed, including name, dose, frequency, action, and possible adverse effects
- Signs and symptoms to discuss with health care provider, including adverse effects
- Oral hygiene measures to minimize gingival hyperplasia
- Possible (though harmless) urine discoloration
- Activity allowances and restrictions, such as avoiding driving and other hazardous activities until drug's effect is known
- Avoidance of alcohol and self-medication with over-the-counter products
- Compliance with therapy, including adherence to regimen, avoidance of abrupt discontinuation, and consistent use of same drug preparation
- Importance of follow-up care, including laboratory tests and primary care visits
- Care during and after a seizure
- Community resources for support and information

Adverse reactions

- Gingival hyperplasia, rare blood dyscrasias, diplopia, nystagmus, ataxia, drowsiness, slurred speech, tremors, nausea and vomiting

Interactions

- Alcohol (long-term use), diazoxide, influenza vaccine, rifampin, and folic acid may decrease phenytoin activity and diminish the drug's effectiveness
- Amiodarone, antihistamines, chloramphenicol, cimetidine, cycloserine, diazepam, disulfiram, isoniazid, oral anticoagulants, phenylbutazone, salicylates, sulfamethizole, and valproate may increase phenytoin activity, leading to phenytoin toxicity
- Oral tube feedings may interfere with absorption of oral phenytoin, diminishing the drug's effectiveness; feedings should be scheduled at least 1 hour before or 2 hours after phenytoin dose
- Phenytoin is incompatible with dextrose and any dextrose-containing solutions

Nursing responsibilities

- Monitor the patient for signs and symptoms of toxicity (ataxia, nystagmus, and dysarthria), hypotension, coma, or unresponsive pupils; treatment for toxicity is nonspecific
- Monitor therapeutic hydantoin, complete blood count, and liver enzyme levels to avoid or detect toxicity
- **When administering phenytoin intravenously (I.V.), dilute in normal saline solution (dextrose solutions cause a precipitate); infuse no faster than 50 mg/minute**

- Teach the patient about the importance of good oral hygiene and regular dental examinations to prevent gingival hyperplasia
- If GI upset occurs, may give drug with food
- Instruct the patient to consult the physician or pharmacist before changing drug brands because bioavailability may differ among brands (for specific teaching tips, see *Teaching about oral hydantoin anticonvulsant therapy*)

BARBITURATES AND DEOXYBARBITURATES

Mechanism of action
- Depress the sensory cortex and motor activity and alter cerebellar function, causing drowsiness, sedation, and hypnosis; in high doses, barbiturates may induce anesthesia

Pharmacokinetics
- Absorption: Absorbed slowly in the GI tract; rate of absorption increases if given on an empty stomach
- Distribution: Protein-bound and well distributed in body tissues
- Metabolism: Metabolized by the liver
- Excretion: Excreted in the urine; primidone is also excreted in breast milk

Drug examples
- mephobarbital (Mebaral), phenobarbital (Luminal), primidone (Mysoline)

Indications
- To treat tonic-clonic (grand mal) seizures, partial seizures, and insomnia
- As adjuncts to anesthesia; may be used as an emergency control for acute convulsive episodes

Contraindications and precautions
- Barbiturates are contraindicated in patients who are sensitive to barbiturates and in pregnant and breast-feeding women
- Also contraindicated in patients with hepatic impairment or severe respiratory disease and in those who have had a previous addiction to a sedative or hypnotic
- Intra-arterial and subcutaneous (S.C.) administrations are contraindicated

Adverse reactions
- dizziness, drowsiness, hypotension, respiratory depression (with high doses), blood dyscrasias

Interactions
- Alcohol may cause additive CNS effects and death
- Phenobarbital toxicity can occur if primidone is given with phenobarbital (primidone is metabolized in the liver to phenobarbital)
- Barbiturates reduce the effectiveness of hormonal contraceptives

Nursing responsibilities
- Assess patient's respiratory status before and during drug therapy
- Discourage alcohol use during drug therapy

Key facts about barbiturates and deoxybarbiturates
- Depress sensory cortex and motor activity and alter cerebellar function, causing drowsiness, sedation, and hypnosis
- May induce anesthesia
- Metabolized by the liver
- Excreted in urine and breast milk

When to use barbiturates and deoxybarbiturates
- Tonic-clonic seizures
- Partial seizures
- Insomnia
- Acute convulsive episodes

When NOT to use barbiturates and deoxybarbiturates
- Hypersensitivity
- Pregnancy
- Breast-feeding
- Hepatic impairment
- Severe respiratory disease
- Previous addiction to sedative or hypnotic

Adverse reactions to watch for
- Dizziness, drowsiness, hypotension, respiratory depression, blood dyscrasias

Key nursing actions

- Assess respiratory status before and during drug therapy.
- Discourage alcohol use during drug therapy.
- Monitor for withdrawal symptoms (anxiety, muscle twitching, hand and finger tremors, weakness, dizziness, nausea and vomiting, convulsions, delirium)
- Notify prescriber immediately if patient develops fever, sore throat, mouth sores, bruising, bleeding, or tiny broken blood vessels under the skin during drug therapy.

Key facts about benzodiazepines

- Action is poorly understood
- Depress CNS at limbic and subcortical levels, suppressing seizure activity
- Metabolized by the liver
- Excreted in urine and breast milk

When to use benzodiazepines

- Absence seizures
- Lennox-Gastaut syndrome
- Akinetic and myoclonic seizures
- Long-term treatment of epilepsy (clonazepam only)
- Partial seizures
- Acute alcohol withdrawal
- Acute status epilepticus
- Anxiety
- Skeletal muscle spasms

When NOT to use benzodiazepines

- Hypersensitivity
- Acute angle-closure glaucoma
- Coma
- Shock
- Acute alcohol intoxication

- Know that barbiturates may be habit-forming; tolerance and psychological and physical dependence may occur, especially following prolonged use at high doses
- Monitor the patient for withdrawal symptoms
  - Minor symptoms may appear 8 to 12 hours after the last dose and include anxiety, muscle twitching, hand and finger tremors, weakness, dizziness, and nausea and vomiting
  - Severe symptoms include convulsions and delirium within 16 hours of last dose and may last up to 5 days after abrupt cessation of these drugs
  - Notify the prescriber immediately if patient develops fever, sore throat, mouth sores, bruising, bleeding, or tiny broken blood vessels under the skin during drug therapy

BENZODIAZEPINES

Mechanism of action

- Although their action is poorly understood, benzodiazepines depress the CNS at the limbic and subcortical levels, suppressing seizure activity

Pharmacokinetics

- Absorption: Absorbed rapidly and completely in the GI tract
- Distribution: Highly protein-bound. Distribution rate varies with each drug
- Metabolism: Metabolized by the liver
- Excretion: Excreted in the urine
  - Benzodiazepines cross the placental barrier and also are excreted in breast milk
  - Half-life is 20 to 100 hours

Drug examples

- clonazepam (Klonopin), clorazepate (Tranxene), diazepam (Valium)

Indications

- Clonazepam is used to treat absence (petit mal) seizures, Lennox-Gastaut syndrome (petit mal variant), and akinetic and myoclonic seizures; only clonazepam is recommended for long-term treatment of epilepsy
- Clorazepate is used as an adjunctive treatment of partial seizures and for acute alcohol withdrawal
- Diazepam is used to treat acute **status epilepticus**, anxiety, and skeletal muscle spasms

Contraindications and precautions

- Contraindicated in patients with hypersensitivity or acute angle-closure glaucoma
- Diazepam also is contraindicated in patients in a coma or shock and in those with acute alcohol intoxication

Adverse reactions

- Ataxia, drug dependence, respiratory and cardiovascular depression (with I.V. diazepam), drowsiness (most common), dizziness, blood dyscrasias

Interactions
- Increase CNS depression if given with CNS depressants, alcohol, or cimetidine
- Increase digoxin levels and digoxin toxicity if given together
- If given with phenobarbital, increases effects of both drugs
- Hormonal contraceptives decrease the metabolism of benzodiazepines

Nursing responsibilities
- Caution the patient not to stop the drug abruptly; doing so could produce status epilepticus or worsen the seizure disorder
- Know that psychological dependence may develop with the use of clonazepam or diazepam
- When administering I.V. diazepam:
  - Administer no faster than 5 mg/minute in adults and over at least 3 minutes in children
  - Avoid giving in small veins
  - Don't mix with other drugs in the same syringe
  - Give by direct I.V. push only; don't give as an infusion

SUCCINIMIDES

Mechanism of action
- Reduce epileptic attacks by suppressing paroxysmal three cycle per second spike and wave activity, depressing the motor cortex, and elevating the threshold of the CNS to convulsive stimuli

Pharmacokinetics
- Absorption: Readily absorbed in the GI tract
- Distribution: Serum levels peak in 3 to 7 hours; therapeutic serum levels range from 40 to 100 mcg/ml
- Metabolism: Metabolized by the liver
- Excretion: Excreted in the urine; half-life is 30 hours in children, 60 hours in adults

Drug examples
- ethosuximide (Zarontin), methosuximide (Celontin), phensuximide (Milontin)

Indications
- To control absence (petit mal) seizures

Contraindications and precautions
- Contraindicated in patients who are hypersensitive to succinimides or its components

Adverse reactions
- Anorexia, nausea, vomiting, blood dyscrasias, drowsiness
- Methsuximide: drowsiness, ataxia, dizziness are the most common.
- Phensuximide: hematuria is common.

Adverse reactions to watch for
- Ataxia, drug dependence, respiratory and cardiovascular depression, drowsiness, dizziness, blood dyscrasias

Key nursing actions
- Caution patient not to stop drug abruptly (could produce status epilepticus or worsen disorder).
- Administer I.V. diazepam no faster than 5 mg/minute in adults and over at least 3 minutes in children.
- Don't mix I.V. diazepam with other drugs in same syringe.

Key facts about succinimides
- Reduce epileptic attacks by suppressing paroxysmal three cycle per second spike and wave activity, depressing the motor cortex, and elevating the threshold of the CNS to convulsive stimuli
- Metabolized in the liver
- Excreted in urine

When to use succinimides
- Absence seizures

When NOT to use succinimides
- Hypersensitivity

Adverse reactions to watch for
- Anorexia, nausea, vomiting, blood dyscrasias, drowsiness, ataxia, dizziness, hematuria

Key nursing actions

- Don't withdraw the drug abruptly.
- If GI upset occurs, give drug with food or milk.
- Monitor for adverse reactions.
- Notify prescriber if rashes, joint pain, unexplained fever, sore throat, unusual bleeding or bruising, drowsiness, dizziness, or blurred vision develops.
- Tell patient to avoid alcohol during therapy.

Key facts about oxazolidinediones

- Affect the brain and nervous system to change seizure patterns
- Metabolized by the liver
- Excreted in urine

When to use oxazolidinediones

- Absence seizures

When NOT to use oxazolidinediones

- Hypersensitivity
- Pregnancy
- Breast-feeding
- Liver disease
- Renal disease
- Diseases affecting the bone marrow
- Optic or retinal diseases

Adverse reactions to watch for

- Dangerous levels of sedation, dizziness, or drowsiness; photosensitivity reaction

Interactions
- Hydantoins: May increase hydantoin levels
- Valproic acid: May increase or decrease succinimide levels
- Primidone: Lowers primidone levels

Nursing responsibilities
- Don't withdraw the drug abruptly because it may precipitate absence (petit mal) seizures
- If GI upset occurs, give the drug with food or milk
- Monitor the patient for adverse reactions
- Notify the prescriber if the patient develops rashes, joint pain, unexplained fever, sore throat, unusual bleeding or bruising, drowsiness, dizziness, or blurred vision because they may be symptoms of overdose
- Notify the prescriber if the patient becomes pregnant
- Tell the patient to avoid alcohol during therapy
- Warn patients taking phensuximide that the drug may cause urine to turn pink, red, or reddish brown, which is common and not harmful

OXAZOLIDINEDIONES

Mechanism of action
- The exact mechanism of action is not well established; affect the brain and nervous system to change seizure patterns

Pharmacokinetics
- Absorption: Readily absorbed in the GI tract
- Distribution: Unknown
- Metabolism: Metabolized by the liver into active metabolites
- Excretion: Excreted in the urine; half-life is 16 to 24 hours

Drug examples
- trimethadione (Tridione)

Indications
- To control absence (petit mal) seizures (as second-line drugs)

Contraindications and precautions
- Contraindicated in those who are hypersensitive to oxazolidinediones
- Contraindicated in pregnant and breast-feeding women
- Contraindicated in patients with liver disease, renal disease, diseases affecting the bone marrow, or optic or retinal diseases

Adverse reactions
- Sedation, photophobia, vomiting, aplastic anemia, allergic reaction

Interactions
- Antidepressants, alcohol, antihistamines, pain relievers, anxiolytics, other seizure medications, and muscle relaxants may cause dangerous levels of sedation, dizziness, or drowsiness
- Sunlight exposure may cause photosensitivity reactions

Nursing responsibilities
- Give drug with food if patient complains of GI upset
- Advise the patient that the drug may cause extreme drowsiness and sedation and to avoid activities requiring mental alertness, coordination, or concentration
- **Notify the prescriber immediately if the patient develops ataxia, fever, sore throat, rash, easy bruising, or visual disturbances because these symptoms may indicate overdose; treatment for overdose is immediate gastric lavage**

Key nursing actions
- Give drug with food if patient complains of GI upset.
- Advise patient that extreme drowsiness and sedation may occur.
- Notify prescriber immediately if ataxia, fever, sore throat, rash, easy bruising, or visual disturbances develop.

SULFONAMIDES

Mechanism of action
- Unknown; however, have been shown to raise the threshold for generalized seizures in rats and to increase dopaminergic and serotonergic neurotransmission
- Have been shown to block sodium channels, stabilize neuronal membranes, and suppress neuronal hypersynchronization

Key facts about sulfonamides
- Raise the threshold for generalized seizures in rats
- Increase dopaminergic and serotonergic neurotransmission
- Block sodium channels
- Stabilize neuronal membranes
- Suppress neuronal hypersynchronization

Pharmacokinetics
- Absorption: Plasma levels peak in 2 to 6 hours; food delays the rate of absorption
- Distribution: 40% of the drug is protein-bound; extensively binds to erythrocytes, so plasma levels are higher in red blood cells than in plasma
- Metabolism: Metabolized in the liver by cytochrome P-450 isoenzyme 3A4
- Excretion: Excreted in the urine

Drug examples
- zonisamide (Zonegran)

Indications
- As adjunctive therapy in the treatment of partial seizures in adults with epilepsy

When to use sulfonamides
- Partial seizures related to epilepsy

Contraindications and precautions
- Contraindicated in patients who are hypersensitive to drug or its components and in patients who have renal failure
- Used in pregnant or breast-feeding women only if the benefits outweigh the risks
- Used cautiously in patients with heat-related disorders and in pediatric patients because of the increased risk of oligohydrosis; monitor for decreased sweating and increased body temperature

When NOT to use sulfonamides
- Hypersensitivity
- Renal failure

Adverse reactions
- Somnolence, agitation, fatigue, ataxia, dizziness, headache, anorexia

Adverse reactions to watch for
- Somnolence, agitation, fatigue, ataxia, dizziness, headache, anorexia

Interactions
- Drugs that induce liver enzymes (CYP-450) increase the metabolism and clearance of zonisamide and decrease its half-life
- Food delays rate of zonisamide absorption

Key nursing actions

- Monitor for adverse reactions.
- If rash or seizures worsen, contact prescriber immediately.
- Also notify the prescriber if the patient develops fever, easy bruising, sore throat, or oral ulcers.

Key facts about other anticonvulsants

- Action largely unknown; may reduce polysynaptic responses and block posttetanic potentiation by blocking voltage-sensitive sodium channels
- Metabolized in the liver
- Excreted in urine

When to use other anticonvulsants

- Tonic-clonic seizures
- Simple and complex partial seizures
- Trigeminal neuralgia
- Neurogenic pain
- Absence seizures
- Postherpetic neuralgia

When NOT to use other anticonvulsants

- Hypersensitivity
- Bone marrow suppression
- Within 14 days of MAO inhibitor therapy
- Pregnancy
- Breast-feeding

Adverse reactions to watch for

- Sedation, refractory absence seizures, photophobia, drowsiness, blood dyscrasias

Nursing responsibilities

- Monitor the patient for adverse reactions; if rash or seizures worsen, contract the prescriber immediately
- **Risk of kidney stones is increased with zonisamide so encourage the patient to drink plenty of fluids to reduce risk of stone formation; notify the prescriber if the patient complains of sudden back pain, abdominal pain, or hematuria**
- Notify the prescriber if the patient develops a fever, easy bruising, sore throat, or oral ulcers

MISCELLANEOUS ANTICONVULSANTS

Mechanism of action

- Largely unknown; however, thought to reduce polysynaptic responses and block posttetanic potentiation by blocking the voltage-sensitive sodium channels

Pharmacokinetics

- Absorption: Rate varies with each drug
- Distribution: Varies with each drug
- Metabolism: Metabolized in the liver
- Excretion: Excreted in the urine

Drug examples

- carbamazepine (Tegretol), divalproex sodium (Depakote), felbamate (Felbatol), gabapentin (Neurontin), lamotrigine (Lamictal), levetiracetam (Keppra), oxcarbazepine (Trileptal), tiagabine (Gabitril), topiramate Topamax), valproate sodium (Depakene)

Indications

- Carbamazepine, lamotrigine, and topiramate are used to treat tonic-clonic seizures, simple and complex partial seizures, trigeminal neuralgia, and neurogenic pain
- Divalproex sodium and valproate sodium are used to treat simple and absence seizures
- Felbamate, gabapentin, levetiracetam, oxcarbazepine, and tiagabine are used as adjunctive therapy in treating partial seizures with or without secondary generalization
- Gabapentin also is used to treat postherpetic neuralgia

Contraindications and precautions

- Contraindicated in patients hypersensitive to the drug or its components
- Contraindicated in patients with bone marrow suppression and within 14 days of MAO inhibitor therapy
- Contraindicated in pregnant and breast-feeding women

Adverse reactions

- Sedation, refractory absence seizures (with paramethadione), photophobia, drowsiness (most common), blood dyscrasias

Interactions

- Anticonvulsants potentiate CNS depressants and alcohol
- Concurrent use with tricyclic antidepressants or phenothiazines lowers the seizure threshold and decreases the effectiveness of anticonvulsants• Many drugs alter the hepatic metabolism of anticonvulsants, leading to either decreased serum anticonvulsant levels and loss of seizure control or excessive serum anticonvulsant levels and toxicity
- Anticonvulsants decrease the effectiveness of hormonal contraceptives

Nursing responsibilities

- Assess seizure characteristics, including location and duration
- Implement seizure precautions, as indicated
- Watch for signs and symptoms of anticonvulsant toxicity, including CNS depression, ataxia, nausea and vomiting, drowsiness, dizziness, visual disturbances, and restlessness
- Consider giving anticonvulsants with food to decrease GI irritation
- Instruct the patient not to discontinue the drug without consulting the prescriber because this may precipitate tonic-clonic seizures
- Warn the patient not to consume alcohol during anticonvulsant therapy to prevent potentiation of CNS depressant effects
- Urge the patient to use caution when driving or performing other activities requiring alertness until the response to the drug is known (typically, the physician gives permission to drive based on adequacy of seizure control)
- Instruct the patient to carry identification describing the disorder and drug regimen
- Encourage the patient on long-term anticonvulsant therapy to comply with periodic blood studies (these determine serum drug levels and detect serious hematologic toxicity)
- Notify the prescriber if the patient develops fever, sore throat, oral ulcers, easy bruising or bleeding, or fatigue because these symptoms may indicate aplastic anemia, which may be fatal

Key nursing actions

- Assess seizure characteristics.
- Implement seizure precautions, as indicated.
- Watch for signs and symptoms of anticonvulsant toxicity.
- Instruct the patient not to discontinue the drug without consulting the prescriber.
- Warn the patient not to consume alcohol during anticonvulsant therapy.
- Instruct the patient to carry identification describing the disorder and drug regimen.
- Notify prescriber if fever, sore throat, oral ulcers, easy bruising or bleeding, or fatigue develops.

ANTIPARKINSONIANS

DOPAMINERGIC AGONISTS

Mechanism of action

- Restore the natural balance of the neurotransmitters acetylcholine and dopamine in the CNS, decreasing signs and symptoms of Parkinson's disease
- In idiopathic Parkinson's disease (parkinsonism), dopamine-containing neurons in the basal ganglia are destroyed or deficient, leading to unopposed cholinergic activity and loss of fine motor control
- In drug-induced parkinsonism, neuroleptics (such as phenothiazines) block dopamine receptors in the CNS, leading to functional loss of dopamine activity

Key facts about dopaminergic agonists

- Restore natural balance of acetylcholine and dopamine in the CNS
- Decrease signs and symptoms of Parkinson's disease
- Metabolized in the brain, periphery, and the liver
- Excreted in urine

- These drugs increase the amount of dopamine available in the CNS or enhance neurotransmission of dopamine
- Levodopa and levodopa-carbidopa restore dopamine levels (levodopa is converted to dopamine by enzymes in the brain); carbidopa is used with levodopa because it makes more levodopa available for transport to the brain, thereby allowing a lower levodopa dosage and reduced adverse effects
- Amantadine increases the amount of dopamine in the brain, either by increasing dopamine release or by blocking dopamine reuptake from the presynaptic neurons
- Bromocriptine, pramipexole, ropinirole, and pergolide activate dopamine receptor sites, producing effects similar to those of dopamine
- Selegiline is thought to inhibit MAO activity, thereby increasing dopaminergic activity

Pharmacokinetics

- Absorption: Rapidly absorbed; food delays absorption
- Distribution: Extensively absorbed throughout the body; pramipexole also is distributed into the red blood cells
- Metabolism: Metabolized in the brain, periphery, and the liver
- Excretion: Primarily excreted in the urine; half-life is 1 to 3 hours but is longer with sustained-release form of the drug

Drug examples

- amantadine (Symmetrel), bromocriptine (Parlodel), levodopa (L-dopa [Dopar]), levodopa-carbidopa (Sinemet), pergolide mesylate (Permax), pramipexole (Mirapex), ropinirole (Requip), selegiline hydrochloride (L-deprenyl hydrochloride [Eldepryl]), tolcapone (Tasmar)

When to use dopaminergic agonists

- Parkinson's disease
- Influenza A
- Hyperprolactinemia
- Cocaine abuse

Indications

- Levodopa, levodopa-carbidopa, ropinirole, and pramipexole are used primarily to treat Parkinson's disease
- Pergolide, selegiline, bromocriptine, and amantadine are used with levodopa-carbidopa to treat Parkinson's disease
- Pergolide permits lower dosages of levodopa-carbidopa with the same effects
- Selegiline enhances the response to levodopa-carbidopa in patients who don't respond to levodopa-carbidopa alone
- Amantadine also is used as an antiviral to prevent and treat influenza A
- Bromocriptine also is used to treat hyperprolactinemia and as an experimental treatment for cocaine abuse

When NOT to use dopaminergic agonists

- Angle-closure glaucoma

Contraindications and precautions

- Levodopa is contraindicated in patients with angle-closure glaucoma
- These drugs should be used with caution in patients with residual arrhythmias after myocardial infarction; in those with a history of peptic ulcer disease, psychosis, or seizure disorders; in those experiencing hallucinations, confusion, or dyskinesia; and in pregnant and breast-feeding women

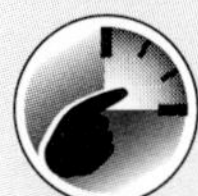

TIME-OUT FOR TEACHING

Teaching about dopaminergic agonists

Make sure to include the following topics in your teaching plan for the patient receiving a dopaminergic agonist.

- Medication prescribed, including name, dose, frequency, duration, and possible adverse effects
- Signs and symptoms to discuss with health care provider, including adverse effects
- Time required for drug to reach maximum effectiveness
- Safety measures, including possible need for assistive devices
- Avoidance of alcohol and self-medication with over-the-counter products
- Compliance with therapy, including adherence to regimen and prescribed dosage; avoidance of discontinuation of therapy if long-term
- Importance of follow-up care

- Levodopa should be used with caution in patients with bronchial asthma, emphysema, or severe CV, pulmonary, renal, hepatic, or endocrine disease and in those who need a sympathomimetic such as epinephrine

Adverse reactions

- Amantadine may cause dizziness, confusion, and mood changes
- Bromocriptine may cause confusion, involuntary body movements, and orthostatic hypotension
- Levodopa, levodopa-carbidopa, ropinirole, pramipexole, and pergolide commonly may cause nausea, vomiting, orthostatic hypotension, involuntary body movements, and dry mouth, altered tastes, tremors, insomnia, agitation, and hallucinations
- Selegiline may cause nausea

Interactions

- MAO inhibitors may precipitate a hypertensive crisis when used with levodopa
- May increase peripheral metabolism of levodopa when levodopa is used with pyridoxine (vitamin B_6), decreasing the amount of levodopa available to the brain

Nursing responsibilities

- Assess for signs and symptoms of parkinsonism (rigidity, tremors, akinesia, and bradykinesia)
- Base patient evaluation on improvement in signs and symptoms of parkinsonism without severe adverse effects
- When administering levodopa, instruct the patient to avoid excessive vitamin B_6 intake to prevent adverse drug interactions (for specific teaching tips, see *Teaching about dopaminergic agonists*).

Topics for patient discussion

- Medication regimen
- Signs and symptoms to discuss with physician
- Time required for drug to reach maximum effectiveness
- Safety measures
- Avoidance of alcohol and over-the-counter drug use
- Follow-up care

Adverse reactions to watch for

- Dizziness, confusion, mood changes, involuntary body movements, orthostatic hypotension, nausea, vomiting, dry mouth, altered tastes, tremors, insomnia, agitation, hallucinations

Key nursing actions

- Assess for signs and symptoms of parkinsonism.
- Base patient evaluation on improvement in signs and symptoms of parkinsonism without severe adverse effects.

Key facts about cholinergic blockers

- Block muscarinic acetylcholine receptors in the CNS, thereby suppressing acetylcholine activity
- Metabolism and excretion unknown

When to use cholinergic blockers

- Parkinson's disease
- Idiopathic Parkinson's disease
- Postencephalitic parkinsonism
- Acute dystonic reactions
- Drug-induced extrapyramidal reactions

When NOT to use cholinergic blockers

- Angle-closure glaucoma
- Pyloric or duodenal obstruction
- Myasthenia gravis
- Stenosing peptic ulcers
- Achalasia
- Megacolon
- Prostatic hypertrophy
- Bladder neck obstructions

Adverse reactions to watch for

- Blurred vision, constipation, dry mouth, urine retention

Key nursing actions

- Assess bowel and urinary function for evidence of adverse effects.
- Instruct patient to consult health care provider or pharmacist before taking nonprescription drugs.
- If GI upset occurs, administer drug with food.

- When administering levodopa, bromocriptine, or pergolide, instruct the patient to change position slowly to minimize orthostatic hypotension

CHOLINERGIC BLOCKERS (ANTICHOLINERGICS)

Mechanism of action
- Block muscarinic acetylcholine receptors in the CNS, thereby suppressing acetylcholine activity

Pharmacokinetics
- Unknown

Drug examples
- benztropine mesylate (Cogentin), biperiden (Akineton), diphenhydramine hydrochloride (Benadryl), trihexyphenidyl hydrochloride

Indications
- To treat Parkinson's disease, idiopathic Parkinson's disease, postencephalitic parkinsonism, acute dystonic reactions, and drug-induced extrapyramidal reactions

Contraindications and precautions
- Angle-closure glaucoma, pyloric or duodenal obstruction, myasthenia gravis, stenosing peptic ulcers, achalasia, megacolon, prostatic hypertrophy, and bladder neck obstructions

Adverse reactions
- Blurred vision, dry mouth, constipation, urine retention

Interactions
- May cause increased anticholinergic effects when used with similar-acting drugs

Nursing responsibilities
- Assess the patient's bowel and urinary function for evidence of adverse effects
- Instruct the patient to consult the health care provider or pharmacist before taking any nonprescription drugs, to prevent adverse drug interactions
- Teach the patient to minimize dry mouth by increasing fluid intake and by using ice chips, hard candy, or gum
- If GI upset occurs, may give the drug with food
- Teach the patient to reduce constipation by increasing fluid and fiber intake
- Use cautiously in hot weather, especially in those who are elderly, chronically ill, or alcoholic, or who have CNS diseases because severe anhidrosis and fatal hyperthermia may occur

ANTIMYASTHENICS (CHOLINERGICS])

Mechanism of action
- Relieve muscle weakness associated with myasthenia gravis by blocking acetylcholine breakdown at the neuromuscular junction

Pharmacokinetics

- Absorption: Usually poorly absorbed in the GI tract; duration of action varies in patients with myasthenia gravis, depending on the physical and emotional stress suffered and the severity of the disease
- Distribution: 15% to 25% is protein-bound; may cross the placental barrier in large doses
- Metabolism: Either undergoes hydrolysis by cholinesterases or is metabolized by the liver
- Excretion: Excreted in the urine

Drug examples

- ambenonium chloride (Mytelase), edrophonium (Tensilon), neostigmine (Prostigmin), pyridostigmine (Mestinon)

Indications

- To treat or diagnose myasthenia gravis
- Neostigmine, ambenonium, and pyridostigmine are used to control myasthenic symptoms
- Edrophonium is used to diagnose myasthenia gravis and to distinguish cholinergic crisis from myasthenic crisis

Contraindications and precautions

- Contraindicated in patients with hypersensitivity
- Edrophonium is contraindicated in patients with bromide allergy

Adverse reactions

- Result from cholinergic overstimulation
- Include abdominal pain, nausea, vomiting, diarrhea, sweating, miosis, increased salivation, increased bronchial secretions, and difficulty breathing

Interactions

- Concurrent use with similar-acting drugs causes additive cholinergic effects
- Concurrent use with guanethidine and other ganglionic blockers may increase myasthenic symptoms and hypertension

Nursing responsibilities

- Assess the patient's neuromuscular status, including reflexes, muscle strength, and gait
- Have emergency resuscitation equipment (suction equipment, oxygen, and mechanical ventilator) on hand if edrophonium is used
- Monitor the patient for signs and symptoms of drug overdose (cholinergic crisis) and underdose (possible myasthenic crisis)
  - Cholinergic crisis usually develops within 1 hour of drug administration; signs and symptoms include muscle weakness, dyspnea, dysphagia, increased respiratory secretions and saliva, nausea, vomiting, cramping, diarrhea, and diaphoresis
  - Myasthenic crisis usually doesn't occur for 3 or more hours after drug administration; signs and symptoms include extreme muscle weakness, dyspnea, and dysphagia

Key facts about antimyasthenics

- Relieve muscle weakness associated with myasthenia gravis by blocking acetylcholine breakdown at the neuromuscular junction
- Undergoes hydrolysis by cholinesterases or metabolized by the liver
- Excreted in urine

When to use antimyasthenics

- Myasthenia gravis
- Myasthenic crisis

When NOT to use antimyasthenics

- Hypersensitivity
- Bromide allergy

Adverse reactions to watch for

- Abdominal pain, nausea, vomiting, diarrhea, sweating, miosis, increased salivation, increased bronchial secretions, difficulty breathing

Key nursing actions

- Assess neuromuscular status.
- Monitor patient for signs and symptoms of drug overdose or underdose.
- Urge patient to carry identification describing the disease and drug regimen.
- Base patient evaluation on improvement of neuromuscular symptoms or strength without cholinergic signs or symptoms

- **Know that atropine is the antidote for cholinergic overdose and increasing the anticholinesterase dosage is the treatment for myasthenic crisis**
- Explain to the patient that antimyasthenic therapy is long-term
- Teach the patient the importance of taking doses according to schedule
  - Timely administration prevents weakness
  - Profound weakness can impair the patient's ability to breathe and swallow
- Urge the patient to carry identification describing the disease and drug regimen
- Base patient evaluation on improvement of neuromuscular symptoms or strength without cholinergic signs or symptoms
- Know that parenteral doses of neostigmine and pyridostigmine should be much smaller than oral doses because absorption increases with the parenteral route

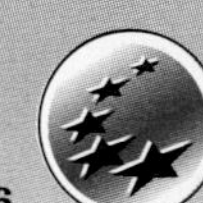

TOP 6

Items to study before your next test on drugs and the CNS

1. Mechanism of action of CNS stimulants, anticonvulsants, antiparkinsonians, and antimyasthenics
2. Common adverse effects of the various CNS stimulants, anticonvulsants, antiparkinsonians, and antimyasthenics
3. Nursing responsibilities when administering CNS stimulants, anticonvulsants, antiparkinsonians, and antimyasthenics
4. Teaching for the patient who is receiving a CNS stimulant, an anticonvulsant, an antiparkinsonian, or an antimyasthenic
5. Differences between dopaminergic and cholinergic blocking drugs
6. Importance of patient compliance with antimyasthenic therapy

NCLEX CHECKS

It's never too soon to begin your NCLEX preparation. Now that you've reviewed this chapter, carefully read each of the following questions and choose the best answer. Then compare your responses to the correct answers.

1. A patient with Parkinson's disease is being treated with levodopa (Dopar). You would be most concerned if the patient develops:

☐ **A.** edema.
☐ **B.** tachycardia.
☐ **C.** blurred vision.
☐ **D.** nausea and vomiting.

2. The health care provider suspects that a patient has myasthenia gravis. Which anticholinesterase can be used to diagnose this disorder?

☐ **A.** Ambenonium (Mytelase)
☐ **B.** Edrophonium (Tensilon)
☐ **C.** Physostigmine (Antilirium)
☐ **D.** Pyridostigmine (Mestinon)

3. A patient prescribed diazepam (Valium), a benzodiazepine, is most likely to experience which adverse reaction?

☐ **A.** Hypertension
☐ **B.** Rash
☐ **C.** Sedation
☐ **D.** Tachycardia

4. The nurse is preparing a female patient with tonic-clonic seizure disorder for discharge. Which instructions should the nurse include about phenytoin (Dilantin)?

Select all that apply:

- ☐ **A.** Monitor for skin rash.
- ☐ **B.** Maintain adequate amounts of fluid and fiber in the diet.
- ☐ **C.** Perform good oral hygiene, including daily brushing and flossing.
- ☐ **D.** Receive necessary periodic blood work.
- ☐ **E.** Report to the physician any problems with walking, coordination, slurred speech, or nausea.
- ☐ **F.** Feel safe about taking this drug, even during pregnancy.

ANSWERS AND RATIONALES

1. CORRECT ANSWER: B

Levodopa is a dopamine agonist. Cardiac adverse reactions such as tachycardia are the most serious adverse reactions to levodopa because they may lead to ventricular tachycardia and death. Edema isn't a common adverse reaction to this drug. Nausea, vomiting, and blurred vision are common adverse reactions but aren't as serious as the cardiovascular effects.

2. CORRECT ANSWER: B

Edrophonium or neostigmine may be used to diagnose myasthenia gravis. Ambenonium and pyridostigmine are used to treat myasthenia gravis, not to diagnose it. Physostigmine is used to reverse the effects of tricyclic antidepressant and anticholinergic poisoning.

3. CORRECT ANSWER: C

Diazepam relieves anxiety. Sedation is the most common adverse reaction, affecting 4% to 12% of all patients taking diazepam. Rash is a less likely effect. Tachycardia and hypertension aren't adverse reactions to this drug.

4. CORRECT ANSWER: A, C, D, E

A rash may occur 10 to 14 days after starting phenytoin. If a rash appears, the patient should notify the physician and discontinue the medication. Because phenytoin may cause gingival hyperplasia, the patient must practice good oral hygiene and see a dentist regularly. Periodic blood work is necessary to monitor complete blood counts, platelet levels, hepatic function, and drug levels. Signs and symptoms of phenytoin toxicity include problems with walking, coordination, slurred speech, and nausea. Other signs of toxicity include lethargy, diplopia, nystagmus, and disturbances in balance. These symptoms must be reported to the physician immediately. While adequate amounts of fluid and fiber are part of a healthy diet, they aren't required for a patient taking phenytoin. Phenytoin must be used cautiously during pregnancy because of the increased incidence of birth defects; phenobarbital is a safer drug to take during pregnancy.

Drugs and pain

LEARNING OBJECTIVES

After studying this chapter, you should be able to:

- Describe the mechanisms of action of opioid and nonopioid analgesics, opioid and opioid-agonist antagonists, and general and local anesthetics.
- Describe nursing responsibilities when administering analgesics.
- Compare the effects of general anesthesia with those of local anesthesia on the patient who undergoes surgery.
- Identify nursing measures that may enhance the therapeutic response to analgesics.
- Identify nursing responsibilities when caring for a patient receiving a general or local anesthetic.
- Discuss appropriate teaching for the patient who is receiving an analgesic and for the patient who is receiving an anesthetic.

CHAPTER OVERVIEW

Effective pain management requires knowledge of analgesic pharmacology and careful evaluation of the patient's response. Nonopioid and opioid analgesics are used for moderate to severe pain, relief of dyspnea in pulmonary edema, and persistent cough. Except during palliative care or in oncology patients, concerns about addiction to opioids must be balanced with the goal of relieving pain and knowledge of drug tolerance, dependence, and abuse. Opioid antagonists are used to reverse effects of the opioid analgesic when respiratory or central nervous system (CNS) depression has occurred. Nonopioid analgesics include salicylates, nonsteroidal anti-inflammatory drugs (NSAIDs), and acetaminophen and are used for relief of mild to moderate pain, inflammation, and fever, and as prophylaxis for thromboembolic disorders. Combining nonopioid and opioid drugs may produce more effective analgesia. Nursing responsibilities include monitoring vital signs and the patient's satisfaction, preventing constipation, and evaluating pain relief.

General anesthetics cause analgesia, muscular relaxation, and a decreased level of consciousness. Local anesthetics block sensation on the skin, in body tissues when infiltrated, and in epidural or spinal blocks. Preparation for surgery and patient teaching will help relieve anxiety and gain cooperation perioperatively. Nursing responsibilities related to anesthetics include maintaining airway patency, having resuscitation equipment on hand, and observing the patient for arrhythmias.

ANATOMY AND PHYSIOLOGY

Anatomy

- Nociceptors
  - Where pain sensation begins
  - Part of the afferent neurons; free nerve endings located primarily in the skin, periosteum, joint surfaces, and arterial walls
  - Two types of nociceptors
    - Myelinated A-delta fibers, which are fast-conducting fibers that signal sharp, well-localized pain
    - Unmyelinated C fibers, which are more numerous, smaller, and slower than the A-delta fibers and signal dull, poorly localized pain
  - Chemical mediators stimulate the nociceptors:
    - Chemical mediators are released or synthesized in response to tissue damage
    - Prostaglandins, histamine, bradykinin, and serotonin are examples of chemical mediators
  - Once the nociceptors are activated, the pain impulse travels to the dorsal horn of the spinal cord, where the nociceptors end
    - Neurotransmitters of the afferent neurons
    - Somatostatin
    - Cholecystokinin
    - Substance P
- Dorsal horn of the spinal cord
  - Where the nociceptors terminate
  - Control center for incoming information from the afferent neurons, for pain impulse regulation, and for descending influences from higher centers in the CNS

Function

- Pain acts as a protective mechanism that indicates an underlying physiologic or psychological problem

A&P highlights

- Nociceptors are where pain begins
- Myelinated A-delta fibers are fast-conducting fibers that signal sharp, well-localized pain
- Unmyelinated C fibers are more numerous, smaller, and slower than the A-delta fibers and signal dull, poorly localized pain
- Dorsal horn of the spinal cord is where nociceptors terminate
- Pain acts as a protective mechanism that indicates an underlying physiologic or psychological problem
- Pain is subjective and varies widely from person to person, based upon a person's perception, emotional state, and ethnic, cultural, or religious influences
- Analgesics may block the effect of these neurotransmitters

- Pain is subjective and varies widely from person to person, based upon a person's perception, emotional state, and ethnic, cultural, or religious influences
- Analgesics may block the effect of these neurotransmitters

Pain theory (Melzack-Wall gate-control theory)

- Most widely accepted pain theory
- Dorsal horn is the regulator between the peripheral fibers and the CNS and acts as the gatekeeper of pain and nonpain signals before sending an impulse to the CNS
- Pain perception may be inhibited by simultaneously activating nonpain signals to the CNS

NONOPIOID ANALGESICS

Key facts about nonopioid analgesics

- Act peripherally to prevent prostaglandin formation in inflamed tissues by two actions:
  - Inhibit stimulation of pain receptors
  - Inhibit prostaglandin synthesis in the CNS and stimulate peripheral vasodilation to reduce fever
- Metabolized in liver
- Excreted in urine, breast milk and kidneys

Mechanism of action

- Act peripherally to prevent prostaglandin formation in inflamed tissues by two actions
  - Inhibiting stimulation of pain receptors
  - Inhibiting prostaglandin synthesis in the CNS and stimulating peripheral vasodilation to reduce fever (antipyretic action)

Pharmacokinetics

- Absorption
  - Salicylate absorption occurs mainly in the upper part of the small intestine through passive diffusion and partly in the stomach; food or sustained or enteric-coated salicylates delay absorption
  - Acetaminophen (para-aminophenol derivatives) are absorbed rapidly and completely in the GI tract and absorbed well from the rectal mucosa
  - NSAIDs are absorbed in the GI tract
- Distribution
  - Salicylates are distributed widely throughout the body, including breast milk and placenta
  - Acetaminophen is distributed widely in body fluids and crosses the placental barrier
  - NSAIDs are distributed widely
- Metabolism
  - Salicylates are metabolized by the liver
  - Acetaminophen is metabolized by the liver
  - NSAIDs are metabolized by the liver
- Excretion
  - Salicylates are excreted in the urine
  - Acetaminophen is excreted in the urine and in breast milk
  - NSAIDs are primarily excreted in the kidneys

Drug examples

- Salicylate analgesics: aspirin (A.S.A.), choline and magnesium salicylates (Trilisate), choline salicylate (Arthropan), diflunisal (Dolobid), and salsalate (Disalcid)
- Para-aminophenol derivative nonopioid analgesics: acetaminophen (Datril, Tempra, Tylenol)
- NSAIDs: diclofenac (Cataflam, Voltaren), fenoprofen calcium (Nalfon), flurbiprofen (Ansaid), ibuprofen (Advil, Haltran, Medipren, Motrin, Nuprin, Rufen, Trendar), ketoprofen (Orudis), ketorolac tromethamine (Toradol), meclofenamate (Meclomen), mefenamic acid (Ponstel), naproxen (Naprosyn), naproxen sodium (Anaprox), piroxicam (Feldene), sulindac (Clinoril), and tolmetin (Tolectin)

Indications

- Acetaminophen, aspirin, choline salicylate, diflunisal, fenoprofen, ibuprofen, naproxen, ketoprofen, ketorolac, magnesium salicylate, meclofenamate, mefenamic acid, and salsalate are used to treat mild to moderate pain
- All drugs, except acetaminophen and mefenamic acid, are used to treat arthritis and osteoarthritis
- Acetaminophen, aspirin, and ibuprofen also are used to reduce fever
- Aspirin, naproxen, and sulindac also are used to reduce inflammation
- Aspirin also is used to prevent transient ischemic attacks and myocardial infarction (MI) by smoothing platelets
- Ibuprofen, ketoprofen, mefenamic acid, naproxen, and naproxen sodium also are used to treat dysmenorrhea
- The type and dose of the analgesic depends on the type and level of pain and the patient's response to previous therapy

Contraindications and precautions

- All these drugs, except acetaminophen, are contraindicated in pregnancy and aspirin hypersensitivity
- Aspirin is contraindicated in bleeding disorders and GI ulcers
- These drugs should be used with caution in patients with asthma or nasal polyps
- Aspirin shouldn't be given to children unless under the supervision of the prescriber because of the increased risk of Reye's syndrome
- Giving more than 4 grams of acetaminophen daily has been associated with serious liver toxicity

Adverse reactions

- These drugs may cause GI pain and upset, nausea, vomiting, diarrhea, heartburn, dizziness, headache, and tinnitus
- Acetaminophen hypersensitivity can produce such signs and symptoms as laryngeal edema, rash, fever, angioneurotic edema, and mucosal lesions
- Aspirin hypersensitivity can produce such signs and symptoms as rash, bronchospasm, rhinitis, and shock

When to use nonopioid analgesics

- Pain
- Arthritis and osteoarthritis
- Fever reduction
- Inflammation reduction
- Prevention of transient ischemic attacks and MI
- Dysmenorrhea

When NOT to use nonopioid analgesics

- Aspirin hypersensitivity
- Bleeding disorders
- Children
- GI ulcers
- Pregnancy

Adverse reactions to watch for

- GI pain and upset, nausea, vomiting, diarrhea, heartburn, dizziness, headache, tinnitus, laryngeal edema, rash, fever, angioneurotic edema, mucosal lesions, bronchospasm, rhinitis, and shock

Key nursing actions

- Administer the drug before meals for a rapid effect and with meals for GI irritation reduction.
- Advise the patient that the CDC warns against giving salicylates to children or adolescents with influenza, varicella, or viral illness.

Key facts about opioid analgesics and agonist-antagonists

- Bind to opiate receptors in the CNS to alter the perception of and emotional response to pain
- May cause withdrawal symptoms in patients with physical dependence on opioids
- Metabolized in liver
- Excreted in urine

Interactions

- Concurrent use with opioid analgesics enhances pain relief
- Concurrent use of NSAIDs with oral anticoagulants prolongs bleeding time and increases anticoagulant effects
- Concurrent use of aspirin with other NSAIDs or corticosteroids may exacerbate the GI adverse effects of aspirin and reduce aspirin effectiveness
- Long-term concurrent use of acetaminophen with NSAIDs increases the risk of renal toxicity or failure
- NSAIDs exacerbate the GI adverse effects of alcohol

Nursing responsibilities

- For a more rapid effect, administer the drug before meals; to reduce GI irritation, administer the drug with meals
- Instruct the patient to inform the physician or dentist of the prescribed drug regimen before undergoing medical or dental treatment or surgery
- Advise the patient that the Centers for Disease Control and Prevention warns against giving salicylates (including aspirin) to children or adolescents with influenza, varicella (chickenpox), or viral illness because these drugs may be linked to Reye's syndrome

OPIOID ANALGESICS AND AGONIST-ANTAGONISTS

Mechanism of action

- Opioid agonists and opioid agonist-antagonists bind to opiate receptors in the CNS to alter the perception of and emotional response to pain
- Opioid agonist-antagonists possess partial antagonist properties (they block further opioid binding at the opiate receptor sites they occupy) and may cause withdrawal symptoms in patients with physical dependence on opioids

Pharmacokinetics

- Absorption: Oral doses are absorbed readily from the GI tract. Intravenous (I.V.) administration produces the most rapid and reliable analgesic effect; absorption is delayed with intramuscular (I.M.) or subcutaneous (S.C.) routes
- Distribution: Distributed widely, with 30% to 35% protein-binding capacity
- Metabolism: Metabolized extensively in the liver
- Excretion: Metabolites are excreted in the urine

Drug examples

- Opioid analgesics: codeine, fentanyl (Sublimaze Duragesic), hydromorphone (Dilaudid), meperidine (Demerol), morphine sulfate (Duramorph, MS Contin, MSIR), oxycodone (OxyContin, Roxicodone), oxycodone with aspirin (Percodan), oxycodone with acetaminophen (Percocet, Tylox) and propoxyphene (Darvon, Darvon-N)
- Opioid agonist-antagonists: buprenorphine (Buprenex), butorphanol (Stadol), nalbuphine (Nubain), and pentazocine (Talwin)

Indications

- To treat pain that is unresponsive to nonopioid analgesics; the type and amount of analgesic depends on the type and level of pain and the patient's response to previous therapy
- Butorphanol, fentanyl, meperidine, morphine, nalbuphine, and pentazocine also are used as adjuncts to anesthesia
- Codeine and hydromorphone also are used to relieve cough
- Morphine also is used to treat the pain caused by an MI or acute pulmonary edema

Contraindications and precautions

- Use cautiously in patients with head injury, hepatic or renal disease, and CNS depression and in pregnant and breast-feeding women; dosage may need to be reduced in these patients
- Use cautiously in elderly or debilitated patients, who may require a decreased dosage

Adverse reactions

- Orthostatic hypotension, sedation, dizziness, light-headedness, dysphoria, hallucinations, constipation, respiratory depression, tolerance, physical dependence, psychological dependence, hypersensitivity reactions

Interactions

- Concurrent use with alcohol, sedating antihistamines, hypnotics, or sedatives causes additive CNS depression
- Opioid agonist-antagonists may cause withdrawal symptoms in patients with physical dependence on opioid analgesics
- Concurrent use with nonopioid analgesics may enhance pain relief

Nursing responsibilities

- Assess the patient's blood pressure, pulse, and respiratory status before administering the drug and periodically throughout analgesic therapy
- Because regular analgesic administration may be more effective than as-needed doses, administer doses before pain becomes severe
- Prolonged use of an opioid analgesic or opioid agonist-antagonist may cause dependence and tolerance; however, this shouldn't preclude administration of adequate analgesia
  - Patients receiving opioids for pain relief rarely develop psychological dependence; however, with long-term therapy they may require progressively higher doses to relieve pain (because of increased drug tolerance)
  - To prevent withdrawal symptoms, discontinue opioid analgesics gradually after long-term use
  - Dependency shouldn't preclude administration of opioids for pain relief in patients with cancer or as palliative treatment in terminally ill patients
  - Naloxone is the antidote for opioid overdose
- Instruct the patient to take oral analgesics with food to minimize GI irritation

When to use opioid analgesics and agonist-antagonists

- Adjuncts to anesthesia
- Cough relief
- Pain due to myocardial infarction or pulmonary edema
- Pain unresponsive to nonopioid analgesics

Adverse reactions to watch for

- Orthostatic hypotension, sedation, light-headedness, dizziness, dysphoria, hallucinations, constipation, respiratory depression, tolerance, physical dependence, psychological dependence, and hypersensitivity reactions

Key nursing actions

- Assess the patient's blood pressure, pulse, and respiratory status before administering the drug and periodically throughout analgesic therapy.
- Prolonged use of an opioid analgesic or opioid agonist-antagonist may cause dependence and tolerance, but this shouldn't preclude administration of adequate analgesia.

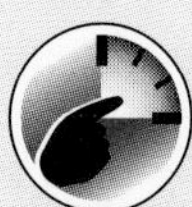

TIME-OUT FOR TEACHING

Teaching about opioid analgesics

Make sure to include the following topics in your teaching plan for the patient receiving an opioid analgesic.

- Medication prescribed, including name, dose, frequency, action, and adverse effects
- Instructions for administering drug before pain becomes severe
- Avoidance of alcohol and other central nervous system depressants
- Measures to prevent constipation
- Alternative pain management strategies
- Signs and symptoms to discuss with physician, including adverse reactions and overdose
- Medical follow-up

Topics for patient discussion

- Medication prescribed
- Administration instructions
- Signs and symptoms, including adverse reactions

- Teach the patient to change position slowly to minimize orthostatic hypotension
- Warn the patient to avoid activities requiring alertness until the response to the drug is known (for specific teaching tips, see *Teaching about opioid analgesics*).
- Discuss ways to minimize dry mouth and constipation (such as sucking on hard candy and increasing fluid intake and consumption of bulk foods high in fiber) and suggest that the prescriber include a stool softener or laxative daily with the patient's pain regimen

Key facts about opioid antagonists

- Competitively block the effects of opioids without producing analgesic effects
- May cause withdrawal symptoms in patient with physical dependence on opioids
- Metabolized in liver
- Excreted in urine

OPIOID ANTAGONISTS

Mechanism of action

- Competitively block the effects of opioids without producing analgesic effects; they may cause withdrawal symptoms in patients with physical dependence on opioids

Pharmacokinetics

- Absorption: Naloxone and nalmefene are administered I.V., I.M. or S.C. Naltrexone is well absorbed orally.
- Distribution: Rapidly distributed to block over 80% of the brain opioid receptors within 5 minutes after I.V. administration; 23% protein-bound after oral administration
- Metabolism: Metabolized by the liver
- Excretion: Excreted in the urine

When to use opioid antagonists

- Opioid overdose
- Adjunct to therapy in treating drug abuse

Drug examples

- nalmefene (Revex), naloxone (Narcan), naltrexone (ReVia)

Indications

- To reverse CNS and respiratory depression in opioid overdose
- Naltrexone is used as an adjunct to therapy to keep detoxified patients drug free, similar to the use of disulfiram (Antabuse) to prevent resumption of alcohol
- Naloxone and nalmefene are used to treat opioid overdose

Contraindications and precautions
- Use cautiously in patients physically dependent on opioids because of the risk of severe withdrawal symptoms

Adverse reactions
- May cause nausea, vomiting, tachycardia, hypotension, hypertension, arrhythmias
- An unconscious patient returning to consciousness abruptly after naloxone administration may hyperventilate and experience tremors

Interactions
- Reverse all opioid effects, including analgesia, when used with an opioid
- Naltrexone causes withdrawal symptoms if given to a patient receiving an opioid agonist or to an opioid addict

Nursing responsibilities
- Assess the patient's respiratory status, blood pressure, pulse, and level of consciousness until the opioid wears off
- Monitor duration of drug effects; repeat doses may be needed if effects of the opioid outlast those of the opioid antagonist
- Because an opioid antagonist reverses analgesia (as well as respiratory depression), the dosage should be adjusted according to the patient's pain level
- Failure of the patient to improve markedly means that signs and symptoms result from disease or from use of CNS depressants other than opioids
- Administer slowly and monitor the patient's respiratory and pain status and level of consciousness at all times. Give only the amount required to reverse respiratory depression or increase mental alertness because total reversal of pain relief will put the patient in undue distress

GENERAL ANESTHETICS

RAPID-ACTING HYPNOTICS

Mechanism of action
- Stabilize neuronal membranes to produce progressive, reversible CNS depression

Pharmacokinetics
- Absorption: Administered I.V
- Distribution: Distributed rapidly into tissues
- Metabolism: Hepatically metabolized
- Excretion: Excretion may be renal or hepatic

Drug examples
- methohexital (Brevital), midazolam hydrochloride (Versed), propofol (Diprivan), thiopental sodium (Pentothal)

Indications
- To induce and maintain anesthesia for short-term procedures
- To prolong anesthesia when used with gaseous anesthetics

Adverse reactions to watch for

- Nausea, vomiting, tachycardia, hypotension, hypertension, arrhythmias, hyperventilation, and tremors

Key nursing actions

- Assess respiratory status, blood pressure, pulse, and level of consciousness until the opioid wears off.
- Opioid dosage should be adjusted according to the patient's pain level.
- Give only the amount required to reverse respiratory depression or increase mental alertness.

Key facts about rapid-acting hypnotics

- Stabilize neuronal membranes to produce progressive, reversible CNS depression
- Metabolized hepatically
- Renal or hepatic excretion

Indications for rapid-acting hypnotics

- Anesthesia induction and maintenance
- Anesthesia extension

Topics for patient discussion

- Type of anesthetic prescribed
- Possible psychomotor function impairment
- Signs and symptoms, including adverse reactions

Adverse reactions to watch for

- Respiratory depression, apnea, hypotension, tachycardia, nausea and vomiting, muscle twitching, tissue necrosis with extravasation

Key nursing actions

- Determine if the patient has allergies before the surgery.
- Assess CV, respiratory, and renal status and level of consciousness before and after surgery

Key facts about inhalation anesthetics

- Depress the CNS
- Metabolized in lungs and liver
- Excreted in urine

TIME-OUT FOR TEACHING

Teaching about general anesthetics

Make sure to include the following topics in your teaching plan for the patient receiving a general anesthetic.

- Type of anesthetic prescribed, including name, dose, frequency, action, and possible adverse effects
- Withholding of food and fluids for at least 8 hours before surgery
- Avoidance of alcohol and other central nervous system depressants for at least 24 hours after receiving anesthetic
- Possible psychomotor function impairment for 24 hours or more after receiving anesthetic
- Signs and symptoms to discuss with the physician, including adverse effects

Contraindications and precautions

- Use cautiously in patients with CV or respiratory instability

Adverse reactions

- Respiratory depression, apnea, hypotension, tachycardia, nausea and vomiting, muscle twitching, tissue necrosis with extravasation

Interactions

- Causes additive CNS depression when used with similar-acting drugs

Nursing responsibilities

- Find out if the patient has any allergies before the surgery or procedure
- Inform the patient as to what to expect before, during, and after the surgery or procedure
- Explain to the patient that no food or fluids will be allowed for at least 8 hours before surgery (for specific teaching tips, see *Teaching about general anesthetics*)
- Assess the patient's CV, respiratory, and renal status and level of consciousness before and after the surgery or procedure

INHALATION ANESTHETICS

Mechanism of action

- Depress the CNS

Pharmacokinetics

- Absorption: Absorbed by the lungs
- Distribution: Distributed to other tissues; distributed rapidly to organs with high blood flow, including the brain, liver, kidneys, and heart
- Metabolism: Eliminated primarily by the lungs, but enflurane and halothane are also metabolized by the liver
- Excretion: Metabolites are excreted in the urine

Drug examples

- desflurane (Suprane), enflurane (Ethrane), halothane (Fluothane), isoflurane (Forane), methoxyflurane (Penthrane), nitrous oxide

Indications

- To produce loss of consciousness, loss of responsiveness to sensory stimulation including pain, and muscle relaxation
- To maintain anesthesia for surgery requiring precise, rapid control of the depth of anesthesia

Contraindications and precautions

- **Use cautiously in elderly or debilitated patients because they are predisposed to an exaggerated response to the drugs**
- **Even smaller-than-normal drugs doses may result in hypotension, prolonged respiratory depression, and longer recovery in elderly and debilitated patients**

Adverse reactions

- Exaggerated response to the normal dose (most common), postanesthesia nausea and vomiting, hypotension, arrhythmias, tachycardia, confusion, agitation, memory loss

Interactions

- If given with labetalol, increases hypotensive effects
- If given with other CNS depressants, increases CNS and respiratory depression and hypotension
- If given with xanthines, such as caffeine or theophylline, increases risk of arrhythmias
- Neuromuscular blockades, including succinylcholine, increases neuromuscular blockade effects and increases risk of malignant hyperthermia
- Enflurane and isoniazid or aminoglycosides increases the risk of nephrotoxicity
- Desflurane given with midazolam or fentanyl decreases anesthetic requirements

Nursing responsibilities

- Find out if patient has any allergies to drugs before surgery
- Advise the patient not to eat or drink anything for at least 8 hours before surgery to prevent aspiration of stomach contents into the lungs during anesthesia
- Inform the patient that psychomotor functions may be impaired for 24 hours or more after inhalation anesthesia
- Monitor the patient for adverse reactions to the inhalation anesthetic during the entire drug administration and during recovery
- **Keep atropine available at all times to reverse possible bradycardia**
- Monitor the patient's temperature frequently; hypothermia occurs frequently and is a common effect of inhalation anesthesia
- **Shivering is normal during recovery; if shivering occurs, keep the patient warm with extra blankets or heat and administer oxygen, as prescribed, to compensate for the increased oxygen demand**

When to use inhalation anesthetics

- Promotion of loss of consciousness, loss of responsiveness to sensory stimulation including pain, and muscle relaxation
- Anesthesia maintenance

Adverse reactions to watch for

- Exaggerated response to the normal dose (most common), postanesthesia nausea and vomiting, hypotension, arrhythmias, tachycardia, confusion, agitation, memory loss

Key nursing actions

- Keep atropine available at all times to reverse possible bradycardia.
- Monitor the patient's temperature frequently.
- Shivering is normal during recovery; if shivering occurs, keep the patient warm with extra blankets or heat and administer oxygen, as prescribed, to compensate for the increased oxygen demand.

INJECTABLE ANALGESIC ANESTHETICS

Mechanism of action
- Depress the CNS

Pharmacokinetics
- Absorption: Administered I.V., thereby bypassing the mechanism that reduces bioavailability
- Distribution: Distributed rapidly; onset of action is rapid and short-acting
- Metabolism: Metabolized by the liver
- Excretion: Excreted in the feces

Drug examples
- Alfentanil (Alfenta), etomidate, fentanyl (Sublimaze), remifentanil (Ultiva), sufentanil (Sufenta)

Indications
- To induce rapid anesthesia (usually for situations requiring anesthesia of short duration, such as outpatient surgery) or conscious sedation
- To decrease pain

Contraindications and precautions
- Contraindicated in patients hypersensitive to these drugs

Adverse reactions
- Possible respiratory depression, arrhythmias, bradycardia, and skeletal and thoracic muscle rigidity
- Alfentanil and fentanyl may cause seizures, asystole, dry mouth, urine retention, and shivering

Interactions
- Verapamil with etomidate may increase anesthetic effect and cause respiratory depression and apnea
- Increases effects of injection anesthetic if given with other opiates, inhalation anesthetics, hypnotics, or sedatives

Nursing responsibilities
- Continuously assess the patient's respiratory status for signs of respiratory depression
- **Only persons experienced in endotracheal intubation should use these drugs; equipment for this procedure should be kept on hand**
- Many injectable drugs are incompatible with other drugs or solutions

NEUROLEPTANESTHETICS

Mechanism of action
- Droperidol and ketamine produce dissociation from the environment during induction of anesthesia by directly acting on the cortex and limbic system
- Droperidol-fentanyl produces pain relief and sedation by directly blocking subcortical receptors

Key facts about injectable analgesic anesthetics
- Depress the CNS
- Metabolized by liver
- Excreted in feces

When to use injectable analgesic anesthetics
- Rapid anesthesia or conscious sedation induction
- Pain

When NOT to use injectable analgesic anesthetics
- Hypersensitivity

Adverse reactions to watch for
- Respiratory depression, arrhythmias, bradycardia, skeletal and thoracic muscle rigidity, seizures, asystole, dry mouth, urine retention, and shivering

Key nursing actions
- Continually assess respiratory status.
- Only those experienced in endotracheal intubation should use these drugs.

Pharmacokinetics

- Absorption: Administered I.V.
- Distribution: Rapidly distribution
- Metabolism: Metabolized in the liver
- Excretion: Excreted in the feces

Drug examples

- Droperidol (Inapsine), droperidol-fentanyl (Innovar), ketamine (Ketalar)

Indications

- To tranquilize and induce analgesia before surgery or diagnostic procedures

Contraindications and precautions

- Ketamine is contraindicated in patients with significant hypertension, severe cardiac decompensation, any condition in which a significant blood pressure increase would endanger the patient, or a history of cerebrovascular accidents, and during surgery of the pharynx, larynx, or bronchial tree (unless used with a muscle relaxant)
- Use droperidol with extreme caution in patients with heart failure, bradycardia, or electrolyte abnormalities

Adverse reactions

- Possible arrhythmias, hypotension, respiratory depression, laryngospasm, cough, and bronchospasms
- Ketamine may cause disturbing dreams or hallucinations during emergence from anesthesia, along with seizures, muscle rigidity, excessive salivation, and shivering
- Droperidol may cause extrapyramidal signs and symptoms, QT interval prolongation, and torsade de pointes

Interactions

- When given with CNS depressants, has additive or potentiating CNS effects
- Epinephrine may paradoxically enhance droperidol-induced hypotension

Nursing responsibilities

- **For the patient who received droperidol-fentanyl, all doses of analgesics and other CNS depressants must be reduced by one-third to one-half during recovery from anesthesia**
- Monitor vital signs and cardiopulmonary status before, during, and after injection
- Minimize environmental stimulation to prevent untoward reactions on emergence from anesthesia
- Inform patient that mental alertness, coordination, and physical dexterity may be impaired for some time after general anesthesia

Key facts about neuroleptanesthetics

- Droperidol and ketamine produce dissociation from the environment during induction of anesthesia
- Droperidol-fentanyl produces pain relief and sedation by directly blocking subcortical receptors
- Metabolized in liver
- Excreted in feces

When to use neuroleptanesthetics

- Analgesia induction

When NOT to use neuroleptanesthetics

- Hypertension
- Cardiac decompensation
- History of cerebrovascular accidents
- Surgery of the pharynx, larynx, or bronchial tree

Adverse reactions to watch for

- Arrhythmias, hypotension, respiratory depression, laryngospasm, cough, bronchospasms, disturbing dreams or hallucinations, seizures, muscle rigidity, excessive salivation, shivering, extrapyramidal signs and symptoms, QT interval prolongation, and torsade de pointes

Key nursing actions

- In droperidol-fentanyl, all doses of analgesics and other CNS depressants must be reduced by one-third to one-half during recovery from anesthesia

Key facts about local anesthetics

- Provide analgesic relief by blocking the conduction of nerve impulses at the point of contact
- Metabolism varies
- Excreted in urine

When to use local anesthetics

- Pain
- Anesthesia, including spinal and epidural

When NOT to use local anesthetics

- Drug hypersensitivity
- Myasthenia gravis
- Severe shock
- Impaired cardiac conduction

Adverse reactions to watch for

- Possible anxiety, restlessness, arrhythmias, bradycardia, hypotension, chills, miosis, tinnitus, hypersensitivity reactions

LOCAL ANESTHETICS

Mechanism of action

- Local anesthetics provide analgesic relief by blocking the conduction of nerve impulses at the point of contact, causing expansion of the nerve-cell membrane and inability of the cell to depolarize, which is necessary for impulse transmission

Pharmacokinetics

- Absorption: Varies widely
- Distribution: Distributed throughout the body
- Metabolism: Esters and amides undergo different types of metabolism
- Excretion: Metabolites are excreted in the urine

Drug examples

- benzocaine (Dermoplast), bupivacaine hydrochloride (Marcaine), chloroprocaine hydrochloride (Nesacaine), cocaine hydrochloride, dibucaine (Nupercainal), lidocaine hydrochloride (Xylocaine Hydrochloride), mepivacaine (Carbocaine), procaine hydrochloride (Novocain), ropivacaine (Naropin), tetracaine hydrochloride (Pontocaine)

Indications

- To prevent or relieve pain from a medical procedure, disease, or injury
- For severe pain unrelieved by topical anesthetics or analgesics
- Bupivacaine, procaine, and tetracaine are used for spinal anesthesia
- Bupivacaine, lidocaine, and mepivacaine are used for epidural anesthesia
- Cocaine, benzocaine, and dibucaine are used on the skin or mucous membranes to provide anesthesia for itching, burning, or short procedures

Contraindications and precautions

- Contraindicated in patients with known hypersensitivity to these drugs and in those with myasthenia gravis, severe shock, or impaired cardiac conduction
- Use these drugs cautiously in patients with hepatic disease, hypotension, or heart block, hyperthyroidism, or other endocrine diseases
- Because these drugs carry a risk of toxicity, use them cautiously, especially in elderly or debilitated patients

Adverse reactions

- Possible anxiety, restlessness, arrhythmias, bradycardia, hypotension, chills, miosis, tinnitus, hypersensitivity reactions
- The higher the dose of local anesthetics, the higher the incidence of adverse reactions

Interactions

- Slows anesthetic absorption and prolongs anesthetic effects when used with epinephrine (deliberate drug combination)
- Increases CNS depression when used with other CNS depressants

Nursing responsibilities

- At onset of drug action, the patient's ability to sense cold, warmth, pain, and touch decreases in the affected area; then, local motor function diminishes
- Postoperatively, assess for return of motor function and sensation in reverse order to that described above.
- Advise the patient to expect transient lack of sensation in the anesthetized area after surgery
- Ensure that the gag reflex has returned before feeding a patient whose throat has been anesthetized

TOPICAL ANESTHETICS

Mechanism of action

- Benzocaine, butacaine, butamben, cocaine, dyclonine, lidocaine, dibucaine, tetracaine, and pramoxine block nerve impulse transmission; they accumulate in the nerve cell membrane, causing it to expand and lose its ability to depolarize
- Benzyl alcohol and clove oil appear to stimulate the nerve endings and interfere with pain perception
- Ethyl chloride and menthol superficially freeze the tissue, stimulating the cold sensation receptors and blocking the nerve endings in the frozen area

Pharmacokinetics

- Absorption: No significant systemic absorption, unless with frequent or high-dose application to the eye or large areas of burned or injured skin
- Distribution: Distributed locally
- Metabolism
  - Tetracaine and other esters are extensively metabolized in the blood and liver
  - Dibucaine, lidocaine, and other amides are metabolized primarily by the liver
- Excretion: Excreted in the urine

Drug examples

- Benzocaine, benzyl oxide, butacaine, butamben, clove oil, cocaine, dyclonine, ethyl chloride, lidocaine, menthol, pramoxine, tetracaine

Indications

- To relieve or prevent pain, especially minor pain, itching, and irritation
- To anesthetize an area before an injection is given
- To numb mucosal surfaces before a tube or catheter is inserted

Contraindications and precautions

- Contraindicated in patients with a known hypersensitivity to the drug or its group
- Dibucaine shouldn't be used in large quantities, especially in denuded or blistered areas

Key nursing actions

- Assess for return of motor function and sensation postoperatively.
- Ensure that the gag reflex has returned before feeding a patient whose throat has been anesthetized.

Key facts about topical anesthetics

- Block nerve impulse transmission
- Stimulate the nerve endings and interfere with pain perception
- Stimulate the cold sensation receptors and block the nerve endings in the frozen area
- Metabolized in blood and liver
- Excreted in urine

When to use topical anesthetics

- Pain
- Anesthesia
- Surface numbing

When NOT to use topical anesthetics

- Drug hypersensitivity

Adverse reactions to watch for

- Hypersensitivity

Key nursing actions

- Assess the area where topical anesthetic is to be applied before, during and after application.
- Don't apply a refrigerated topical anesthetic to broken skin or mucous membranes.

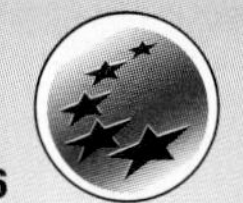

TOP 6

Items to study before your next test on drugs and pain

1. Mechanisms of action of opioid and nonopioid analgesics, opioid and opioid-agonist antagonists, and general and local anesthetics
2. Nursing responsibilities when administering analgesics
3. Effects of general anesthesia and local anesthesia on a patient who undergoes surgery
4. Nursing measures that may enhance the therapeutic response to analgesics.
5. Nursing responsibilities when caring for a patient receiving a general or local anesthetic
6. Appropriate teaching for the patient who is receiving an analgesic or anesthetic

- Dyclonine must be used cautiously in areas with traumatized mucosa or localized sepsis
- Butacaine and cocaine should be used cautiously in patients with CV disease or hyperthyroidism
- Butacaine also should be used cautiously in patients with open lesions
- Lidocaine should be used cautiously in elderly patients and patients with large areas of broken skin or mucous membranes

Adverse reactions
- Hypersensitivity reaction (including rash, pruritus, and breathing difficulty)

Interactions
- Lidocaine shouldn't be used with beta blockers or cimetidine because it may increase the risk of lidocaine toxicity

Nursing responsibilities
- Assess the area where the topical anesthetic is to be applied before, during, and after drug administration
- **Don't apply a refrigerated topical anesthetic (such as ethyl chloride) to broken skin or mucous membranes**
- Watch for signs of localized frostbite in patients receiving a refrigerant (such as ethyl chloride) or for skin irritation with other topical anesthetics
- Discontinue drug if a rash develops

NCLEX CHECKS

It's never too soon to begin your NCLEX preparation. Now that you've reviewed this chapter, carefully read each of the following questions and choose the best answer. Then compare your responses to the correct answers.

1. A patient is hospitalized with terminal cancer. For the past 3 weeks, she has been receiving morphine sulfate, 5 mg I.V., every 4 hours, and has experienced relief from pain. She now says pain is still present, even after receiving the drug. You recognize that this patient:

- ☐ **A.** has become dependent on the drug.
- ☐ **B.** has developed a tolerance to the opioid.
- ☐ **C.** resents that the nurse is healthy and she isn't.
- ☐ **D.** is seeking attention for herself because of poor self-image.

2. Which of the following symptoms would you observe in an adult patient developing salicylism?

- ☐ **A.** Rash and bronchial wheezing
- ☐ **B.** Respiratory depression and acidosis
- ☐ **C.** Respiratory alkalosis and tachypnea
- ☐ **D.** Bleeding from the gums and blood in the urine

3. A patient in the intensive care unit has just been given an accidental overdose of morphine. He lost consciousness and has slow, shallow respirations at a rate of 8 breaths/minute. What drug should be given?

- [ ] **A.** Flumazenil (Romazicon)
- [ ] **B.** Naloxone (Narcan)
- [ ] **C.** Naltrexone (ReVia)
- [ ] **D.** Norepinephrine (Levophed)

4. A patient taking the nonsteroidal anti-inflammatory drug (NSAID) naproxen (Naprosyn) for his osteoarthritis has recently started taking a thiazide diuretic for moderate hypertension. You should teach the patient which of the following actions?

- [ ] **A.** Stick to the therapeutic regimen.
- [ ] **B.** Watch for GI bleeding.
- [ ] **C.** Have regular blood pressure checks.
- [ ] **D.** Increase dietary fiber to avoid constipation.

5. The use of naproxen with oral anticoagulants or corticosteroids may increase the risk of GI bleeding. During a thoracotomy, a patient received halothane and nitrous oxide. After the surgery, you monitor him closely. Which adverse reaction to inhalation anesthetics is most common?

- [ ] **A.** Respiratory distress
- [ ] **B.** Nausea and vomiting
- [ ] **C.** Hypersensitivity reaction
- [ ] **D.** Exaggerated response to a normal dose

6. A physician orders a topical anesthetic to relieve a child's pain from a knee abrasion. When instructing the child's parents about the drug, tell them to be alert for which of the following reactions?

- [ ] **A.** Minor pain
- [ ] **B.** Arrhythmias
- [ ] **C.** Risk of infection
- [ ] **D.** Rash, pruritus, and breathing difficulty

7. The nurse is assessing a client with a history of multiple substance abuse. The client reports that he's been experiencing nausea, vomiting, and diarrhea. The nurse observes flushing, piloerection (hair erection), increased lacrimation (secretion of tears), and rhinorrhea. These signs and symptoms most likely indicate withdrawal from what category of drugs?

____

ANSWERS AND RATIONALES

1. CORRECT ANSWER: B
Long-term use of central nervous system drugs can lead to tolerance, which means that increased doses of the drug are needed to achieve the same effect. Patients being treated with opioids for chronic pain may require higher doses of the drug for effective pain relief. Dependency is usually not an issue in treating terminally ill cancer patients. Lack of relief also does not necessarily indicate dependency. You can't conclude that the patient has a poor self-image or feels resentful based upon the information given.

2. CORRECT ANSWER: C
Salicylate (aspirin) levels directly stimulate the respiratory centers in the central nervous system, thereby resulting in tachypnea and respiratory alkalosis. Rash and bronchial wheezing are symptoms of an allergic reaction to salicylates. Respiratory depression and acidosis aren't associated commonly with high salicylate levels. Bleeding is an adverse reaction to salicylates.

3. CORRECT ANSWER: B
Morphine is an opiate and the patient needs an opiate receptor antagonist. Naloxone is a rapid-acting parenteral opiate antagonist. Flumazenil is a benzodiazepine antagonist. Naltrexone is available only in oral form and is too slow-acting for this patient. Norepinephrine isn't involved in the mechanism of action of opiates and would be ineffective.

4. CORRECT ANSWER: C
NSAIDs taken with thiazide diuretics can cause reduced antihypertensive and diuretic effects, so blood pressure must be checked regularly and the patient should be alert for signs of fluid retention. The use of naproxen with other drugs has no effect on bowel pattern.

5. CORRECT ANSWER: D
Because the patient is receiving two inhaled drugs, the most common adverse reaction would be an exaggerated response to the normal dose, most likely because of predisposing medical conditions before surgery. Hypersensitivity is a potential adverse reaction that is more common with injection anesthetics. Nausea, vomiting, and respiratory distress may occur postoperatively, but aren't considered the most common.

6. CORRECT ANSWER: D
Rash, pruritus, and breathing difficulty indicate a hypersensitivity reaction and can be caused by a topical anesthetic. Minor pain should be relieved with, not caused by, the use of topical anesthetics. Arrhythmias are common with inhalation or injection anesthetics. The risk of infection is always present with an injury or surgery.

7. CORRECT ANSWER: OPIOID
Typical symptoms of opioid addiction and withdrawal include flushing, piloerection, nausea, vomiting, abdominal cramps, increased lacrimation, and rhinorrhea. The nurse must be aware of symptoms of opioid withdrawal due to an increase in abuse of opioids, such as heroine and hydrocodone.

5 Drugs and mood alteration

LEARNING OBJECTIVES

After studying this chapter, you should be able to:

- Identify medications commonly used as sedative-hypnotics, anxiolytics, antipsychotics, antidepressants, and antimanics.
- Describe the mechanism of action of sedative-hypnotics, anxiolytics, antipsychotics, antidepressants, and antimanics.
- Name the indications for sedative-hypnotics, anxiolytics, antipsychotics, antidepressants, and antimanics.
- Describe precautions the nurse must take when administering sedative-hypnotics, anxiolytics, antipsychotics, antidepressants, or antimanics.
- List the common adverse effects of sedative-hypnotics, anxiolytics, antipsychotics, antidepressants, and antimanics.
- Identify nursing responsibilities when administering sedative-hypnotics, anxiolytics, antipsychotics, antidepressants, or antimanics.
- Discuss appropriate teaching for a patient receiving a sedative-hypnotic, an anxiolytic, an antipsychotic, an antidepressant, or an antimanic.

CHAPTER OVERVIEW

Sedatives, anxiolytics, hypnotics, antipsychotics (or neuroleptics), and antidepressants all depress the central nervous system (CNS). The degree of CNS depression is dose dependent. Sedatives and anxiolytics are prescribed for their calming effect and ability to reduce anxiety. Hypnotics are prescribed to produce drowsiness and induce sleep. These drugs can produce physiologic and psychological dependence and tolerance. Many are controlled substances and have the potential for abuse; therefore, they are generally prescribed for short-term use. Nursing responsibilities include assessing for relief of anxiety without excessive sedation, improving the patient's sleep without "hangover" effect, and instructing the patient not to consume alcohol, take other CNS depressants, or perform hazardous activities while taking these preparations.

Antipsychotics are used to manage schizophrenia and psychotic depression and to treat bipolar disorder (a group of illnesses characterized by periods of euphoria and excessive activity, depression, or both) unresponsive to lithium. These drugs are useful for controlling psychotic symptoms, including thought disturbances, hallucinations, and delusions. Chlorpromazine and droperidol are used to treat nausea and vomiting; droperidol is combined with fentanyl as an adjunct to anesthesia. Nursing responsibilities consist of monitoring drug response, including affect, anxiety, and hallucinations. Patient teaching includes interventions to assist with compliance, measures to relieve or prevent dry mouth and constipation, and monitoring for agranulocytosis (with clozapine use). Anticipatory teaching for patients and families should include information on extrapyramidal symptoms and the dangers of noncompliance when feeling better.

Antidepressants are used to treat depression, a mood disorder characterized by sadness, hopelessness, worthlessness, agitation, or anxiety. These drugs inhibit the reuptake of norepinephrine, leaving more available to the CNS. Nursing responsibilities include assessing mood, sleep patterns, appetite, and suicidal ideation. Teaching focuses on safety related to dizziness or drowsiness, interventions for adverse effects, and dietary restrictions with monoamine oxidase inhibitors.

The antimanic agents lithium carbonate and lithium citrate are the treatment of choice for bipolar disorder, although certain anticonvulsants also may be used. The nurse must exercise extreme caution when administering lithium to patients with renal disease, cardiovascular disease, or sodium depletion and to patients receiving diuretic therapy. Nursing responsibilities include monitoring serum lithium levels and teaching patients and families to watch for and report signs and symptoms of lithium toxicity.

A&P highlights

- Psychopathology is affected by psychosocial and biological factors.
- Neurotransmitters are released from the presynaptic neuron and relay impulses across the synapse to receptors on the postsynaptic neuron.
- The neurotransmitter then binds to the receptors; subsequent physiologic responses indirectly affect behavior.
- Psychoactve drugs provide symptomatic relief of psychotic disorders by altering neurotransmission in the CNS.

ANATOMY AND PHYSIOLOGY

Anatomy

- In addition to psychosocial factors, psychopathology is affected by biological factors
- Abnormal neurotransmission occurs among several neurotransmitters
  - Acetylcholine
  - Dopamine
  - Gamma-aminobutyric acid (GABA)
  - Glutamate
  - Serotonin
  - Norepinephrine
- Neuronal signaling occurs in the CNS

- **Physiology**
  - Neurotransmitters usually are released from the presynaptic neuron and relay impulses across the synapse to the receptors on the postsynaptic neuron
  - Once the neurotransmitter is released, it binds to the receptors and subsequent physiologic responses indirectly affect behavior
- **Function**
  - Psychoactive drugs aren't intended to cure psychiatric disorders
  - Psychoactive drugs provide symptomatic relief of psychotic disorders
  - Psychopharmacology alters neurotransmission in the CNS, which subsequently influences behavior

SEDATIVE-HYPNOTICS AND ANXIOLYTICS

BARBITURATES

- **Mechanism of action**
  - The exact mechanism of action of barbiturates is unknown
  - The drugs are believed to cause generalized CNS depression by mimicking or enhancing the effects of GABA in the brain
- **Pharmacokinetics**
  - Absorption: Rapidly absorbed in the GI tract
  - Distribution: Rapidly and widely distributed in the tissues, primarily in the brain
  - Metabolism: Metabolized by the liver
  - Excretion: Excreted in the feces
- **Drug examples**
  - Rapid-acting barbiturates include thiopental sodium (Pentothal)
  - Short-acting barbiturates include pentobarbital (Nembutal) and secobarbital sodium (Seconal sodium)
  - Long-acting barbiturates include phenobarbital (Luminal)
- **Indications**
  - Rapid-acting barbiturates are used to induce anesthesia
  - Short-acting barbiturates are used to treat insomnia and as adjuncts to anesthesia
  - Long-acting barbiturates are used to treat insomnia and seizures
- **Contraindications and precautions**
  - These drugs are contraindicated in pregnancy, in uncontrolled pain, and in patients with a history of acute intermittent porphyria and preexisting CNS depression
  - Use cautiously in patients who are suicidal or who have a history of drug addiction
  - Use cautiously in elderly patients, who may require a decreased dosage

Key facts about barbiturates

- Believed to cause generalized CNS depression by mimicking or enhancing the effects of GABA in the brain
- Metabolized by the liver
- Excreted in the feces

When to use barbiturates

- Anesthesia
- Insomnia
- Seizures

When NOT to use barbiturates

- Pregnancy
- Uncontrolled pain
- History of acute intermittent porphyria and CNS depression

Adverse reactions to watch for

- Hangover feeling, slurred speech, paradoxical excitement

Key nursing actions

- Assess patient's sleep patterns.
- Administer I.V. doses slowly.
- Know that many sedative-hypnotics are controlled substances.
- Limit amount of medication available to patient.
- Know that long-term use of these drugs may cause physical and psychological dependence.
- Monitor patient's respiratory status.

Topics for patient discussion

- Therapy regimen
- Signs and symptoms of possible adverse reactions
- Activity restrictions
- Safety measures
- Avoidance of alcohol and over-the-counter antihistamines and other CNS depressants
- Notification of physician before using other prescription drugs
- Possibility of dependence and tolerance
- Need for compliance with therapy and medical follow-up

Adverse reactions

- These drugs may cause hangover feeling, slurred speech, and paradoxical excitement in the elderly and those in severe pain

Interactions

- These drugs may increase metabolism and decrease effectiveness of many concurrently used drugs, including warfarin and hormonal contraceptives
- Herbal preparations, such as valerian and kava, have additive CNS effects

Nursing responsibilities

- Assess the patient's sleep patterns; barbiturates reduce rapid-eye-movement sleep
- Administer I.V. doses slowly; rapid administration may cause respiratory and cardiovascular depression
- Base patient evaluation on decreased insomnia without excessive daytime sedation
- Know that many sedative-hypnotics are controlled substances
- Limit the amount of medication available to the patient to prevent hoarding of the drug, especially when risk of suicide exists
- Know that the long-term use of sedative-hypnotics may cause tolerance and physical and psychological dependence
- Inform the patient that the dosage should be decreased gradually after long-term use to prevent withdrawal symptoms
- Caution the patient to avoid driving and other activities requiring alertness until the response to the drug is known (for specific teaching tips, see *Teaching about sedative-hypnotics*)
- Warn the patient to avoid alcohol and other CNS depressants
- Monitor the patient's respiratory status to detect respiratory depression
- Institute safety precautions to prevent injury

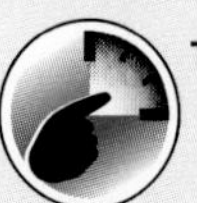

TIME-OUT FOR TEACHING

Teaching about sedative-hypnotics

Include these topics in your teaching plan for the patient receiving a sedative-hypnotic.

- Medication therapy regimen, including drug name, dose, frequency, duration, and possible adverse effects
- Signs and symptoms of possible adverse effects and when to notify the physician
- Activity restrictions, such as motor vehicle operation or other hazardous activities
- Safety measures
- Avoidance of alcohol and self-medication with over-the-counter products containing alcohol, antihistamines, or other central nervous system depressants
- Notification of the physician before using other prescription drugs, such as tranquilizers, opioids, or pain relievers
- Possibility of dependence and tolerance
- Compliance with therapy and medical follow-up

BENZODIAZEPINES

Mechanism of action

- These drugs cause generalized CNS depression by mimicking or enhancing the effects of GABA by antagonizing a protein that inhibits GABA binding to its receptors

Pharmacokinetics

- Absorption: Well absorbed in the GI tract; I.M. absorption can vary and be erratic
- Distribution: Highly lipophilic and protein-bound; widely and rapidly distributed into the tissues, especially to the brain
- Metabolism: Metabolized by the liver
- Excretion: Excreted in the urine

Drug examples

- Alprazolam (Xanax, Xanax XR), chlordiazepoxide hydrochloride (Librium), clonazepam (Klonopin), clorazepate (Tranxene), diazepam (Valium), estazolam (ProSom), flurazepam (Dalmane), lorazepam (Ativan), midazolam (Versed), oxazepam (Serax), prazepam (Centrax), quazepam (Doral), temazepam (Restoril), triazolam (Halcion)

Indications

- Alprazolam, chlordiazepoxide, clorazepate, diazepam, lorazepam, oxazepam, and prazepam are used to treat anxiety
- Chlordiazepoxide, clorazepate, diazepam, lorazepam, and oxazepam are used to treat alcohol withdrawal
- Diazepam, lorazepam, and midazolam are used preoperatively to induce sedation and amnesia
- Estazolam, flurazepam, quazepam, temazepam, and triazolam are used to treat insomnia
- Clonazepam and diazepam are used to treat seizures
- Diazepam is used to produce skeletal muscle relaxation

Contraindications and precautions

- These drugs are contraindicated in pregnancy, uncontrolled pain, preexisting CNS depression, and acute angle-closure glaucoma
- They are also contraindicated in patients who are suicidal or who have a history of substance abuse
- These drugs should be used with caution in elderly patients, who may require a decreased dosage, and in patients with renal or hepatic impairment

Adverse reactions

- These drugs commonly cause drowsiness, ataxia, temporary memory impairments, and reactions of rage, excitement, or hostility
- Increased depression, confusion, headaches, vertigo, GI disturbances, menstrual irregularities, and changes in libido also may occur

Key facts about benzodiazepines

- Cause generalized CNS depression by mimicking or enhancing the effects of GABA
- Metabolized by the liver
- Excreted in the urine

When to use benzodiazepines

- Anxiety
- Alcohol withdrawal
- Preoperative sedation and amnesia
- Insomnia
- Seizures
- Skeletal muscle relaxation

When NOT to use benzodiazepines

- Pregnancy
- Uncontrolled pain
- Preexisting CNS depression
- Acute angle-closure glaucoma

Adverse reactions to watch for

- Drowsiness, ataxia, temporary memory impairments, reactions of rage, excitement, or hostility

Interactions

- Herbal preparations, such as valerian and kava, will have additive CNS effects
- Antacids may decrease absorption of benzodiazepines
- Cimetidine, erythromycin, hormonal contraceptives, and some antidepressants may increase the plasma levels of the benzodiazepine
- Carbamazepine may decrease benzodiazepine levels
- Antihistamines, barbiturates, MAO inhibitors, and other cyclic antidepressants and alcohol increase CNS depression
- Cigarette smoking decreases the effectiveness of the benzodiazepine

Nursing responsibilities

- Administer I.V. doses slowly to prevent respiratory depression or apnea
- Instruct the patient to notify the physician if the dose becomes ineffective after a few weeks — but *not* to increase the dosage unless instructed by the physician

Key nursing actions

- Administer I.V. doses slowly.
- Instruct patient to notify physician if dose becomes ineffective after a few weeks.
- Advise patient not to increase dosage unless instructed by physician.

NONBARBITURATE SEDATIVE-HYPNOTICS AND ANXIOLYTICS

Mechanism of action

- These drugs cause generalized CNS depression

Pharmacokinetics

- Absorption: Rapidly absorbed
- Distribution: Widely distributed into the tissues
- Metabolism: Metabolized by the liver
- Excretion: Excreted in the feces

Key facts about nonbarbiturate sedative-hypnotics and anxiolytics

- Cause generalized CNS depression
- Metabolized by the liver
- Excreted in the feces

Drug examples

- Buspirone (BuSpar), chloral hydrate (Noctec), diphenhydramine (Benadryl, Sominex), hydroxyzine (Atarax, Vistaril), meprobamate (Miltown), promethazine hydrochloride (Anergan 50, Phenergan), propofol (Diprivan), zaleplon (Sonata), zolpidem (Ambien)

Indications

- Buspirone, hydroxyzine, and meprobamate are used to treat anxiety
- Chloral hydrate is used to treat insomnia and to induce preoperative sedation
- Hydroxyzine and promethazine are used for sedation and as adjuncts to opioid analgesics
- Propofol is used as a general anesthetic
- Zolpidem is used to treat insomnia

When to use nonbarbiturate sedative-hypnotics and anxiolytics

- Anxiety
- Insomnia
- Preoperative sedation
- As adjuncts to opioid analgesics
- General anesthesia

Contraindications and precautions

- These drugs are contraindicated in pregnancy, uncontrolled pain, and preexisting CNS depression
- They must be used with caution in patients who are suicidal or who have a history of drug addiction

- These drugs should be used with caution in elderly patients, who may require a decreased dosage

Adverse reactions
- Drowsiness
- Respiratory depression

Interactions
- These drugs may potentiate CNS depression and can prove lethal when used concurrently with alcohol, antidepressants, antihistamines, or phenothiazines
- These drugs may have additive effects if used with herbal preparations, such as valerian or kava
- Use of diphenhydramine with other products that contain diphenhydramine (including topical agents) increases the drug's additive effects and the risk of adverse reactions

Nursing responsibilities
- When administering hydroxyzine I.M., use the Z-track method of injection to prevent tissue irritation
- Administer chloral hydrate after meals to minimize gastric irritation
- Know that diphenhydramine is an ingredient in over-the-counter hypnotics

When NOT to use nonbarbiturate sedative-hypnotics and anxiolytics
- Pregnancy
- Uncontrolled pain
- Preexisting CNS depression

Adverse reactions to watch for
- Drowsiness, respiratory depression

Key nursing actions
- Use Z-track method of injection (hydroxyzine).
- Administer after meals (chloral hydrate).

ANTIPSYCHOTICS

PHENOTHIAZINES

Mechanism of action
- These drugs block the neurotransmitter dopamine in the limbic system, inhibiting transmission of neural impulses (antipsychotic action)
- These drugs also inhibit the chemoreceptor trigger zone in the medulla of the brain

Pharmacokinetics
- Absorption: Readily absorbed orally and parenterally; absorbed over weeks with long-acting depot I.M. administration
- Distribution: widely distributed; highly lipophilic and protein-bound, crossing the blood-brain barrier
- Metabolism: Metabolized by the liver
- Excretion: Excreted mostly in the urine

Drug examples
- Chlorpromazine (Thorazine), fluphenazine (Prolixin), mesoridazine (Serentil), perphenazine (Trilafon), prochlorperazine (Compazine), promazine (Sparine), thioridazine hydrochloride (Mellaril), thiothixene (Navane), trifluoperazine (Stelazine)

Key facts about phenothiazines
- Block the neurotransmitter dopamine in the limbic system, inhibiting transmission of neural impulses
- Inhibit the chemoreceptor trigger zone in the medulla of the brain
- Metabolized in the liver
- Excreted mostly in the urine

When to use phenothiazines

- Psychosis, schizophrenia, schizoaffective disorder, depression with psychotic features, psychotic symptoms associated with organic brain syndrome
- Nausea and vomiting

When NOT to use phenothiazines

- Angle-closure galucoma
- CNS depression
- Pregnancy (first trimester)
- Coma
- Risk of suicide

Adverse reactions to watch for

- Extrapyramidal symptoms, tardive dyskinesia, neuroleptic malignant syndrome, sedation, blurred vision, dry mouth, constipation, blood dyscrasias, photosensitivity reaction, sunburn, heat intolerance

Key nursing actions

- Tell patient that phenothiazines may discolor urine to pink or red-brown.
- Instruct patient to call physician before taking over-the-counter or herbal preparations.
- Monitor QT interval in patient taking thioridazine.

Indications

- Fluphenazine, mesoridazine, perphenazine, prochlorperazine, promazine, thioridazine, thiothixene, and trifluoperazine are used to treat psychosis, schizophrenia, schizoaffective disorder, depression with psychotic features, and psychotic symptoms associated with organic brain syndrome
- Chlorpromazine, perphenazine, prochlorperazine, and thiethylperazine are used to treat nausea and vomiting

Contraindications and precautions

- These drugs are contraindicated in angle-closure glaucoma and CNS depression, in pregnant women in their first trimester, in patients who are comatose or likely to experience significant CNS depression from other substances or medications, and in patients at risk for suicide
- These drugs must be withheld 48 hours before and 24 hours after myelography with metrizamide because they may reduce the seizure threshold
- These drugs should be used with caution in elderly patients and in those with acute myocardial infarction (MI), heart disease, benign prostatic hyperplasia, orthostatic hypotension, or respiratory distress (including asthma and emphysema)
- Thioridizine prolongs the QT interval and is contraindicated in patients with cardiac arrhythmias and in patients taking fluvoxamine, propanolol, pindolol, fluoxetine, or any other drug that prolongs the QT interval

Adverse reactions

- Extrapyramidal symptoms (such as akathisia, dystonia, and parkinsonism), tardive dyskinesia, neuroleptic malignant syndrome, sedation, blurred vision, dry mouth, constipation, blood dyscrasias, photosensitivity reaction (which may cause temporary blue-gray skin pigmentation on exposed surfaces), sunburn, heat intolerance
- Extrapyramidal symptoms are the major concern with antipsychotic therapy

Interactions

- These drugs potentiate alcohol and CNS depressants
- Concurrent use with antihypertensives and nitrates causes additive hypotension
- Antacids decrease absorption of antipsychotics
- Neuroleptics decrease the seizure threshold; therefore, increased doses of anticonvulsants may be needed
- Concurrent use of antipsychotics with anticholinergics, including antihistamines, antiparkinsonians, and antidepressants, may increase anticholinergic side effects

Nursing responsibilities

- Inform the patient that phenothiazines may discolor urine to pink or red-brown, and reassure him that the color change is harmless
- Instruct the patient to consult his health care provider before taking any over-the-counter or herbal preparations during drug therapy

- Monitor the QT interval in patients taking thioridazine hydrochloride (Mellaril)

BUTYROPHENONES

Mechanism of action
- These drugs block the neurotransmitter dopamine in the limbic system, inhibiting transmission of neural impulses (antipsychotic action)
- These drugs also inhibit the chemoreceptor trigger zone in the medulla of the brain

Pharmacokinetics
- Absorption: Readily absorbed orally and parenterally; absorbed over weeks with long-acting depot I.M. administration
- Distribution: Widely distributed; highly lipophilic and protein-bound, crossing the blood-brain barrier
- Metabolism: Metabolized by the liver
- Excretion: Excreted mostly in the urine

Drug examples
- Droperidol (Inapsine), haloperidol (Haldol)

Indications
- Droperidol is used to treat nausea and vomiting during surgery and diagnostic procedures and in combination with fentanyl as an adjunct to anesthesia
- Haloperidol is used to treat psychosis; Tourette syndrome; behavioral problems in children with combative, explosive hyperexcitability; and hyperactivity in hyperactive children

Contraindications and precautions
- These drugs are contraindicated in angle-closure glaucoma and CNS depression
- These drugs must be withheld 48 hours before and 24 hours after myelography with metrizamide because they may reduce the seizure threshold
- These drugs should be used with caution in acute MI, heart disease, benign prostatic hyperplasia, and orthostatic hypotension
- Droperidol is contraindicated in patients with known or suspected QT prolongation

Adverse reactions
- Extrapyramidal symptoms, tardive dyskinesia, neuroleptic malignant syndrome, sedation, blurred vision, dry mouth, constipation, blood dyscrasias, photosensitivity reaction (which may cause temporary blue-gray skin pigmentation on exposed surfaces), sunburn, heat intolerance

Interactions
- These drugs potentiate alcohol and CNS depressants

Key facts about butyrophenones
- Block the neurotransmitter dopamine in the limbic system, inhibiting the transmission of neural impulses
- Inhibit the chemoreceptor trigger zone in the medulla of the brain
- Metabolized in the liver
- Excreted mostly in the urine

When to use butyrophenones
- Nausea and vomiting during surgery and diagnostic procedures
- As adjunct to anesthesia
- Psychosis, Tourette syndrome, behavioral problems in children with explosive hyperexcitability, hyperactivity in hyperactive children

When NOT to use butyrophenones
- Angle-closure glaucoma
- CNS depression

Adverse reactions to watch for
- Extrapyramidal symptoms, tardive dyskinesia, neuroleptic malignant syndrome, sedation, blurred vision, dry mouth, constipation, blood dyscrasias, photosensitivity reaction, sunburn, heat intolerance

Key nursing actions

- Tell patient to avoid driving or other hazardous activities until CNS effects of drug are known.
- Advise patient to avoid alcohol and other CNS depressants during therapy.

Key facts about atypical antipsychotics

- Block the neurotransmitter dopamine in the limbic system, inhibiting the transmission of neural impulses
- Inhibit the chemoreceptor trigger zone in the medulla of the brain
- Metabolized by the liver
- Excreted mostly in the urine

When to use atypical antipsychotics

- Psychotic disorders, such as schizophrenia and schizoaffective disorders
- Obsessive-compulsive disorder
- Bipolar disorder
- Risk of suicidal behavior

When NOT to use atypical antipsychotics

- Angle-closure glaucoma
- CNS depression

- Concurrent use with antihypertensives and nitrates causes additive hypotension
- Antacids decrease absorption of antipsychotics
- Neuroleptics decrease the seizure threshold; therefore, increased doses of anticonvulsants may be needed

Nursing responsibilities

- Tell the patient to avoid driving or performing other hazardous activities until CNS effects are known
- Tell the patient to avoid alcohol or other CNS depressants during drug therapy because of possible additive effects and hypotension

ATYPICAL ANTIPSYCHOTICS

Mechanism of action

- These drugs block the neurotransmitter dopamine in the limbic system, inhibiting transmission of neural impulses (antipsychotic action)
- These drugs also inhibit the chemoreceptor trigger zone in the medulla of the brain

Pharmacokinetics

- Absorption: Readily absorbed orally and parenterally; absorbed over weeks with long-acting depot I.M. administration
- Distribution: Widely distributed; highly lipophilic and protein-bound, crossing the blood-brain barrier
- Metabolism: Metabolized by the liver
- Excretion: Excreted mostly in the urine

Drug examples

- Clomipramine (Anafranil), clozapine (Clozaril), loxapine (Loxitane), molindone (Moban), olanzapine (Zyprexa), quetiapine (Seroquel), risperidone (Risperdal), ziprasidone hydrochloride (Geodon)

Indications

- These atypical antipsychotics are used to manage psychotic disorders, such as schizophrenia and schizoaffective disorders
- Clomipramine is used in treating obsessive-compulsive disorder
- Olanzapine and risperidone also are used to treat bipolar disorder
- Clozapine is also used to reduce the risk of recurrent suicidal behavior in patients with schizophrenia and schizoaffective disorders

Contraindications and precautions

- These drugs are contraindicated in angle-closure glaucoma and CNS depression
- These drugs must be withheld 48 hours before and 24 hours after myelography with metrizamide because they may reduce the seizure threshold
- These drugs should be used with caution in acute MI, heart disease, benign prostatic hyperplasia, and orthostatic hypotension

Adverse reactions

- Extrapyramidal symptoms, tardive dyskinesia, neuroleptic malignant syndrome, sedation, blurred vision, dry mouth, constipation, blood dyscrasias, photosensitivity reaction (which may cause temporary blue-gray skin pigmentation on exposed surfaces), sunburn, heat intolerance.
- Clozapine can cause agranulocytosis, which necessitates close monitoring of the patient's white blood cell count
- Quetiapine may cause cataract development and may increase liver function test values
- Ziprasidone and risperidone may increase the QT interval and prolactin levels

Interactions

- These drugs potentiate the effects of alcohol and CNS depressants
- Concurrent use with antihypertensives and nitrates causes additive hypotension
- Antacids decrease absorption of antipsychotics
- Neuroleptics decrease the seizure threshold; increased doses of anticonvulsants may be needed

Nursing responsibilities

- Assess the patient's mental status; loss of contact with reality may signal noncompliance
- Monitor the patient for extrapyramidal symptoms and other adverse effects such as tardive dyskinesia, which is irreversible
- With antiemetic use, assess for nausea and vomiting
- If the patient is recovering from anesthesia with droperidol or fentanyl, decrease opioid analgesic dosages to one-quarter to one-third of normal
- After parenteral doses, monitor the patient for orthostatic hypotension
- Know that the patient who receives long-term antipsychotic therapy should undergo regular evaluation of red and white blood cell counts to detect blood dyscrasias
- Know that the drug should be discontinued gradually
- Teach the patient about the importance of complying with therapy because these drugs may take several weeks to produce desired effects (for specific teaching tips, see *Teaching about antipsychotics,* page 82)
- Warn the patient not to consume alcohol or take other CNS depressants while taking these drugs
- Caution the patient to avoid driving and other activities requiring alertness until the response to the drug is known
- Instruct the patient not to take antacids within 1 hour of taking these drugs
- Discuss ways to minimize dry mouth and constipation
- Urge the patient to use a sunscreen and protective clothing (to prevent photosensitivity reaction) and to avoid temperature extremes (to prevent heat intolerance)

Adverse reactions to watch for

- Extrapyramidal symptoms, tardive dyskinesia, neuroleptic malignant syndrome, sedation, blurred vision, dry mouth, constipation, blood dyscrasias, photosensitivity reaction, sunburn, heat intolerance

Key nursing actions

- Assess patient's mental status.
- Monitor patient for extrapyramidal symptoms and other adverse reactions.
- If patient is recovering from anesthesia with droperidol or fentanyl, decrease opioid analgesic dosages to one-quarter to one-third of normal.
- After parenteral doses, monitor patient for orthostatic hypotension.
- Know that patient receiving long-term antipsychotic therapy should undergo regular evaluation of red and white blood cell counts.
- Don't give antacids within 1 hour of administering these drugs.
- Know that drug should be discontinued gradually.
- Teach patient to:
  - comply with therapy
  - avoid alcohol and other CNS depressants
  - avoid driving and hazardous activities until CNS effects of drug are known
  - use sunscreen and wear protective clothing.

Topics for patient discussion

- Therapy regimen
- Signs and symptoms of possible adverse reactions
- Time required for drug to reach maximum effectiveness
- Safety measures
- Avoidance of alcohol and CNS depressants
- Need for compliance with therapy and medical follow-up

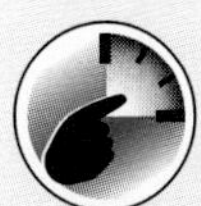

TIME-OUT FOR TEACHING

Teaching about antipsychotics

Include these topics in your teaching plan for the patient receiving an antipsychotic.

- Medication therapy regimen, including drug name, dose, frequency, duration, and possible adverse effects
- Signs and symptoms of possible adverse effects, including extrapyramidal effects and tardive dyskinesia, and when to notify the physician
- Time required for the drug to reach maximum effectiveness
- Safety measures
- Avoidance of central nervous system depressants
- Need for compliance with therapy and medical follow-up

- Base patient evaluation on improved interaction with others and greater participation in activities of daily living (or on resolution of nausea and vomiting with antiemetic use)

ANTIDEPRESSANTS

TRICYCLIC, SECOND-GENERATION, AND MISCELLANEOUS ANTIDEPRESSANTS AND SSRIs

Key facts about tricyclic, second-generation, and miscellaneous antidepressants and SSRIs

- Tricyclic and second-generation antidepressants increase the amount of norepinephrine, serotonin, or both through reuptake inhibition, thus normalizing the receptor site associated with depression
- SSRIs block the reuptake of serotonin into the presynaptic cells, thus increasing serotonin levels at the synapse
- Metabolized by the liver
- Tricyclic antidepressants excreted mostly in the urine as metabolites

Mechanism of action

- Tricyclic and second-generation antidepressants increase the amount of norepinephrine, serotonin, or both through reuptake inhibition, thus normalizing the hyposensitive receptor site associated with depression
- Selective serotonin reuptake inhibitors (SSRIs) block the reuptake of serotonin into the presynaptic cells, thereby increasing serotonin levels at the synapse

Pharmacokinetics

- Absorption: Tricyclic and second-generation antidepressants are completely absorbed after oral administration; SSRIs are well absorbed in the GI tract
- Distribution: Antidepressants are widely distributed in the tissues because they are extremely fat-soluble, but second-generation antidepressants aren't distributed to cardiac tissue; SSRIs are highly protein-bound
- Metabolism: Metabolized by the liver; SSRIs undergo hepatic metabolism by the cytochrome P-450 enzyme
- Excretion: Tricyclic antidepressants are excreted primarily in the urine as metabolites

Drug examples

- Tricyclic antidepressants include amitriptyline hydrochloride (Endep), amoxapine (Asendin), clomipramine (Anafranil), desipramine (Norpramin), doxepin (Sinequan), imipramine (Tofranil), and nortriptyline (Pamelor)
- Second-generation and miscellaneous antidepressants include bupropion hydrochloride (Wellbutrin), fluoxetine hydrochloride (Prozac, Prozac Weekly, Sarafem), maprotiline (Ludiomil), nefazodone (Serzone), trazodone hydrochloride (Desyrel), and venlafaxine hydrochloride (Effexor)
- SSRIs include citalopram (Celexa), escitalopram (Lexapro), fluoxetine (Prozac), fluvoxamine (Luvox), paroxetine (Paxil), and sertraline (Zoloft)

Indications

- These drugs are used to treat endogenous depression; tricyclic antidepressants are the drugs of choice for episodes of major depression
- Second-generation antidepressants are used to treat the same major depressive episodes as the tricyclic antidepressants and have the same degree of effectiveness; however, they have fewer side effects
- Imipramine also is used to treat enuresis
- Doxepin also is used to treat anxiety
- Amitriptyline, doxepin, imipramine, nortriptyline, and trazodone also are used to treat neurogenic pain (unlabeled use)
- SSRIs may be used to treat generalized anxiety disorder, depression, and obsessive-compulsive disorder; they also may be useful in treating bulimia nervosa
- Fluoxetine and bupropion also may be used for smoking cessation
- Fluoxetine also may be used to treat premenstrual dysphoric disorder
- Clomipramine was the first drug to be approved to treat obsessive-compulsive disorder

Contraindications and precautions

- Concurrent use of fluoxetine and MAO inhibitors is contraindicated
- These drugs may reduce the seizure threshold
- They should be discontinued 48 hours before and 24 hours after myelography involving metrizamide to prevent lowering the seizure threshold
- Older patients are at increased risk for adverse effects from tricyclic antidepressants, but they tolerate SSRIs better
- Nefazodone is contraindicated in those with active liver disease
- SSRIs should be used cautiously in elderly patients and in patients with hepatic or renal failure
- SSRIs should be discontinued by gradually tapering the drug

Adverse reactions

- Tricyclic antidepressants may cause orthostatic hypotension, tachycardia, blurred vision, dry mouth, constipation, seizure, and rash; they may exacerbate heart failure or an existing bundle-branch block
- Second-generation antidepressants may cause seizures, insomnia, and nausea; some may cause anticholinergic effects

When to use tricyclic, second-generation, and miscellaneous antidepressants and SSRIs

- Endogenous depression; episodes of major depression
- Enuresis
- Anxiety
- Neurogenic pain (unlabeled use)
- Generalized anxiety disorder
- Obsessive-compulsive disorder
- Depression
- Bulimia nervosa
- Smoking cessation
- Premenstrual dysphoric disorder

When NOT to use tricyclic, second-generation, and miscellaneous antidepressants and SSRIs

- MAO inhibitor therapy
- Active liver disease

Adverse reactions to watch for

- Orthostatic hypotension, tachycardia, blurred vision, dry mouth, constipation, seizures, rash, exacerbation of heart failure or bundle-branch block
- Insomnia, nausea, anticholinergic effects
- Somnolence, drowsiness, fatigue, tremor, asthenia, sexual disturbances

Key nursing actions

- Know that these drugs should be discontinued gradually.
- Know that these drugs may take several weeks to produce desired effects.
- Teach patient to:
- – avoid alcohol and nonprescription drugs
- – avoid driving and other hazardous activities until CNS effects of drug are known
- – take daily dose of tricyclic antidepressants at bedtime
- – take fluoxetine or paroxetine early in day
- – not crush controlled-release tablets, but to swallow them whole.

- **Bupropion is distinguishable from all other tricyclic antidepressants because it doesn't cause drowsiness and has fewer cardiovascular and anticholinergic side effects**
- SSRIs may cause insomnia, somnolence, drowsiness, fatigue, tremor, asthenia, or seizures; they may also cause sexual disturbances, such as delayed ejaculation and anorgasmia

Interactions

- These drugs may reduce the effectiveness of antihypertensives
- Concurrent use with alcohol, antihistamines, and other CNS depressants causes additive CNS depression
- **Antidepressant use with MAO inhibitors may cause hypertensive crisis and seizures**
- **SSRIs and MAO inhibitors or other serotonergic agents, such as clomipramine or buspirone, may cause serotonin syndrome**
- **Serotonin syndrome symptoms include fever, agitation, hypertension, hyperthermia, rigidity, and myoclonus and can result in seizures, coma, or death**
- **Five weeks should elapse after starting fluoxetine and starting MAO inhibitor therapy. A 2-week "washout" period should follow discontinuation of other SSRIs before MAO inhibitor therapy begins**
- These drugs shouldn't be used with St. John's wort because it may cause additive CNS depression
- Tricyclic antidepressants cause photosensitivity; advise the patient to wear protective clothing and to use sunblock when exposed to sunlight for a prolonged period
- Bupropion should be used cautiously with other drugs that affect hepatic metabolism
- Use of paroxetine with tryptophan can produce adverse reactions, such as headache, nausea, sweating, and dizziness
- Trazodone may produce additive effects when combined with other drugs

Nursing responsibilities

- Know that these drugs should be discontinued gradually
- **Teach the patient about the importance of complying with therapy; these drugs may take several weeks to produce desired effects**
  - **Tricyclics may take up to 30 days to reach their full therapeutic response**
  - **Amitriptyline may produce a therapeutic effect within 10 to 14 days**
  - **SSRIs may begin to take effect in 1 to 4 weeks**
- Warn the patient to avoid alcohol and nonprescription drugs to prevent adverse drug interactions
- Caution the patient to avoid driving and other activities requiring alertness until the effects of the drug are known
- **Instruct the patient taking fluoxetine or paroxetine to take the drug early in the day to avoid interference with sleep; otherwise, suggest**

that the patient taking any other tricyclic antidepressant take the daily dosage at bedtime to avoid sedation or anticholinergic effects

- Tell the patient not to crush controlled-release tablets, but to swallow them whole

MONOAMINE OXIDASE (MAO) INHIBITORS

Mechanism of action

- These drugs impair inactivation of norepinephrine, serotonin, or both, thus prolonging their presence in CNS synapses and increasing their concentrations in the body

Pharmacokinetics

- Absorption: Although information is limited, MAO inhibitors are well absorbed rapidly and completely from the GI tract following oral administration
- Distribution: Widely distributed
- Metabolism: Metabolized in the liver by acetylation
- Excretion: Excreted mainly in the feces and partly in the urine, mostly as metabolites

Drug examples

- Isocarboxazid (Marplan), phenelzine sulfate (Nardil), tranylcypromine sulfate (Parnate)

Indications

- To treat depression in patients who can't tolerate other forms of therapy, such as psychotherapy
- To treat bulimia (in the form of atypical depression) and panic disorder with associated agoraphobia and globus hystericus syndrome (unlabeled uses)

Contraindications and precautions

- Contraindicated in patients with a known hypersensitivity to the drugs or their components
- Also contraindicated in patients with pheochromocytomas, heart failure, liver disease or abnormal liver function test results, renal impairment, confirmed or suspected cerebrovascular accident, cardiovascular disease, hypertension, and history of headaches
- Concurrent administration with other MAO inhibitors, tricyclic antidepressants, anesthetics, CNS depressants, antihypertensives, caffeine, cheeses, or other foods high in tyramine content is also contraindicated
- Use cautiously in pregnant and breast-feeding women and in patients with diabetes or epilepsy
- Safety and efficacy haven't been established in children younger than age 16

Key facts about MAO inhibitors

- Impair inactivation of norepinephrine, serotonin, or both, thus prolonging their presence in CNS synapses and increasing their concentrations in the body
- Metabolized in the liver
- Excreted mainly in the feces and partly in the urine

When to use MAO inhibitors

- Depression
- Bulimia (unlabeled use)
- Panic disorder with associated agoraphobia and globus hystericus syndrome (unlabeled use)

When NOT to use MAO inhibitors

- Hypersensitivity to MAO inhibitors or their components
- Pheochromocytomas, heart failure, liver disease or abnormal liver function test results, renal impairment, confirmed or suspected cerebrovascular accident, cardiovascular disease, hypertension, history of headaches
- With other MAO inhibitors, tricyclic antidepressants, anesthetics, CNS depressants, antihypertensives, caffeine, cheeses, or other foods high in tyramine

Adverse reactions to watch for

- Restlessness, insomnia, dizziness, drowsiness, headache, orthostatic hypotension, anorexia, blurred vision, peripheral edema, constipation, dry mouth, nausea, and vomiting
- Hypertensive crisis

Key nursing actions

- Don't administer these drugs in the evening.
- Assess patient's mental status for mood changes and suicidal tendencies.
- Know that it may take several weeks for these drugs to produce desired effects.
- Be alert for suicide attempts when depression begins to lift and energy improves.
- Monitor patient for signs and symptoms of hypertensive crisis.
- Teach patient to:
  - avoid alcohol and foods containing tyramine
  - carry identification describing disorder and drug regimen.

Adverse reactions

- The most serious adverse reaction to MAO inhibitors is hypertensive crisis, which can lead to death
- The most common adverse reactions to MAO inhibitors are restlessness, insomnia, dizziness, drowsiness, headache, orthostatic hypotension, anorexia, blurred vision, peripheral edema, constipation, dry mouth, nausea, and vomiting

Interactions

- MAO inhibitors interact with most other drugs
- Concurrent use with amphetamines, antidepressants, dopamine, epinephrine, guanethidine, levodopa, methyldopa, nasal decongestants, norepinephrine, reserpine, tyramine-containing foods, and vasoconstrictors may cause hypertensive crisis
- Concurrent use with opioid analgesics may cause hypertension, hypotension, coma, or seizures; MAO inhibitors should be discontinued several weeks before surgery
- Concurrent use with high doses of tranylcypromine may cause dependence and addiction

Nursing responsibilities

- Don't administer these drugs in the evening because they may cause insomnia
- Assess the patient's mental status for mood changes and suicidal tendencies
- Teach the patient that it may take 1 to 4 weeks for antidepressant effects to occur
- Be alert for suicide attempts when depression begins to lift and energy improves
- Discontinue these drugs gradually
- Teach the patient about the importance of complying with therapy; these drugs may take several weeks to produce desired effects (for specific teaching tips, see *Teaching about MAO inhibitors*)
- Caution the patient to avoid alcohol and foods containing tyramine (red wine, beer, aged cheeses, yeast, avocados, bananas, yogurt, smoked or pickled fish, chocolate, overripe fruit, and beverages containing caffeine) to prevent hypertensive crisis
- Monitor the patient for signs and symptoms of hypertensive crisis, such as increased blood pressure, severe headache, palpitations, neck stiffness or soreness, nausea, and vomiting
- Instruct the patient to carry identification describing the disorder and the drug regimen

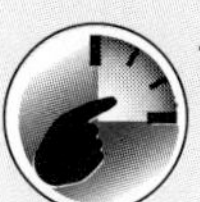

TIME-OUT FOR TEACHING

Teaching about MAO inhibitors

Include these topics in your teaching plan for the patient receiving a monoamine oxidase (MAO) inhibitor.

- Medication therapy regimen, including drug name, dose, frequency, duration, and possible adverse effects
- Signs and symptoms of possible adverse effects and when to notify the physician
- Signs and symptoms of hypertensive crisis
- Dietary restrictions
- Need to inform other health care providers about MAO therapy
- Need for compliance with therapy and medical follow-up

ANTIMANICS (LITHIUM)

Mechanism of action

- Lithium competes with calcium, magnesium, potassium, and sodium in body tissues and at the binding site and alters the sodium transport in nerve and muscle cells
- Although its specific mechanism of action is unknown, lithium affects the synthesis, storage, release, and reuptake of central monoamine neurotransmitters
- Lithium's antimanic effects may result from increases in norepinephrine reuptake and serotonin sensitivity

Pharmacokinetics

- Absorption: Readily absorbed from the GI tract
- Distribution
  - Widely distributed in most body tissues and fluid and levels peak within 6 to 10 hours; concentrations are higher in the bones
  - Lithium crosses the blood-brain and placental barriers and appears in breast milk
- Metabolism: Lithium isn't metabolized
- Excretion: Excreted almost entirely in the urine

Drug examples

- Lithium carbonate (Eskalith, Lithane, Lithobid, Lithonate, Lithotabs), lithium citrate (Cibalith-S)

Indications

- Lithium is used to treat mania and bipolar affective disorders (also known as bipolar disorder)
- Carbamazepine (Tegretol) and valproic acid (Depakene, Depakote) may be used as alternative treatment for mania

Topics for patient discussion

- Therapy regimen
- Signs and symptoms of possible adverse effects
- Signs and symptoms of hypertensive crisis
- Dietary restrictions
- Need to inform other health care providers about MAO inhibitor therapy
- Need for compliance with therapy and medical follow-up

Key facts about lithium

- Alters the sodium transport in nerve and muscle cells
- Affects synthesis, storage, release, and reuptake of central monoamine neurotransmitters
- Antimanic effects may result from increases in norepinephrine reuptake and serotonin sensitivity
- Excreted mostly in the urine

When to use lithium

- Mania
- Bipolar affective disorders

When NOT to use lithium

- Renal or cardiovascular disease
- Breast-feeding
- Severe dehydration
- Severe sodium depletion
- Severe debilitation

Adverse reactions to watch for

- Hand tremors, transient muscle weakness, hypertonia, nausea, vomiting, bloating, diarrhea, anorexia, abdominal pains, mild thirst, polyuria, polydipsia, nephrogenic diabetes insipidus

Key nursing actions

- Know that tolerance for lithium is high in acute phase of mania and decreases as mania subsides.
- Assess for suicidal tendencies and institute suicide precautions, as necessary.
- Assess patient for signs and symptoms of lithium toxicity, including vomiting, diarrhea, slurred speech, decreased coordination, drowsiness, muscle weakness, and twitching.
- Teach patient to:
  - drink 2 to 3 L of fluid daily; maintain adequate salt intake; avoid excessive amounts of coffee, tea, and cola; and avoid activities that cause excess sodium loss
  - avoid driving and other hazardous activities until CNS effects of drug are known
  - consult physician before taking nonprescription drugs.

Contraindications and precautions

- Lithium is contraindicated in patients with renal or cardiovascular disease, in breast-feeding women, and in patients with severe dehydration, sodium depletion, or debilitation because the risk of toxicity is increased
- Use cautiously in elderly patients and those with thyroid disease
- Use in pregnant women only when the benefits outweigh the risks to the fetus

Adverse reactions

- Mild nausea and general discomfort might occur during the first few days, but these symptoms usually subside with continued treatment or temporary reduction or cessation of the drug
- The most common adverse reactions involve the CNS, the GI tract, and the kidneys and include hand tremors, transient muscle weakness, hypertonia, nausea, vomiting, bloating, diarrhea, anorexia, abdominal pains, mild thirst, polyuria, polydipsia, and nephrogenic diabetes insipidus
- Antimanics may cause hypothyroidism

Interactions

- Concurrent use of lithium with diuretics, fluoxetine, methyldopa, or nonsteroidal anti-inflammatory drugs increases lithium reabsorption by the kidney or inhibits lithium excretion, either of which increases the risk of lithium toxicity
- Acetazolamide, aminophylline, sodium bicarbonate, and an increased sodium intake may increase renal excretion of lithium, reducing its effectiveness
- Antimanics interfere with norepinephrine and may reduce the effects of antihypertensives
- Antipsychotics, such at phenothiazines and haloperidol, may increase lithium levels and cause neurotoxicity
- Antipsychotics, when combined with lithium, have also been associated with acute encephalopathic syndrome (consisting of weakness, lethargy, fever, confusion, disorientation, and adverse extrapyramidal reactions)
  - This syndrome may be similar to or the same as neuroleptic malignant syndrome (NMS)
  - NMS is also an adverse effect of antipsychotics

Nursing responsibilities

- Monitor serum lithium levels to evaluate drug effectiveness and prevent toxicity
- **Know that the therapeutic range for long-term lithium use ranges from 0.6 to 1.2 mEq/L**
- **Be aware that tolerance for lithium is high in the acute phase of mania and then decreases as the mania subsides; effective lithium levels will range from 1 to 1.5 mEq/L during acute mania and then the dosage will be readjusted**
- Assess for suicidal tendencies and institute suicide precautions, as necessary
- Administer the drug with food to minimize GI irritation

- Monitor the patient's renal function before drug therapy begins and regularly thereafter because lithium is excreted renally
- **Know that lithium toxicity can occur despite normal lithium levels; assess the patient for signs and symptoms of toxicity, such as vomiting, diarrhea, slurred speech, decreased coordination, drowsiness, muscle weakness, and twitching**
- Know that lithium depletes sodium reabsorption, causing sodium depletion in the body, which in turn increases the risk of lithium toxicity
- **To help the patient avoid lithium toxicity, instruct him to drink 2 to 3 L of fluid daily; maintain adequate salt intake; avoid excessive amounts of coffee, tea, and cola (which have a diuretic effect); and avoid activities that cause excess sodium loss**
- Instruct the patient to consult the physician or pharmacist before taking nonprescription drugs to prevent adverse drug interactions
- Know that lithium can cause drowsiness, blackouts, and confusion; caution the patient to avoid hazardous activities or driving until CNS effects are known

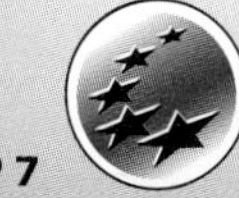

TOP 7

items to study before your next test on drugs and mood alteration

1. Medications commonly used as sedative-hypnotics, anxiolytics, antipsychotics, antidepressants, and antimanics
2. Mechanism of action of sedative-hypnotics, anxiolytics, antipsychotics, antidepressants, and antimanics
3. Indications for sedative-hypnotics, anxiolytics, antipsychotics, antidepressants, and antimanics
4. Precautions the nurse must take when administering sedative-hypnotics, anxiolytics, antipsychotics, antidepressants, or antimanics
5. Common adverse effects of sedative-hypnotics, anxiolytics, antipsychotics, antidepressants, and antimanics
6. Nursing responsibilities when administering sedative-hypnotics, anxiolytics, antipsychotics, antidepressants, or antimanics
7. Appropriate teaching for a patient receiving a sedative-hypnotic, an anxiolytic, an antipsychotic, an antidepressant, or an antimanic

NCLEX CHECKS

It's never too soon to begin your NCLEX preparation. Now that you've reviewed this chapter, carefully read each of the following questions and choose the best answer. Then compare your responses to the correct answers.

1. A patient taking a barbiturate such as pentobarbital sodium (Nembutal) should be taught to:

- ☐ **A.** decrease the drug gradually rather than stop it abruptly.
- ☐ **B.** decrease the dose if drowsiness occurs.
- ☐ **C.** drink alcohol only in moderation.
- ☐ **D.** avoid driving a car while taking the drug.

2. Which of the following agents are believed to work by stimulating the inhibitory neurotransmitter gamma-aminobutyric acid (GABA)?

- ☐ **A.** Barbiturates
- ☐ **B.** Benzodiazepines
- ☐ **C.** Selective serotonin reuptake inhibitors (SSRIs)
- ☐ **D.** Tricyclic antidepressants

3. Which of the following descriptions of the anxiolytic buspirone (BuSpar) is accurate?

- ☐ **A.** It has a rapid onset of action.
- ☐ **B.** It has a high potential for abuse.
- ☐ **C.** It has more adverse reactions than benzodiazepines.
- ☐ **D.** It doesn't have any interaction with alcohol.

4. A patient with schizophrenia has been taking chlorpromazine (Thorazine) for several months and wants to attend a picnic on the 4th of July. You would be most concerned about which of the drug's adverse reactions?

☐ A. Constipation
☐ B. Hypotension
☐ C. Increased appetite
☐ D. Photosensitivity

5. A patient began taking haloperidol (Haldol) yesterday for schizophrenia. Today, he says that his neck feels stiff and he's having trouble walking. You note that his eyes are rolled slightly upward. Which of the following changes would you expect the physician to make to this patient's drug regimen?

☐ A. Change the drug to fluoxetine (Prozac)
☐ B. Add diazepam (Valium) to the regimen
☐ C. Change the drug to fluphenazine (Prolixin)
☐ D. Add benztropine (Cogentin), 1 mg twice daily

6. A postmenopausal woman who has developed major depression is started on fluoxetine (Prozac) therapy. Which is the most important point to include in her discharge instructions?

☐ A. The daily dose of fluoxetine can be taken either in the morning or in the evening.
☐ B. A rash or itching may develop when the drug is first started, but it will go away later.
☐ C. There are no restrictions on driving or other hazardous activities because the drug is nonsedating.
☐ D. Over-the-counter (OTC) or other prescription drugs are safe because few drug interactions occur with fluoxetine.

7. A patient is being discharged with a prescription for amitriptyline (Endep). Which of the following statements is most important to tell this patient?

☐ A. The drug will help reduce the symptoms of depression.
☐ B. The patient should have no anxiety when the drug becomes effective.
☐ C. Pulmonary function studies should be performed periodically.
☐ D. Long-term use of the drug causes extrapyramidal adverse reactions.

8. When teaching a patient prescribed a monoamine oxidase (MAO) inhibitor, you should instruct him to avoid foods containing which of the following substances?

☐ A. Pyridoxine
☐ B. Riboflavin
☐ C. Thiamine
☐ D. Tyramine

9. A patient started taking lithium for bipolar disorder. Which of the following signs or symptoms would alert you that his serum level of lithium is too high?

☐ A. Rash
☐ B. Hypothyroidism
☐ C. Fine hand tremor
☐ D. Elevated white blood cell count

10. A physician prescribes lithium for a patient diagnosed with bipolar disorder. The nurse needs to provide appropriate education for the patient on this drug. Which of the following topics should the nurse cover?

Select all that apply:

☐ A. Potential for addiction
☐ B. Signs and symptoms of drug toxicity
☐ C. Potential for tardive dyskinesia
☐ D. Information regarding a low-tyramine diet
☐ E. Need to monitor blood levels consistently
☐ F. Timeframe (7 to 21 days) in which mood changes will take place

ANSWERS AND RATIONALES

1. CORRECT ANSWER: A

Barbiturates should be tapered gradually. Stopping the drug may cause withdrawal symptoms, such as nausea, vomiting, muscle twitches, hallucinations, or seizures. The patient shouldn't drink alcohol during drug therapy because alcohol will potentiate central nervous system depressant effects. Drowsiness is an expected adverse reaction of barbiturates. Driving a car isn't contraindicated during drug therapy; however, the patient needs to know the drug's effects on mental alertness before operating a motor vehicle.

2. CORRECT ANSWER: B

Benzodiazepines, which stimulate GABA, are used primarily as sedatives and hypnotics. Examples of benzodiazepines include diazepam, flurazepam, and lorazepam. Barbiturates are general central nervous system depressants. SSRIs inhibit the neurotransmitter serotonin, not GABA. Tricyclic antidepressants inhibit norepinephrine and serotonin.

3. CORRECT ANSWER: D

BuSpar is unlike any other anxiolytic because it doesn't interact with alcohol or other central nervous system depressants. It has a slow onset of action, is less sedating, and has a lower chance of being abused than other anxiolytics.

4. CORRECT ANSWER: D

Thorazine may cause photosensitivity. July 4th is usually a hot time of the year, with bright sunlight. Because of the photosensitivity caused by the drug, the patient may burn easily when exposed to the sun. Constipation shouldn't be a concern at the picnic. Hypotension is an occasional adverse reaction that usually occurs early in the treatment. Increased appetite is also an occasional adverse reaction, but isn't of concern in this instance.

5. CORRECT ANSWER: D

The patient's symptoms are extrapyramidal reactions induced by the antipsychotic haloperidol. Adding an anticholinergic like benztropine will reverse extrapyramidal reactions. Fluoxetine isn't effective for psychosis. There are no indications that the patient would benefit from diazepam, a benzodiazepine. Fluphenazine has the same risk for this adverse reaction as haloperidol.

6. CORRECT ANSWER: B

Some of the less serious adverse effects of fluoxetine, such as rash and itching, occur when the drug is first taken, but these are easily controlled with antihistamines or corticosteroids and usually will subside with continued therapy. The drug should be taken in the morning; evening doses may cause insomnia. Fluoxetine is less sedating than many other psychotropic drugs; however, some patients experience dizziness and drowsiness when first starting the drug, so driving and performing other hazardous activities should be avoided. The drug interacts with many other drugs, so the patient should be encouraged to check with the prescriber before taking any OTC medications.

7. CORRECT ANSWER: A

Amitriptyline is a tricyclic antidepressant that increases the levels of serotonin and norepinephrine in the neurons, thereby reducing the symptoms of depression. It usually isn't possible to be completely anxiety-free. Liver and renal function and blood counts, not pulmonary function, should be monitored for patients on long-term therapy. Extrapyramidal adverse reactions occur from long-term use of phenothiazine, not amitriptyline.

8. CORRECT ANSWER: D

Patients receiving MAO inhibitors should avoid foods containing tyramine because of the risk of a hypertensive crisis. Tyramine is contained in many foods, such as aged cheese, coffee, avocados, bananas, ales, red wines, and other undistilled beverages. The need for a restrictive diet makes the use of MAO inhibitors difficult. These drugs also may interact adversely with other drugs, further limiting their use. MAO inhibitors usually are prescribed in dire situations when other drugs don't work. The intake of thiamine, riboflavin, and pyridoxine (water-soluble vitamins) isn't limited with MAO inhibitors.

9. CORRECT ANSWER: C

Although all of the above choices are potential adverse reactions to lithium, only the hand tremor occurs as a result of an increase in serum lithium level. Rash, hypothyroidism, and elevated white blood cell count aren't dose related and can occur even at low lithium serum levels.

10. CORRECT ANSWER: B, E, F

Patient teaching should cover the signs and symptoms of drug toxicity as well as the need to report them to the physician. The patient should be instructed to monitor his lithium levels on a regular basis to avoid toxicity. The nurse should explain that 7 to 21 days may pass before the patient notes a change in his mood. Lithium does not have addictive properties. Tyramine is a potential concern to patients taking monoamine-oxidase inhibitors.

6

Drugs and the musculoskeletal system

LEARNING OBJECTIVES

After studying this chapter, you should be able to:

- Describe the mechanisms of action of antigout drugs, antarthritics, and skeletal muscle relaxants.
- List the indications for antigout drugs, antarthritics, and skeletal muscle relaxants.
- Describe common adverse effects of antigout drugs, antarthritics, and skeletal muscle relaxants.
- Identify nursing responsibilities when administering antigout drugs, antarthritics, and skeletal muscle relaxants.
- Discuss patient teaching related to antigout drugs, antarthritics, and skeletal muscle relaxants.

CHAPTER OVERVIEW

Gout is a disorder of purine metabolism that causes uric acid to accumulate in the blood. The uric acid may precipitate into joints, skin, and other tissues, producing inflammation and tenderness. Antigout drugs work by either decreasing uric acid production or enhancing renal excretion of the uric acid. Nursing responsibilities focus on promoting fluid intake, restricting purines and alcohol in the diet, and avoiding aspirin.

Rheumatoid arthritis, a chronic, systemic disease that causes joint inflammation, is treated with various anti-inflammatories. Although nonsteroidal anti-inflammatory drugs (NSAIDs) are generally effective for mild to moderate rheumatoid arthritis, gold salts are indicated for severe rheumatoid arthritis unresponsive to other drug therapies. Nursing responsibilities focus on monitoring the patient for gold toxicity, preventing stomatitis, evaluating the patient for improved range of motion, and taking measures to relieve pain and swelling.

Skeletal muscle relaxants are used to decrease spasticity caused by various spinal cord lesions or to relieve painful musculoskeletal problems. Nursing responsibilities include measures to ensure patient safety.

ANATOMY AND PHYSIOLOGY

Anatomy

- The musculoskeletal system is made up of bones, joints, ligaments, tendons, and muscles
- There are three types of muscle: smooth, cardiac, and skeletal
  - Skeletal muscle is attached to the skeleton
  - The human body has approximately 600 skeletal muscles
  - These muscles contract rapidly and vigorously for short periods
  - Skeletal muscle fibers consist of threadlike structures called myofibrils, which are composed of thick and thin filaments
    - Thick filaments are composed of myosin
    - Thin filaments are composed of actin

Physiology

- Skeletal muscle is under voluntary control; it contracts in response to impulses transmitted from the central nervous system (CNS) by motor nerves
- Each skeletal muscle is innervated by sensory neurons from the somatic (voluntary) nervous system and at least one motor nerve
  - Sensory (afferent) neurons receive impulses concerning the degree of muscle contraction and transmit these impulses to the CNS, coordinating muscle activity
  - Motor (efferent) neurons convey impulses from the CNS to the muscle, triggering muscle contraction
- Muscle contraction occurs when thick and thin filaments slide over each other, forming structures called cross bridges
- For contraction to occur, calcium ions diffuse into the surrounding structures of the filaments, changing the position of these structures and keeping the thick and thin filaments from binding together

Function

- Skeletal muscles move body parts or the body as a whole
- Skeletal muscles are responsible for voluntary and reflex movements
- Contractions generate the most body heat because much of the body is composed of skeletal muscle

A&P highlights

- The musculoskeletal system consists of bones, joints, ligaments, tendons, and muscles.
- There are three types of muscle: smooth, cardiac, and skeletal.
- Skeletal muscle is under voluntary control.
- Each skeletal muscle is innervated by sensory neurons from the somatic nervous system and at least one motor nerve.
- Muscle contraction occurs when thick and thin filaments slide over each other, forming structures called cross bridges.
- Skeletal muscles move body parts or the body as a whole.
- Skeletal muscles are responsible for voluntary and reflex movements.
- Contractions generate the most body heat.
- Spasticity is caused by injury to muscles, joints, tendons, or ligaments or by CNS damage.

- **Spasticity**
  - Caused by injury to muscles, joints, tendons, or ligaments or by CNS damage (such as cerebral palsy, multiple sclerosis, poliomyelitis, spinal cord injury or tumors, or tetanus)
  - Occurs when an excessive number of motor impulses pass to the periphery from the spinal cord
  - Results from an increase in excitatory influences or a decrease in inhibitory influences

ANTIGOUT DRUGS

- **Mechanism of action**
  - Antigout drugs work by decreasing inflammation, reducing uric acid production, or increasing uric acid excretion
  - Allopurinol decreases uric acid production
  - Colchicine reduces the inflammatory process by interfering with polymorphonuclear leukocyte activity
  - Probenecid and sulfinpyrazone enhance renal excretion of uric acid, thereby reducing the serum urate level
- **Pharmacokinetics**
  - Absorption: Well absorbed from the GI tract
  - Distribution: Highly protein-bound
  - Metabolism: Metabolized in the liver
  - Excretion: Excreted primarily by the kidneys
- **Drug examples**
  - Allopurinol (Lopurin, Zyloprim), colchicine, probenecid (Benemid), sulfinpyrazone (Anturane)
- **Indications**
  - Colchicine is used to treat active gout, especially if adequate doses are given early in the attack
  - I.V. colchicine is used when a rapid response is needed during an acute attack
  - Allopurinol, probenecid, and sulfinpyrazone are used to prevent recurrent attacks of gout or gouty arthritis (allopurinol isn't intended for asymptomatic hyperuricemia)
  - Probenecid should be used only after an acute gouty attack has subsided; however, if an acute gouty attack occurs during therapy, probenecid may be continued
- **Contraindications and precautions**
  - Probenecid is contraindicated in patients taking salicylates and in those who are hypersensitive to probenecid or sulfonamides (probenecid is a sulfonamide) or have blood dyscrasias or uric acid kidney stones
  - Probenecid is also contraindicated in children younger than age 2

Key facts about antigout drugs

- Decrease uric acid production
- Reduce inflammatory process
- Enhance renal excretion of uric acid
- Metabolized by the liver
- Excreted primarily by the kidneys

When to use antigout drugs

- Active gout
- Prevention of recurrent attacks of gout or gouty arthritis
- After acute gouty attack

When NOT to use antigout drugs

- Hypersensitivity to these drugs or to sulfonamides or phenylbutazone or other pyrazoles
- Blood dyscrasias
- Salicylate therapy, uric acid kidney stones, children younger than age 2
- Active peptic ulcer disease, symptoms of GI inflammation or ulceration
- Serious GI, renal, hepatic, or cardiac disorders

- Sulfinpyrazone is contraindicated in patients with active peptic ulcer disease, symptoms of GI inflammation or ulceration, hypersensitivity to phenylbutazone or other pyrazoles, or blood dyscrasias
- Allopurinol shouldn't be used in patients with previous severe reaction to the drug
- Colchicine is contraindicated in patients hypersensitive to colchicine and in those with blood dyscrasias or serious GI, renal, hepatic, or cardiac disorders
- Use allopurinol, probenecid, and sulfinpyrazone cautiously in patients with GI, renal, and hepatic disease

Adverse reactions to watch for

- Diarrhea, nausea, vomiting, abdominal pain, bone marrow depression

Adverse reactions

- The most common adverse reactions are GI disturbances, such as diarrhea, nausea, vomiting, and abdominal pain
- These drugs may also cause bone marrow depression
- Allopurinol also may cause rash, drowsiness, acute attacks of gout, and kidney stones
- Probenecid also may cause rash, headache, and uric acid kidney stones
- Sulfinpyrazone also may cause headache and uric acid kidney stones
- Colchicine also may cause myopathy, neuropathy, and malabsorption of vitamin B_{12}

Interactions

- Probenecid and sulfinpyrazone cause sustained increases in serum levels of many drugs, such as penicillin, antineoplastics, ketoprofen, and dapsone
- Allopurinol increases the risk of azathioprine and mercaptopurine toxicity, enhances the effects of oral hypoglycemics, and increases the half-life of anticoagulants, thereby increasing the risk of bleeding
- Use of sulfinpyrazone with aspirin may increase uric acid levels

Nursing responsibilities

- Give these drugs with food or milk to reduce adverse GI reactions
- Assess the involved joints for pain and immobility
- **Know that the patient who is receiving an antigout drug should maintain a fluid intake of 64 to 96 ounces daily to avoid kidney stones**
- Teach the patient about the importance of complying with therapy; explain that irregular administration of antigout drugs may cause elevated uric acid levels and trigger a gout attack
- Instruct the patient to follow the physician's recommendations concerning weight loss, dietary measures, and alcohol restriction
- Caution the patient not to take aspirin with antigout drugs; this could trigger a gout attack (for additional teaching tips, see *Teaching about antigout drugs*)

Key nursing actions

- Give drugs with food or milk.
- Assess joints for pain and immobility.
- Teach patient to:
  - maintain fluid intake of 64 to 96 ounces daily
  - follow physician's recommendations concerning weight loss, dietary measures, and alcohol restriction
  - avoid taking aspirin with antigout drugs.

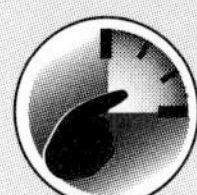

TIME-OUT FOR TEACHING

Teaching about antigout drugs

Include these topics in your teaching plan for the patient receiving an antigout drug.

- Medication regimen, including the drug's name, dose, frequency, duration, and possible adverse effects
- Signs and symptoms to discuss with the physician
- Avoidance of products containing aspirin
- Dietary restrictions
- Safety measures
- Compliance with therapy
- Need to notify the physician of any over-the-counter or herbal drugs
- Follow-up care, including laboratory tests and physician visits

ANTARTHRITICS

Mechanism of action

- Some antarthritics (also called gold salts) inhibit prostaglandin synthesis, thereby reducing inflammation
- The mechanism of action of gold salts and methotrexate for the treatment of rheumatoid arthritis isn't well understood

Pharmacokinetics

- Absorption: Auranofin is absorbed from the GI tract; aurothioglucose and gold sodium thiomalate are administered I.V.
- Distribution: Bound to erythrocytes and distributed mainly intracellularly
- Metabolism: Unknown
- Excretion: Excreted slowly, with about 70% excreted in the urine and the remainder in the feces

Drug examples

- Auranofin (Ridaura), aurothioglucose (Solganal), gold sodium thiomalate (Myochrysine), infliximab (Remicade), leflunomide (Arava), methotrexate (Rheumatrex)

Indications

- Antarthritics and leflunomide are used to treat rheumatoid arthritis
- Infliximab is used to treat rheumatoid arthritis and Crohn's disease
- Methotrexate is used to treat rheumatoid arthritis, psoriasis, and acute lymphocytic leukemia

Contraindications and precautions

- Antarthritics are contraindicated in patients with severe renal or hepatic dysfunction, uncontrolled diabetes mellitus, heart failure, systemic lupus erythematosus, or recent radiation therapy

Topics for patient discussion

- Therapy regimen
- Signs and symptoms to discuss with physician
- Avoidance of products containing aspirin
- Dietary restrictions
- Safety measures
- Need for compliance with therapy
- Need to report use of any over-the-counter or herbal products
- Need for follow-up care

Key facts about antarthritics

- Also called gold salts
- Inhibit prostaglandin synthesis, thereby reducing inflammation
- Excreted slowly, with about 70% excreted in the urine and the remainder in the feces

When to use antarthritics

- Rheumatoid arthritis
- Crohn's disease
- Psoriasis
- Acute lymphocytic leukemia

- Infliximab is contraindicated in patients hypersensitive to any murine protein; use extreme caution in patients with heart failure; latent tuberculosis infection should be treated before infliximab is started
- Methotrexate is contraindicated in pregnant or breast-feeding women, in alcoholics, and in those with alcoholic liver disease or other chronic liver disease, immunodeficiency disease, or blood dyscrasias
- Use antarthritics cautiously in patients with GI, renal, and hepatic disease

Adverse reactions

- Use of gold salts for treating rheumatoid arthritis in patients who don't respond to glucocorticoids, NSAIDs, or salicylates is limited because of toxic adverse effects (such as pruritus, rash, metallic taste, stomatitis, diarrhea, and bone marrow suppression [marked by thrombocytopenia, aplastic anemia, and agranulocytosis])
- Gold salts may cause dizziness, rash, dermatitis, stomatitis, diarrhea, abdominal pain, metallic taste, bone marrow suppression, photosensitivity reactions, and gold toxicity
- Leflunomide may cause hypertension, dizziness, alopecia, and respiratory tract infection
- Infliximab may cause nausea and vomiting, respiratory tract infection, headache, and hypersensitivity reactions (including urticaria, dyspnea, and hypotension occurring within 2 hours of infliximab infusion)
- Methotrexate may cause liver toxicity, nausea and vomiting, bone marrow depression, and methotrexate-induced lung disease

Interactions

- Antarthritics cause additive bone marrow depression when used concurrently with drugs that cause bone marrow depression
- **Food delays methotrexate absorption; administer the drug on an empty stomach**

Nursing responsibilities

- Know that most patients require concurrent therapy with glucocorticoids, NSAIDs, or salicylates, especially during the first few months of therapy
- **Be aware that the signs and symptoms of gold toxicity include pruritus, rash, metallic taste, stomatitis, and diarrhea; if toxicity occurs, the physician may prescribe dimercaprol (BAL in oil) to enhance gold excretion**
- Instruct the patient to report signs and symptoms of toxicity promptly
- Teach the patient about the importance of maintaining good oral hygiene to prevent stomatitis
- Instruct the patient to use sunscreen and wear protective clothing to prevent photosensitivity reactions
- Methotrexate is given in a once-weekly dose; monitor the patient for 30 minutes after administration for vasomotor response
- Know that the therapeutic response to methotrexate usually occurs within 3 to 6 weeks of the start of therapy, and the patient may continue to improve for another 12 weeks or more

When NOT to use antarthritics

- Severe renal or hepatic dysfunction, uncontrolled diabetes mellitus, heart failure, systemic lupus erythematosus, recent radiation therapy
- Hypersensitivity to any murine protein
- Pregnancy, breast-feeding, alcoholism, alcoholic or other chronic liver disease, immunodeficiency disease, blood dyscrasias

Adverse reactions to watch for

- Dizziness, rash, dermatitis, stomatitis, diarrhea, abdominal pain, metallic taste, bone marrow suppression, photosensitivity reaction, gold toxicity

Key nursing actions

- Know signs and symptoms of gold toxicity: pruritus, rash, metallic taste, stomatitis, and diarrhea.
- Be aware that leflunomide requires loading dose and frequent liver tests.
- Know that tuberculin test will likely be ordered before start of infliximab therapy.
- Teach patient to:
  - report signs and symptoms of toxicity promptly
  - maintain good oral hygiene
  - use sunscreen and wear protective clothing.

- Know that leflunomide requires a loading dose and frequent liver tests to assess for toxicity
- Be aware that a tuberculin skin test will likely be ordered before the start of infliximab therapy because tuberculosis has occurred in patients receiving infliximab

SKELETAL MUSCLE RELAXANTS

Mechanism of action
- Skeletal muscle relaxants work directly by acting on the neuromuscular junction or indirectly by acting on the central nervous system (CNS)
- Centrally acting drugs (baclofen, carisoprodol, chlorzoxazone, cyclobenzaprine, diazepam, and methocarbamol) block polysynaptic pathways in the spinal cord, inhibiting nerve-impulse transmission
- Direct-acting drugs (dantrolene) interfere with calcium release in muscle fibers, interfering with muscle contraction at the neuromuscular junction

Pharmacokinetics
- Absorption: Absorbed from the GI tract
- Distribution: Widely distributed throughout the body
- Metabolism: Metabolized in the liver
- Excretion: Excreted by the kidneys

Drug examples
- Baclofen (Lioresal), carisoprodol (Rela, Soma), chlorzoxazone (Parafon Forte DSC), cyclobenzaprine hydrochloride (Flexeril), dantrolene (Dantrium), diazepam (Valium), methocarbamol (Robaxin)

Indications
- Baclofen and dantrolene are used to treat spasticity associated with spinal cord disease or lesions
- Carisoprodol, chlorzoxazone, cyclobenzaprine, diazepam, and methocarbamol are used as adjunctive therapy in acute, painful musculoskeletal conditions
- Dantrolene also is used to prevent and treat malignant hyperthermia

Contraindications and precautions
- Baclofen and oral dantrolene are contraindicated in patients who use spasticity to maintain posture and balance
- Carisoprodol is contraindicated in patients with acute intermittent porphyria or hypersensitivity to the drug; use this drug cautiously in pregnant or breast-feeding women and in patients with impaired renal or hepatic function
- Cyclobenzaprine is contraindicated in patients with hypersensitivity to the drug, arrhythmias, heart block or conduction disturbances, heart failure, or hyperthyroidism; it's also contraindicated during the acute recovery phase of a myocardial infarction and within 14 days of monoamine oxidase (MAO) inhibitor therapy

Key facts about skeletal muscle relaxants

- Work directly by acting on the neuromuscular junction or indirectly by acting on the CNS
- Block polysynaptic pathways in the spinal cord, inhibiting nerve-impulse transmission
- Interfere with calcium release in muscle fibers, thus interfering with muscle contraction at the neuromuscular junction
- Metabolized in the liver
- Excreted by the kidneys

When to use skeletal muscle relaxants

- Spasticity associated with spinal cord disease or lesions
- As adjunct in acute, painful musculoskeletal conditions
- Malignant hyperthermia

When NOT to use skeletal muscle relaxants

- Hypersensitivity to these drugs
- Spasticity to maintain posture and balance
- Acute intermittent porphyria
- Arrhythmias, heart block or conduction disturbances, heart failure, hyperthyroidism, acute recovery phase of MI
- Within 14 days of MAO inhibitor therapy
- Pregnancy, breast-feeding, hepatic disease

- Dantrolene is contraindicated in pregnant or breast-feeding women and in patients with hepatic disease; use cautiously in women, in patients older than age 35, and in those with impaired pulmonary, cardiac, or hepatic function
- Use baclofen cautiously in breast-feeding women, in elderly patients, and in patients with cerebrovascular accident or other brain disorder
- Use these drugs cautiously in patients with GI, renal, or hepatic disease

Adverse reactions to watch for

- Transient dizziness, drowsiness, ataxia, dry mouth, nausea, GI upset

Adverse reactions

- Skeletal muscle relaxants may cause transient dizziness, drowsiness, ataxia, dry mouth, nausea, and GI upset
- Diazepam also may cause physical and psychological dependence
- Dantrolene also may cause muscle weakness

Interactions

- Concurrent use with other CNS depressants or alcohol causes additive CNS depression
- Concurrent use of baclofen or cyclobenzaprine with MAO inhibitors may cause hypertensive crisis, seizures, and death
- Concurrent use of cyclobenzaprine with antidepressants or antihistamines causes additive anticholinergic effects

Key nursing actions

- Give these drugs with meals or milk.
- Assess involved joints for pain and immobility.
- Keep emergency equipment nearby to treat respiratory depression.
- Don't discontinue these drugs abruptly.
- Teach patient to:
  - avoid activities requiring alertness until CNS effects of drug are known.
  - avoid alcohol and CNS depressants.

Nursing responsibilities

- Give skeletal muscle relaxants with meals or milk to prevent GI distress
- Assess the involved joints for pain and immobility
- Instruct the patient to avoid activities requiring alertness until the response to the drug is known
- Teach the patient to avoid alcohol and CNS depressants
- Keep emergency equipment nearby to treat respiratory depression
- Don't discontinue skeletal muscle relaxants abruptly, especially Lioresal, Soma, and Flexeril; to do so may cause hallucinations, seizures, or acute exacerbations of spasticity

NCLEX CHECKS

It's never too soon to begin your NCLEX preparation. Now that you've reviewed this chapter, carefully read each of the following questions and choose the best answer. Then compare your responses to the correct answers.

1. A patient is experiencing malignant hyperthermic crisis. Which peripherally acting skeletal muscle relaxant is used to treat this condition?

☐ **A.** Baclofen (Lioresal)
☐ **B.** Cyclobenzaprine hydrochloride (Flexeril)
☐ **C.** Dantrolene (Dantrium)
☐ **D.** Diazepam (Valium)

2. You're monitoring a patient for adverse reactions to his antigout medication. Expect to pay particular attention to adverse reactions involving which body system?

☐ A. Cardiac
☐ B. GI
☐ C. Renal
☐ D. Respiratory

3. The gold salt aurothioglucose (Solganal) is ordered for a patient as treatment for rheumatoid arthritis. Aurothioglucose relieves the symptoms of rheumatoid arthritis by:

☐ A. acting as an analgesic.
☐ B. relaxing skeletal muscles.
☐ C. reversing arthritic deformities.
☐ D. decreasing liposomal enzyme release.

4. A patient takes probenecid (Benemid) for treatment of gouty arthritis. He asks why he shouldn't take aspirin with probenecid. You respond that aspirin:

☐ A. increases uric acid excretion.
☐ B. interferes with uric acid excretion.
☐ C. decreases the effects of probenecid.
☐ D. increases the effects of probenecid.

5. While admitting a patient, you note he's allergic to diazepam (Valium). The physician has ordered clonazepam (Klonopin), 1.5 mg P.O. three times daily, for this patient. Your best action would be to:

☐ A. give the drug as ordered.
☐ B. hold the drug and notify the physician.
☐ C. give a trial dose of 0.75 mg and monitor the patient for effect.
☐ D. give the drug but watch closely for any adverse reactions.

6. A patient is prescribed gold salts for her rheumatoid arthritis. You want to warn the patient about gold toxicity. Which signs and symptoms should you tell the patient to look for?

Select all that apply:

☐ A. Rash
☐ B. Itching
☐ C. Diarrhea
☐ D. Shortness of breath
☐ E. Metallic taste
☐ F. Headaches

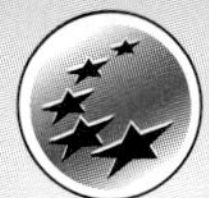

TOP 5

Items to study before your next test on drugs and the musculoskeletal system

1. Mechanisms of action of antigout drugs, antarthritics, and skeletal muscle relaxants
2. Indications for antigout drugs, antarthritics, and skeletal muscle relaxants
3. Common adverse effects of antigout drugs, antarthritics, and skeletal muscle relaxants
4. Nursing responsibilities when administering antigout drugs, antarthritics, and skeletal muscle relaxants
5. Patient teaching related to antigout drugs, antarthritics, and skeletal muscle relaxants

ANSWERS AND RATIONALES

1. CORRECT ANSWER: C

Diazepam, baclofen, dantrolene, and cyclobenzaprine are all used for muscle spasm and spasticity. However, I.V. dantrolene is the only drug used to treat malignant hyperthermic crisis. Oral dantrolene may be given prophylactically (2 to 3 days before anesthesia) for patients with a history of malignant hyperthermia or a family history of the disorder.

2. CORRECT ANSWER: B

Patients typically take antigout medication with food because GI distress is the most common adverse reaction to antigout medications. Cardiac, renal, and respiratory adverse reactions are rare with antigout medications.

3. CORRECT ANSWER: D

Gold salts such as aurothioglucose relieve the symptoms of rheumatoid arthritis by decreasing liposomal enzyme release, thereby altering immune response. Gold salts don't act as analgesics, relax skeletal muscles, or reverse rheumatoid arthritis deformation.

4. CORRECT ANSWER: C

Aspirin decreases but doesn't inactivate the action of probenecid. Aspirin has no effect on the rate of uric acid excretion.

5. CORRECT ANSWER: B

Cross-allergies among benzodiazepines are common, so clonazepam (a benzodiazepine) shouldn't be given to a patient who is allergic to diazepam (another benzodiazepine). Holding the drug and notifying the physician are the most appropriate actions. Because of the possibility of an allergic reaction, the drug shouldn't be given. It's illegal to give trial doses without an order.

6. CORRECT ANSWER: A, B, C, E

Signs and symptoms of gold salt toxicity include bone marrow suppression, diarrhea, stomatitis, pruritus (itching), rash, and a metallic taste. Shortness of breath and headaches are not signs or symptoms of gold toxicity.

Drugs and the respiratory system

LEARNING OBJECTIVES

After studying this chapter, you should be able to:

- Describe the mechanisms of action of bronchodilators, anti-inflammatory inhalants, antitussives, expectorants, mucolytics, and decongestants.
- Describe the rationale for using bronchodilators, anti-inflammatory inhalants, antitussives, expectorants, mucolytics, and decongestants.
- Name common adverse effects of bronchodilators, anti-inflammatory inhalants, antitussives, expectorants, mucolytics, and decongestants.
- Identify nursing responsibilities when administering bronchodilators, anti-inflammatory inhalants, antitussives, expectorants, mucolytics, and decongestants.
- Discuss patient teaching related to bronchodilators, anti-inflammatory inhalants, antitussives, expectorants, mucolytics, and decongestants.

CHAPTER OVERVIEW

Bronchodilators are used to prevent or terminate bronchospasm caused by pulmonary disease, allergy, exercise, or emotional factors. Inhaled anti-inflammatories are used to decrease bronchial inflammation and airway edema. These drugs are useful in treating chronic obstructive pulmonary disease (COPD) and asthma. When inhaled, the drugs act directly on lung tissue, avoiding or minimizing systemic adverse effects. Nursing responsibilities include assessing breath sounds, monitoring vital signs and serum drug levels, and observing for signs and symptoms of dyspnea and drug toxicity. Patient teaching includes instruction on proper inhaler technique and information about adverse effects and mouth care.

Antitussives, expectorants, mucolytics, and nasal decongestants are used to control cough, facilitate secretion removal, and liquefy tenacious mucus in the airways. Antitussives, which can be opioid or nonopioid, are used to suppress dry, nonproductive cough. Expectorants increase secretions in the respiratory tract and may decrease viscosity of thick mucus secretions to allow for expectoration in COPD, pneumonia, and other disorders. Mucolytics break down chemical bonds in tenacious mucus and allow for its removal by coughing or suctioning. Acetylcysteine, a mucolytic, also may be given to decrease hepatotoxicity in acetaminophen overdose. Nasal decongestants shrink swollen mucous membranes, promoting nasal drainage and improving nasal ventilation and breathing. Nursing responsibilities include protecting the airway when secretions are expelled, assessing breath sounds, promoting fluid intake, and providing humidity. Patient teaching focuses on promoting compliance, warning about the dangers of dependency with opioid drugs, and encouraging smoking cessation.

A&P highlights

- The respiratory system consists of the upper and lower airways and the lungs.
- Upper airways include the nose, pharynx, and larynx.
- Lower airways include the trachea and bronchi.
- Lungs are paired, cone-shaped organs that fill the pleural division of the thoracic cavity and extend from the root of the neck to the diaphragm.
- The diaphragm and intercostal muscles produce the normal inspiratory and expiratory movements of the lungs and ribs.
- Movement of oxygen and carbon dioxide between the alveoli, blood, and tissues depends on the concentrations and pressures of these gases; they diffuse from an area with a high partial pressure of the gas to one with a low partial pressure.

ANATOMY AND PHYSIOLOGY

Anatomy

- The respiratory system consists of the upper and lower airways and the lungs
- Upper airways include the nose, pharynx, and larynx
- Lower airways include the trachea and bronchi, which lead into the lungs
  - The primary bronchi branch from the trachea and lead into the lungs
  - The primary bronchi divide into smaller secondary bronchi
  - The secondary bronchi branch into even smaller tertiary bronchi and eventually become bronchioles
    - Bronchioles end in clusters known as alveolar sacs
    - Alveoli are tiny, grapelike clusters of air sacs at the ends of the bronchioles surrounded by an extensive network of capillaries (see *Bronchioles and alveoli*)
- Lungs are paired, cone-shaped organs that fill the pleural division of the thoracic cavity and extend from the root of the neck to the diaphragm

Physiology

- The diaphragm and intercostal muscles produce the normal inspiratory and expiratory movements of the lungs and ribs, which allows for ventilation
- Movement of oxygen and carbon dioxide (gas exchange) between the alveoli, blood, and tissues depends on the concentrations and pressures of these gases; they diffuse from an area with a high partial pressure of the gas to one with a low partial pressure

Bronchioles and alveoli

This illustration shows bronchioles branching into progressively smaller tubes that eventually become alveolar ducts. The alveoli are the basic functional units of the respiratory system; gas exchange (exchange of oxygen and carbon dioxide) between the lungs and bronchi occurs here.

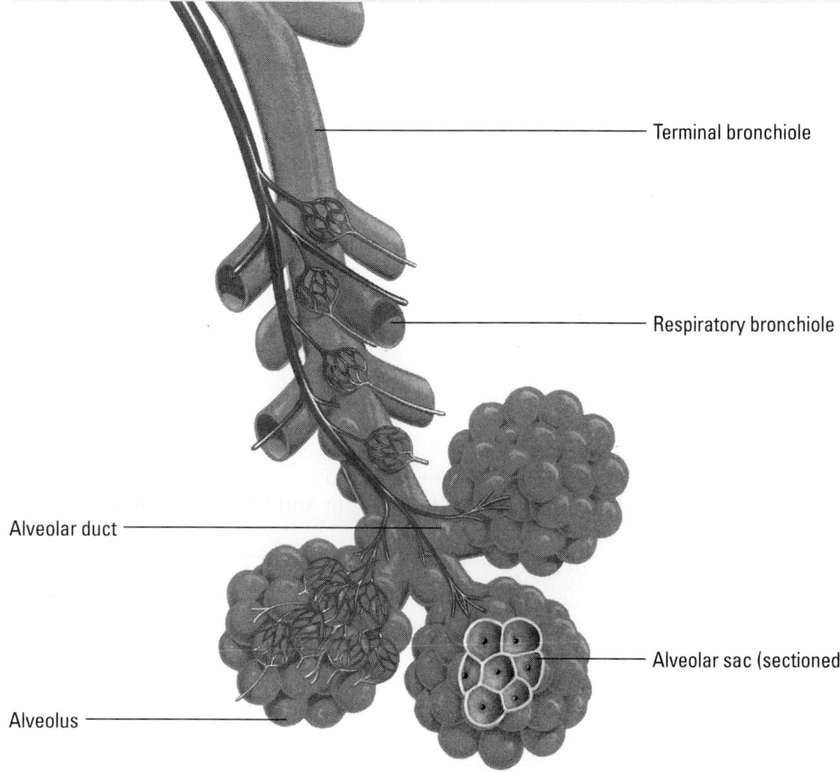

Function

- The main functions of the respiratory system are to supply body tissues with oxygen and to remove carbon dioxide
- The main function of the bronchi is to distribute air to the lungs
- The main function of the alveoli is to perform gas exchange, exchanging oxygen and carbon dioxide by diffusion

BRONCHODILATORS

ADRENERGIC-AGONIST BRONCHODILATORS

Key facts about adrenergic-agonist bronchodilators

- Produce bronchodilation by stimulating cAMP production
- Metabolized by the liver
- Excreted in the urine and feces

Mechanism of action

- Produce bronchodilation by stimulating cyclic adenosine monophosphate (cAMP) production; cAMP is believed to be a bronchodilator

Pharmacokinetics

- Absorption: Absorbed from the respiratory tract; well absorbed from the GI tract when given orally
- Distribution: Cross the blood-brain and placental barriers
- Metabolism: Metabolized by the liver
- Excretion: Drug and its metabolites are excreted in the urine and feces

When to use adrenergic-agonist bronchodilators

- Bronchospasms

Drug examples

- Albuterol (Proventil, Ventolin), ephedrine sulfate (Kondon's Nasal, Pretz-D), epinephrine (Bronkaid Mist, Primatene Mist), ipratropium/albuterol (Combivent), isoetharine (Bronkosol), isoproterenol (Isuprel, Norisodrine), metaproterenol (Alupent, Metaprel), pirbuterol (Maxair), salmeterol xinafoate (Serevent Diskus), terbutaline (Brethine, Bricanyl)

Indications

- Bronchospasms

When NOT to use adrenergic-agonist bronchodilators

- Uncontrolled arrhythmias

Contraindications and precautions

- Contraindicated in patients with uncontrolled arrhythmias
- Prolonged and sustained use of albuterol (such as in continuous nebulization) may cause hypokalemia

Adverse reactions

- May cause anxiety, nervousness, tremor, shaking, headache, palpitations, tachycardia, hypertension, and arrhythmias

Adverse reactions to watch for

- Anxiety, nervousness, tremor, shaking, headache, palpitations, tachycardia, hypertension, arrhythmias

Interactions

- Concurrent use with theophylline preparations causes additive effects
- Beta-adrenergic blockers antagonize the effects of adrenergic agonists

Nursing responsibilities

- Monitor the patient's blood pressure, pulse, respiratory rate, and breath sounds
- Administer the prescribed drug around the clock, as ordered
- If an inhalation drug has been prescribed, teach the patient how to use it
- Instruct the patient to maintain a fluid intake of 2,000 to 3,000 ml/day to make secretions less viscous (for additional teaching tips, see *Teaching about inhaled bronchodilators*)
- Advise the patient to consult the physician or pharmacist before taking any nonprescription drugs to prevent adverse drug interactions
- Instruct the patient to avoid respiratory irritants, such as smoke, dust, and strong scents

Key nursing actions

- Monitor patient's blood pressure, pulse, respiratory rate, and breath sounds.
- Administer drug around the clock, as ordered.
- Teach patient to:
  - maintain fluid intake of 2,000 to 3,000 ml/day
  - consult physician before taking nonprescription drugs
  - avoid respiratory irritants.

METHYLXANTHINE BRONCHODILATORS

Mechanism of action

- Produce bronchodilation by inhibiting cAMP breakdown and blocking adenosine receptors

Pharmacokinetics

- Absorption

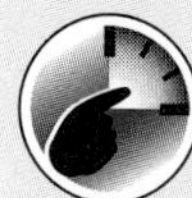

TIME-OUT FOR TEACHING

Teaching about inhaled bronchodilators

Include these topics in your teaching plan for the patient receiving an inhaled bronchodilator.

- Medication regimen, including the drug's name, dose, frequency, duration, and possible adverse effects
- Signs and symptoms to discuss with the physician, including adverse effects
- Proper method for administration, including care of a metered-dose inhaler
- Peak flow monitoring, if indicated
- Information about the patient's disease, including signs and symptoms of exacerbations
- Fluid needs
- Concomitant use of an inhaled bronchodilator and an inhaled anti-inflammatory
- Avoidance of possible allergens or irritants
- Emergency measures
- Compliance with therapy, including taking the drug as prescribed
- Follow-up care, including laboratory tests and physician visits

  - Oral theophylline is absorbed rapidly and completely
  - Suppository form is absorbed erratically
  - Slow-release form depends on gastric pH
  - Food delays absorption
- Distribution
  - Theophylline is not well distributed in fat tissues, so dosage is based on the patient's ideal or actual body weight, whichever is less
  - Theophylline is about 60% protein-bound, crosses the placental barrier, and appears in breast milk
- Metabolism: Metabolized primarily in the liver
- Excretion: Excreted in the urine

Drug examples

- Aminophylline (Phyllocontin, Truphylline), caffeine, theophylline (Constant-T, Elixophyllin, Slo-bid, Slo-Phyllin, Theobid)

Indications

- To prevent or treat bronchospasm.
- To treat asthma, bronchitis, emphysema, and neonatal apnea

Contraindications and precautions

- Contraindicated in patients with hypersensitivity to any xanthine, peptic ulcer disease, and untreated seizure disorders
- Aminophylline is also contraindicated in patients who are hypersensitive to ethylenediamine and who have an infection or irritation of the rectum or lower colon

Topics for patient discussion

- Therapy regimen
- Signs and symptoms to discuss with the physician
- Proper method for administration
- Peak flow monitoring
- Information about the disease
- Concomitant use of inhaled bronchodilator and inhaled anti-inflammatory
- Avoidance of possible allergens or irritants
- Emergency measures
- Compliance with therapy
- Follow-up care

Key facts about methylxanthine bronchodilators

- Produce bronchodilation by inhibiting cAMP breakdown and blocking adenosine receptors
- Metabolized primarily in the liver
- Excreted in the urine

When to use methylxanthine bronchodilators

- Bronchospasm
- Asthma, bronchitis, emphysema, neonatal apnea

- Use cautiously in neonates, in elderly patients, and in those with heart disease, hypoxemia, hepatic disease, hypertension, heart failure, and alcoholism
- **These conventional bronchodilators are not indicated for status asthmaticus, a medical emergency that requires administration of I.V. medication in an ICU setting**

Adverse reactions

- May cause headache, irritability, restlessness, anxiety, insomnia, dizziness, shock, seizures, nausea, vomiting, abdominal cramping, epigastric pain, anorexia, diarrhea, active peptic ulcer, liver failure, rectal irritation or bleeding (aminophylline suppositories), tachycardia, palpitations, arrhythmias, hypotension, hypertension, tachypnea, respiratory arrest, and proteinuria

Interactions

- Beta-adrenergic blockers partially antagonize the effect of methylxanthines and alter the rate of their metabolism, increasing the methylxanthine concentration
- Sympathomimetics and cardiac glycosides potentiate the adverse effects of methylxanthines
- Diuretics potentiate the diuretic effects of methylxanthines
- Phenobarbital, phenytoin, rifampin, cigarette smoking, and charcoal-broiled foods may shorten the half-life of methylxanthines, reducing their effectiveness
- Methylxanthines increase lithium clearance, reducing the effectiveness of lithium
- Erythromycin may increase the half-life of methylxanthines, increasing the risk of methylxanthine toxicity

Nursing responsibilities

- Assess for signs and symptoms of toxicity, such as arrhythmias and seizures
- Monitor serum drug levels to detect toxicity
- **Know that the therapeutic serum theophylline level should range from 10 to 20 mcg/ml**
- Instruct the patient to reduce consumption of xanthine-containing foods and beverages (such as cola, coffee, and chocolate) to prevent toxicity
- Emphasize the importance of routine laboratory studies to determine serum drug levels

When NOT to use methylxanthine bronchodilators

- Hypersensitivity to any xanthine or ethylenediamine
- Peptic ulcer disease
- Untreated seizure disorders
- Infection or irritation of the rectum or lower colon

Adverse reactions to watch for

- Headache, irritability, restlessness, anxiety, insomnia, dizziness, shock, seizures, nausea, vomiting, abdominal cramping, epigastric pain, anorexia, diarrhea, active peptic ulcer, liver failure, rectal irritation or bleeding, tachycardia, palpitations, arrhythmias, hypotension, hypertension, tachypnea, respiratory arrest, and proteinuria

Key nursing actions

- Assess for signs and symptoms of toxicity.
- Know that therapeutic serum theophylline level ranges from 10 to 20 mcg/ml.
- Instruct patient to reduce consumption of xanthine-containing foods and beverages.
- Emphasize importance of routine lab studies.

ANTI-INFLAMMATORY INHALANTS

Mechanism of action

- Prevent the release of or counteract the biochemical mediators (kinins, serotonin, histamine) that cause the tissue inflammation responsible for edema and airway narrowing

Pharmacokinetics

- Absorption: Well absorbed from the GI and respiratory tracts; some of the drug is absorbed systemically
- Distribution: Not widely distributed into tissues; highly protein-bound
- Metabolism: Metabolized primarily by the liver and GI tract by hydrolysis; partially metabolized by the respiratory tract
- Excretion: Eliminated in the feces and urine

Drug examples

- Beclomethasone (Vanceril), budesonide (Pulmicort), cromolyn sodium (Intal Aerosol Spray), dexamethasone (Decadron Phosphate Respihaler), flunisolide (AeroBid), fluticasone (Flovent), mometasone (Nasonex), triamcinolone (Azmacort)

Indications

- Beclomethasone is used to treat chronic bronchitis
- Dexamethasone, flunisolide, and triamcinolone are used to control bronchial asthma in patients with steroid-dependent asthma
- Cromolyn sodium and mometasone are used to treat allergic rhinitis; they are also used as adjunctive treatment for severe perennial asthma and as a prophylactic drug in exercise-induced asthma

Contraindications and precautions

- Anti-inflammatory inhalants are contraindicated for acute bronchospasms
- Use cautiously in patients who are immunosuppressed and in those taking prednisone or other corticosteroid
- Use with extreme caution in patients with clinical tuberculosis or viral respiratory infections

Adverse reactions

- Beclomethasone, dexamethasone, flunisolide, and triamcinolone may cause hoarseness, oropharyngeal irritation, and candidal infection
- Cromolyn sodium may cause coughing, throat irritation, and bronchospasm after inhalation of dry powder

Interactions

- None reported

Nursing responsibilities

- **Instruct the patient who is receiving both a bronchodilator and a glucocorticoid inhaler to use the bronchodilator several minutes before the glucocorticoid; this ensures penetration of the glucocorticoid into the airways**
- Instruct the patient to rinse his mouth after using inhaled steroids
- Inform the patient who is receiving cromolyn that this drug is ineffective during acute bronchospasm attacks; explain that frequent daily use over a prolonged period helps decrease the severity or frequency of attacks
- Instruct the patient on the proper use and care of the inhaler and spacer

Key facts about anti-inflammatory inhalants

- Prevent the release of or counteract the biochemical mediators that cause the tissue inflammation responsible for edema and airway narrowing
- Metabolized primarily by the liver and GI tract; partially metabolized by the respiratory tract
- Excreted in the feces and urine

When to use anti-inflammatory inhalants

- Chronic bronchitis
- Bronchial asthma
- Allergic rhinitis
- As adjuncts for perennial asthma
- As prophylaxis for exercise-induced asthma

When NOT to use anti-inflammatory inhalants

- Acute bronchospasms

Adverse reactions to watch for

- Hoarseness, oropharyngeal irritation, candidal infection, coughing, bronchospasm

Key nursing actions

- Know that cromolyn is ineffective during acute bronchospasm attacks.
- Teach patient to:
  - use bronchodilator several minutes before glucocorticoid inhaler
  - rinse mouth after using inhaled steroids
  - use and care for inhaler properly.

ANTITUSSIVES, EXPECTORANTS, MUCOLYTICS, AND DECONGESTANTS

ANTITUSSIVES

Mechanism of action

- Antitussives suppress the cough reflex by acting on the cough center in the medulla
- Benzonatate acts by anesthetizing cough receptors of vagal afferent fibers throughout the bronchi, alveoli, and pleura

Pharmacokinetics

- Absorption: Well absorbed through the GI tract
- Distribution: Unknown
- Metabolism: Metabolized in the liver
- Excretion: Excreted in the urine

Drug examples

- Opioid antitussives include codeine phosphate and codeine sulfate (Codeine) and hydrocodone (Hycodan)
- Nonopioid antitussives include benzonatate (Tessalon), dextromethorphan (Pertussin, Robitussin DM), and diphenhydramine (Benadryl, Benylin)

Indications

- Antitussives are used to treat nonproductive cough and cough that interferes with sleep or daily activities

Contraindications and precautions

- These drugs are contraindicated in patients who are hypersensitive, pregnant, or breast-feeding
- Use these drugs cautiously in patients with benign prostatic hyperplasia, debilitation, thoracotomy, laparotomy, or a history of drug or alcohol abuse

Adverse reactions

- Opioid antitussives may cause drowsiness, drying of respiratory secretions, and constipation
- Nonopioid antitussives may cause drowsiness and dizziness

Interactions

- These drugs may potentiate antitussive effects when used with alcohol, sedatives, monoamine oxidase inhibitors, anticholinergics, or tranquilizers

Nursing responsibilities

- Instruct the patient taking benzonatate to swallow the drug whole
- Maintain airway patency; provide suction, if necessary
- Assess the patient's breath sounds, evaluate cough for characteristics (such as productive or nonproductive) and frequency, and assess characteristics of bronchial secretions
- Tell the patient to maintain a fluid intake of 2,000 to 3,000 ml/day

Key facts about antitussives

- Suppress the cough reflex
- Anesthetize cough receptors of vagal afferent fibers throughout bronchi, alveoli, and pleura
- Metabolized in the liver
- Excreted in the urine

When to use antitussives

- Nonproductive cough
- Cough that interferes with sleep or daily activities

When NOT to use antitussives

- Hypersensitivity to these drugs
- Pregnancy
- Breast-feeding

Adverse reactions to watch for

- Drowsiness, drying of respiratory secretions, constipation, dizziness

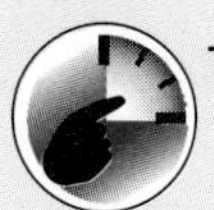

TIME-OUT FOR TEACHING

Teaching about antitussives

Include these topics in your teaching plan for the patient receiving an antitussive.

- Medication regimen, including the drug's name, dose, frequency, duration, and possible adverse effects
- Signs and symptoms to discuss with the physician, including persistent cough and adverse effects
- Safety measures
- Fluid needs
- Possible physical dependency if a narcotic drug is used
- Avoidance of alcohol and other over-the-counter products
- Compliance with therapy, including taking the drug as prescribed
- Follow-up care, including laboratory tests and physician visits

- Advise the patient with a nonproductive cough to minimize talking, stop smoking, maintain adequate environmental humidity, and use chewing gum or sugarless candy to reduce coughing (for additional teaching tips, see *Teaching about antitussives*)
- Instruct the patient to consult the physician if the cough lasts more than 1 week or is accompanied by fever or chest pain
- Instruct the patient not to consume liquids within 30 minutes of taking an antitussive because liquids may negate soothing local effects
- Tell the patient to check with his health care provider before taking any over-the-counter or herbal medications
- **Administer codeine with caution to a patient who is receiving a central nervous system depressant because this combination can be fatal; closely monitor the patient's level of consciousness and respiratory status**

EXPECTORANTS

Mechanism of action

- Decrease the viscosity of tenacious secretions by increasing fluid in the respiratory tract (however, the efficacy of these drugs is questionable)

Pharmacokinetics

- Absorption: Absorbed through the GI tract
- Distribution: Unknown
- Metabolism: Metabolized in the liver
- Excretion: Excreted primarily in the urine

Drug example

- Guaifenesin (Humibid L.A., Robitussin, Tussin)

Topics for patient discussion

- Therapy regimen
- Signs and symptoms to discuss with physician
- Safety measures
- Fluid needs
- Possible physical dependency
- Avoidance of alcohol and other over-the-counter products
- Compliance with therapy
- Follow-up care

Key nursing actions

- Maintain airway patency.
- Assess breath sounds, cough, and bronchial secretions.
- Administer codeine cautiously if patient is receiving CNS depressant.
- Teach patient to:
  - maintain fluid intake of 2,000 to 3,000 ml/day
  - minimize talking, stop smoking, use chewing gum or sugarless candy
  - consult physician if cough lasts more than 1 week or fever or chest pain occurs
  - avoid liquids within 30 minutes of taking drug
  - check with health care provider before taking over-the-counter or herbal products.

Key facts about expectorants

- Decrease the viscosity of tenacious secretions by increasing fluid in the respiratory tract
- Metabolized in the liver
- Excreted primarily in the urine

When to use expectorants

- Cough associated with the common cold and upper respiratory tract infections
- Dry, hacking cough

When NOT to use expectorants

- Hypersensitivity to these drugs

Adverse reactions to watch for

- Vomiting, diarrhea, nausea, drowsiness, abdominal pain

Key nursing actions

- Maintain airway patency.
- Assess breath sounds, cough, and bronchial secretions.
- Teach patient to:
  - maintain fluid intake of 2,000 to 3,000 ml/day
  - check with health care provider before taking over-the-counter or herbal products
  - avoid taking guaifenesin for persistent cough associated with smoking, asthma, emphysema, or excessive secretions.

Key facts about mucolytics

- Decrease mucus viscosity by breaking or altering chemical bonds of glycoprotein complexes in the mucus
- Metabolized by the liver
- About 70% excreted nonrenally

Indications
- To treat cough associated with the common cold and upper respiratory tract infections (questionable efficacy), such as minor bronchial irritations, bronchitis, influenza, sinusitis, emphysema, and bronchial asthma
- To relieve dry, hacking cough

Contraindications and precautions
- These drugs are contraindicated in patients with hypersensitivity
- Use these drugs cautiously in patients with ineffective cough reflex or respiratory insufficiency and in those who are pregnant or breast-feeding

Adverse reactions
- May cause vomiting (if taken in large doses), diarrhea, nausea, drowsiness, and abdominal pain

Interactions
- These may increase the risk of bleeding when administered with anticoagulants

Nursing responsibilities
- **Maintain airway patency; provide suction, if necessary**
- Assess the patient's breath sounds, evaluate cough for characteristics (such as productive or nonproductive) and frequency, and assess characteristics of bronchial secretions
- Tell the patient to maintain a fluid intake of 2,000 to 3,000 ml/day; an increased fluid intake may enhance the effects of expectorants by making secretions less viscous
- Tell the patient to check with his health care provider before taking any over-the-counter or herbal medications
- **Caution the patient not to take guaifenesin for a persistent cough associated with smoking, asthma, emphysema, or excessive secretions**

MUCOLYTICS

Mechanism of action
- Decrease mucus viscosity by breaking or altering the chemical bonds of the glycoprotein complexes in the mucus

Pharmacokinetics
- Absorption: Absorbed from the pulmonary epithelium
- Distribution: About 50% is protein-bound
- Metabolism: Metabolized by the liver
- Excretion: About 70% is excreted nonrenally

Drug example
- Acetylcysteine (Mucomyst)

Indications
- To treat abnormal, viscid, or thick and hard mucus
- As an antidote for acetaminophen overdose

- **Contraindications and precautions**
  - Acetylcysteine is contraindicated in patients with known hypersensitivity
  - Use acetylcysteine cautiously in elderly, debilitated, pregnant, or breast-feeding patients and in those with asthma
- **Adverse reactions**
  - May cause stomatitis, nausea, vomiting, drowsiness, and severe rhinorrhea
  - Bronchospasms may occur, especially in asthmatic patients
- **Interactions**
  - Activated charcoal decreases acetylcysteine's effectiveness
  - Acetylcysteine is incompatible with amphotericin B, chlortetracycline, erythromycin, oxytetracycline, iodized oil, hydrogen peroxide, chymotrypsin, and trypsin
- **Nursing responsibilities**
  - **Maintain airway patency; provide suction, if necessary**
  - Assess the patient's breath sounds, evaluate cough for characteristics (such as productive or nonproductive) and frequency, and assess characteristics of bronchial secretions
  - Tell the patient to maintain a fluid intake of 2,000 to 3,000 ml/day
  - Tell the patient to check with his health care provider before taking any over-the-counter or herbal medications
  - Warn the patient about the "rotten egg" smell of acetylcysteine
  - Be prepared to administer a beta$_2$-adrenergic agonist by aerosol if the patient experiences bronchospasms

DECONGESTANTS

- **Mechanism of action**
  - Directly, decongestants act on alpha-adrenergic receptors in the nasal mucosa and elsewhere, causing contraction of sphincters and constriction of secretory cells
  - Indirectly, decongestants result in norepinephrine release; together with the direct action on receptors, these drugs cause vasoconstriction and nasal decongestion
- **Pharmacokinetics**
  - Absorption: Readily absorbed in the GI tract when taken orally; otherwise, absorbed from the respiratory tract
  - Distribution: Widely distributed throughout the body and into the various tissues and fluids, including breast milk and the placenta
  - Metabolism: Metabolized by the liver
  - Excretion: Excreted largely unchanged in the urine
- **Drug examples**
  - Ephedrine sulfate (Pretz-D), oxymetazoline hydrochloride (Afrin), phenylephrine, hydrochloride (Afrin Children's, Neo-Synephrine), pseudoephedrine hydrochloride (Sudafed), and pseudoephedrine sulfate (Drixoral)

When to use mucolytics

- Abnormal, viscid, or thick and hard mucus
- As antidote for acetaminophen overdose

When NOT to use mucolytics

- Hypersensitivity to these drugs

Adverse reactions to watch for

- Stomatitis, nausea, vomiting, drowsiness, severe rhinorrhea, bronchospasms

Key nursing actions

- Maintain patent airway.
- Assess breath sounds, cough, and bronchial secretions.
- Be prepared to administer beta$_2$-adrenergic agonist if bronchospasm occurs.
- Teach patient to:
  - maintain fluid intake of 2,000 to 3,000 ml/day
  - check with health care provider before taking over-the-counter or herbal products
  - be aware of "rotten smell" of acetylcysteine.

Key facts about decongestants

- Cause contraction of sphincters and constriction of secretory cells
- Cause vasoconstriction and nasal decongestion
- Metabolized in the liver
- Excreted largely unchanged in the urine

Indications

- For temporary relief of nasal congestion due to the common cold, hay fever or other upper respiratory tract allergies, and sinusitis
- To promote nasal or sinus drainage

When to use decongestants

- Temporary relief of nasal decongestion
- Nasal or sinus drainage

Contraindications and precautions

- Contraindicated in patients taking a monoamine oxidase (MAO) inhibitor and in those hypersensitive to the drugs' ingredients
- Use cautiously in patients with thyroid disease, cardiovascular disease, coronary artery disease, hypertension, intraocular pressure, or peripheral vascular disease and in those who have difficulty urinating because of an enlarged prostate
- Use cautiously in patients older than age 60; they are more likely to experience adverse reactions
- Increasing dosage frequency and the amount of a dose may cause toxicity and rebound congestion
- A topical (nasal) decongestant shouldn't be used for more than 3 days; an oral decongestant shouldn't be used for more than 7 days because prolonged use will result in rebound congestion

When NOT to use decongestants

- MAO inhibitor therapy
- Hypersensitivity to these drugs

Adverse reactions

- These drugs may cause arrhythmias, palpitations, tachycardia, bradycardia, hypertension, headache, dizziness, light-headedness, drowsiness, insomnia, nervousness, giddiness, psychological disturbances, and hypersensitivity reactions, including rash, urticaria, and leukopenia

Adverse reactions to watch for

- Arrhythmias, palpitations, tachycardia, bradycardia, hypertension, headache, dizziness, lightheadedness, drowsiness, insomnia, nervousness, giddiness, psychological disturbances, hypersensitivity reactions, including rash, urticaria, and leukopenia

Interactions

- Nasal decongestants given with other sympathomimetic amines may increase central nervous system stimulation
- MAO inhibitors given concurrently with a nasal decongestant may cause severe hypertension or a hypertensive crisis
- Don't give pseudoephedrine with alkalinizing agents because it may decrease urinary excretion of pseudoephedrine, increasing its effects

Nursing responsibilities

- Teach the patient the proper method for using decongestant sprays, inhalers, and drops
- Tell the patient not to share the container with other people and not to allow the tip of the container to touch the nasal passage to avoid contamination
- Notify the prescriber if the patient experiences insomnia, dizziness, weakness, tremor, or irregular heartbeat
- Monitor the patient's blood pressure, pulse rate, and ECG during therapy
- Tell the patient not to exceed the prescribed frequency of dosage or the amount of each dose; doing so may increase the risk of toxicity and cause rebound congestion

Key nursing actions

- Notify prescriber if insomnia, dizziness, weakness, tremor, or irregular heartbeat occurs.
- Monitor blood pressure, pulse rate, and ECG.
- Teach patient to:
  - use medication properly
  - avoid sharing medication
  - take medication as prescribed.

NCLEX CHECKS

It's never too soon to begin your NCLEX preparation. Now that you've reviewed this chapter, carefully read each of the following questions and choose the best answer. Then compare your responses to the correct answers.

1. A patient is receiving theophylline (Theo-Bid). Which of the following assessment findings indicates the patient is responding positively to the drug?

- ☐ **A.** Easy, unlabored respirations
- ☐ **B.** Heart rate of 92 beats/minute
- ☐ **C.** Urine output of 450 ml/shift
- ☐ **D.** Blood pressure of 138/82 mm Hg

2. You're checking for adverse reactions in a patient who has just been given metaproterenol (Alupent) for asthma. Which of the following adverse reactions is likely in a patient who has taken a dose of this drug?

- ☐ **A.** Edema, moon face
- ☐ **B.** Tachycardia, shaking
- ☐ **C.** Bleeding peptic ulcer, vomiting
- ☐ **D.** Moderate hypotension, dizziness

3. You're instructing a patient about the use of albuterol (Proventil) and beclomethasone dipropionate (Vanceril) inhalation therapy at home. You should teach the patient to:

- ☐ **A.** use the glucocorticoid followed by the bronchodilator.
- ☐ **B.** use the bronchodilator followed by the glucocorticoid.
- ☐ **C.** alternate the order of use each time to prevent clearance.
- ☐ **D.** rinse the mouth both before and after use to prevent gum breakdown.

4. A patient comes into the ambulatory care clinic with an upper respiratory tract infection, evidenced by nasal stuffiness, low-grade fever, and a productive cough. She reports difficulty coughing up the mucus. The chest examination is consistent with bronchitis. She would like cough syrup. Which ingredient commonly included in cough syrups is most appropriate for her?

- ☐ **A.** Codeine
- ☐ **B.** Dextromethorphan
- ☐ **C.** Diphenhydramine (Benadryl)
- ☐ **D.** Guaifenesin (Robitussin)

5. A patient who had an upper respiratory tract infection has been using oxymetazoline hydrochloride (Afrin) nasal spray twice daily for 10 days. Although she gets some relief after using it, she says she has to use more and more, and if she doesn't use it, the congestion comes back. What is the most likely explanation for this problem?

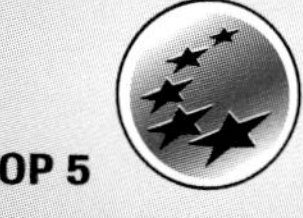

TOP 5

Items to study for your next test on drugs and the respiratory system

1. Mechanisms of action of bronchodilators, anti-inflammatory inhalants, antitussives, expectorants, mucolytics, and decongestants
2. Rationale for using bronchodilators, anti-inflammatory inhalants, antitussives, expectorants, mucolytics, and decongestants
3. Common adverse effects of bronchodilators, anti-inflammatory inhalants, antitussives, expectorants, mucolytics, and decongestants
4. Nursing responsibilities when administering bronchodilators, anti-inflammatory inhalants, antitussives, expectorants, mucolytics, and decongestants
5. Patient teaching related to bronchodilators, anti-inflammatory inhalants, antitussives, expectorants, mucolytics, and decongestants

☐ **A.** She's used the oxymetazoline for too long.
☐ **B.** The twice-daily dosing interval is too short for oxymetazoline.
☐ **C.** A viral infection has probably become a secondary bacterial infection.
☐ **D.** She's developed a tolerance to the pharmacologic effect of oxymetazoline.

6. You're assessing the serum theophylline level in a patient with asthma. Which of the following serum theophylline levels represents the therapeutic range for treating asthma?

☐ **A.** 1 to 5 mcg/ml
☐ **B.** 5 to 10 mcg/ml
☐ **C.** 10 to 20 mcg/ml
☐ **D.** 20 to 25 mcg/ml

7. A prescriber orders theophylline (Slo-bid) for his patient. The nurse knows that theophylline is indicated for which of the following disorders?

Select all that apply:

☐ **A.** Bronchospasm
☐ **B.** Status asthmaticus
☐ **C.** Emphysema
☐ **D.** Bronchitis
☐ **E.** Asthma

ANSWERS AND RATIONALES

1. CORRECT ANSWER: A

Theophylline, like other methylxanthines, commonly is used to treat chronic obstructive pulmonary disease and asthma. The goal of treatment is a normal respiratory rate and easy, unlabored respirations. Theophylline has no effect on urine output. It may increase heart rate and blood pressure, but these aren't indications that the drug is effective.

2. CORRECT ANSWER: B

Alupent stimulates beta receptors to dilate the bronchioles and stimulates the cardiovascular system. This results in tachycardia and shaking. Edema and moon face are usually seen with corticosteroid therapy. Bleeding ulcer and vomiting are usually associated with nonsteroidal anti-inflammatory therapy. Bronchodilators can cause hypertension rather than hypotension.

3. CORRECT ANSWER: B

Albuterol, a bronchodilator, should be used first to open the airways so that the steroid (beclomethasone) can better penetrate the lungs. Taking the steroid first would reduce the therapeutic effects of the steroid. Alternating the order of use would also reduce the therapeutic effect. Gum breakdown is not a concern with the use of these drugs.

4. CORRECT ANSWER: D

Guaifenesin is an expectorant that will help get secretions out of her airways, which will reduce the urge to cough. The other drugs are antitussives, which will reduce only the frequency of the cough, not help expectorate secretions from a productive cough.

5. CORRECT ANSWER: A

The patient is describing classic rebound congestion (also known as rhinitis medicamentosa) that occurs when topical decongestants are used for too long (over 3 days). This doesn't indicate tolerance in the pharmacologic sense, which would involve receptor changes. There are no signs of bacterial infection. Twice daily is the correct dosing interval for this drug.

6. CORRECT ANSWER: C

To treat a respiratory disease such as asthma, the therapeutic serum theophylline level should range from 10 to 20 mcg/ml. A lower serum level may not produce a therapeutic response; a higher level may lead to adverse reactions.

7. CORRECT ANSWER: A, C, D, E

Theophylline and other xanthine derivative bronchodilators are used to treat and prevent bronchospasms, asthma, emphysema, bronchitis, and neonatal apnea. Status asthmaticus is considered a medical emergency that requires the use of parenteral medication in an intensive care setting and the use of conventional bronchodilators, such as oral theophylline alone, would be inadequate and inappropriate as treatment.

8

Drugs and the cardiovascular system

LEARNING OBJECTIVES

After studying this chapter, you should be able to:

- Understand the different indications for inotropic drugs, antiarrhythmics, antihypertensives, and antianginals.
- Describe the general mechanisms of action of cardiac drugs and antilipemics.
- Name common adverse effects of cardiac drugs and antilipemics.
- Identify nursing responsibilities when administering a cardiac drug or an antilipemic.
- Discuss appropriate teaching for the patient who is receiving a cardiac drug or an antilipemic.

CHAPTER OVERVIEW

Because inotropic drugs increase the force of myocardial contraction, they're used to treat symptoms of heart failure and manage atrial arrhythmias. These drugs increase stroke volume and cardiac output, slow conduction, and cause diuresis by increasing blood flow to the kidney. Digoxin, the major inotropic drug, has a very narrow therapeutic margin. Nursing responsibilities include monitoring the patient's apical pulse, cardiac rhythm, and serum drug levels and assessing for signs and symptoms of drug toxicity. Patient teaching focuses on taking a pulse and recognizing symptoms of drug toxicity, worsening heart failure, and arrhythmia. Inamrinone and milrinone are inotropic drugs used in the critically ill patient to increase cardiac output and decrease preload and afterload. Careful observation for arrhythmias and assessment of hemodynamic parameters are indicated for the patient taking inamrinone or milrinone.

Antiarrhythmics are used to suppress or regulate atrial and ventricular conduction disturbances resulting from myocardial infarction and other causes. Most antiarrhythmics have proarrhythmic properties, meaning they can precipitate or aggravate an arrhythmia. The nurse establishes outcomes based on the arrhythmia's etiology and the patient's signs and symptoms. Many antiarrhythmics must be administered in a critical care unit with continuous cardiac monitoring and an infusion pump to control or titrate the drug. Nursing interventions focus on monitoring the patient's rhythm, cardiac output, and blood pressure and providing patient safety. Patient teaching involves fostering compliance and giving instructions on taking the pulse, avoiding caffeine (which may exacerbate the arrhythmia), and reporting episodes of syncope, dizziness, or arrhythmias.

Hypertension, a frequently asymptomatic elevation of blood pressure, is often called the silent killer. If not treated, hypertension may result in such illnesses as myocardial infarction, stroke, and renal failure. The major reasons hypertension complications occur include lack of awareness of the condition and problems with compliance. Antihypertensives lower blood pressure by inhibiting the central or peripheral nervous system, the renin-angiotensin mechanism, or sodium and chloride reabsorption in the renal tubules. Antihypertensives are prescribed based on the cause of the problem. Nursing responsibilities focus on monitoring blood pressure and observing for vascular complications. Patient teaching should cover the importance of compliance, the danger of stopping the drug when feeling better, the need for rising slowly, and observation for swelling when taking calcium channel blockers. Smoking cessation, weight loss, exercise, and restrictions on salt and caffeine intake also may help manage hypertension.

Antianginals reduce myocardial oxygen demand and increase blood flow to ischemic areas of the myocardium. They terminate acute anginal attacks and prevent angina from occurring. Acute angina is managed with a short-acting nitrate, such as nitroglycerin sublingual tablets or spray. Nitroglycerin may be used intravenously for unrelieved chest pain during acute myocardial infarction. Angina prevention is managed with one or more drugs, including nitrates, beta-adrenergic blockers, and calcium channel blockers. Nursing responsibilities focus on monitoring blood pressure and evaluating the location, quality, and duration of chest pain. Patient teaching includes instructions about rising slowly, avoiding alcohol, and notifying the physician of changes in the chest pain pattern or pain that isn't relieved by three nitroglycerin tablets.

Antilipemics are used to prevent and treat atherosclerosis. Because of the adverse effects of antilipemics, dietary modification, weight loss, exercise, and smoking cessation are considered first-line treatment. Antilipemic therapy may be indicated if these measures are ineffective. Nursing responsibilities include encouraging dietary compliance and supplementation of fat-soluble vitamins, as necessary, and monitoring lipid and liver enzyme levels and bowel function. Patient teaching involves timing of doses, proper preparation of powders, reporting intolerance to the drug, and the importance of follow-up blood tests, especially liver function studies.

A&P highlights

- The cardiovascular system consists of the heart and blood vessels and includes the cardiac circulation, pulmonary circulation, systemic circulation, and hepatic circulation.
- The heart pumps blood through the blood vessels.
- Events that occur during a single systole and diastole of the atria and ventricles make up the cardiac cycle; they also produce heart sounds and a pulse.
- The cardiac conduction system sends impulses and controls the heartbeat.
- Blood pressure refers to the pressure of the blood in the systemic circulation.
- Starling's law, baroreceptors and chemoreceptors in major arteries, and hormones secreted by the kidneys control cardiac output and blood pressure.
- The cardiovascular system moves blood throughout the body, helps maintain proper body pH and electrolyte composition, and helps regulate body temperature.

ANATOMY AND PHYSIOLOGY

Anatomy

- The cardiovascular system consists of the heart and blood vessels
- It includes the cardiac circulation, pulmonary circulation, systemic circulation, and hepatic circulation; in pregnant women, the fetal circulation also is included
- Blood vessels include arteries, arterioles, capillaries, venules, and veins

Physiology

- The heart pumps blood through the blood vessels
- The heart's upper chambers (atria) communicate with the lower chambers (ventricles) via the atrioventricular (AV) valves
- Events that occur during a single systole (contraction) and diastole (relaxation) of the atria and ventricles make up the cardiac cycle; they also produce heart sounds and a pulse
- The cardiac conduction system sends impulses and controls the heartbeat
- The cardiac conduction system consists of the sinoatrial (SA) node and internodal tracts, AV node, bundle of His, and Purkinje fibers
- Impulses generated by the conduction system cause synchronized contractions of the atria and ventricles
- Blood pressure refers to the pressure of the blood in the systemic circulation; pressure is highest when the blood is ejected during systole (systolic pressure) and lowest during diastole (diastolic pressure)
- Starling's law (the force of heart muscle contraction is proportional to its initial length), baroreceptors and chemoreceptors in major arteries, and hormones secreted by the kidneys control cardiac output and blood pressure
- The cyclic flow of fluid from the interstitial space to the capillaries and back into the interstitial space depends on capillary hydrostatic pressure, capillary permeability, osmotic pressure, and open lymphatic channels
- Edema (excess fluid in the interstitial space) may result from any disturbance in this fluid transfer

Function

- The cardiovascular system moves blood throughout the body
- It helps maintain proper body pH and electrolyte composition
- It also helps regulate body temperature

DIGOXIN

Mechanism of action

- Digoxin is a cardiac glycoside derived from the digitalis plant; it is the only cardiac glycoside in common use

- Digoxin is known as an inotropic drug because it has a positive inotropic action (that is, it increases the force of myocardial contraction)
- Digoxin also has a negative chronotropic action, by which it depresses the SA node, reduces conduction velocity of the impulse through the AV node, and slows the heart rate

Pharmacokinetics

- Absorption: Varies with the different forms of the drug
- Distribution: Distributed widely throughout the body; extensively bound to skeletal muscles and albumin
- Metabolism: Metabolized by the liver and GI flora
- Excretion: Excreted unchanged in the urine

Drug examples

- Digoxin (Lanoxicaps, Lanoxin, Digitek)

Indications

- To treat heart failure; it commonly is given with diuretics
- To control the ventricular rate in atrial fibrillation, atrial flutter, and paroxysmal atrial tachycardia

Contraindications and precautions

- Digoxin is contraindicated in uncontrolled ventricular arrhythmias, idiopathic hypertrophic subaortic stenosis, constrictive pericarditis, and complete heart block
- The risk of digoxin toxicity is increased in patients with hypercalcemia, hypokalemia, hypomagnesemia, hypothyroidism, or renal failure
- Elderly patients may be at greater risk for toxicity because they are more sensitive to the drug's effects; anorexia may be an early warning sign of toxicity
- Digoxin increases the risk of arrhythmias and should be used with caution in patients with acute myocardial infarction (MI)

Adverse reactions

- May cause bradycardia, fatigue, weakness, nausea, vomiting, and diarrhea
- May cause digoxin toxicity (as evidenced by anorexia, nausea, vomiting, visual disturbances, confusion, bradycardia, heart block, premature ventricular contractions, and tachyarrhythmias)

Interactions

- Potassium-wasting diuretics and other drugs causing potassium loss increase the risk of digoxin toxicity
- Amiodarone, benzodiazepines, bepridil, cyclosporine, diclofenac, diltiazem, macrolides (erythromycin, clarithromycin), nifedipine, quinidine, quinine, spironolactone, tetracyclines, and verapamil increase the serum digoxin level and may cause toxicity
- Beta blockers, calcium channel blockers, I.V. calcium, succinylcholine, sympathomimetics, and diuretics may cause bradycardia and other enhanced digoxin effects

Key facts about digoxin

- A cardiac glycoside derived from the digitalis plant
- Known as an inotropic drug because it has a positive inotropic action (increases the force of myocardial contraction)
- Slows the heart rate
- Metabolized by the liver and GI flora
- Excreted unchanged in the urine

When to use digoxin

- Heart faillure
- Atrial fibrillation
- Atrial flutter
- Paroxysmal atrial tachycardia

When NOT to use digoxin

- Uncontrolled ventricular arrhythmias
- Idiopathic hypertrophic subaortic stenosis
- Constrictive pericarditis
- Complete heart block

Adverse reactions to watch for

- Bradycardia, fatigue, weakness, nausea, vomiting, diarrhea, digoxin toxicity

- Aminoglycosides, antacids, antineoplastics, activated charcoal, cholestyramine, colestipol, kaolin/pectin, metoclopramide, penicillamine, rifampin, and sulfasalazine decrease GI absorption of digoxin
- Foods with high bran content may decrease the oral absorption of digoxin

Key nursing actions

- Before administering digoxin, assess patient's apical pulse, serum drug and electrolyte levels, and renal function; withhold drug and notify physician if pulse rate is below 60 beats/minute or minimum specified by physician.
- Continuously monitor serum digoxin level and watch for signs and symptoms of toxicity.
- Don't alternate dosage forms.
- Know that dosage must be reduced in patients with renal impairment.
- Teach patient to:
  - take prescribed drug properly
  - consult physician before discontinuing drug
  - count his pulse before taking each dose
  - recognize signs and symptoms of digoxin toxicity and heart failure.

Nursing responsibilities

- **Before administering digoxin, assess the patient's apical pulse, serum drug and electrolyte levels, and renal function; withhold the drug and notify the physician if the pulse rate is below 60 beats/minute or the minimum specified by the physician**
- Continuously monitor the patient's serum digoxin level and watch for signs and symptoms of toxicity, especially in elderly patients and during digitalization
- **Don't alternate dosage forms because bioavailability of capsules doesn't equal that of tablets or elixir**
- **Know that digoxin immune FAB (Digibind, DigiFab) is used as an antidote in extreme toxicity**
- Be aware that hypokalemia places the patient receiving digoxin at risk for drug toxicity
- Teach the patient how to take the prescribed drug; warn the patient *not* to take a double dose after missing a dose
- Advise the patient to consult the physician before discontinuing the drug
- Teach the patient to count his pulse before taking each dose; instruct him to notify the physician if his pulse rate is below 60 or above 100 beats/minute
- Teach the patient how to recognize signs and symptoms of digoxin toxicity and heart failure (for specific teaching tips, see *Teaching about cardiac glycosides*)

Topics for patient discussion

- Therapy regimen
- Signs and symptoms of possible adverse reactions and when to notify physician
- Procedure for taking and monitoring pulse
- Dietary restrictions
- Weight monitoring
- Need for compliance with therapy
- Follow-up care

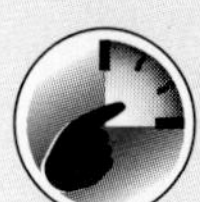

TIME-OUT FOR TEACHING

Teaching about cardiac glycosides

Include these topics in your teaching plan for the patient receiving a cardiac glycoside.

- Medication therapy regimen, including the drug's name, dose, frequency, duration, and possible adverse effects
- Signs and symptoms of possible adverse effects, especially heart failure and toxicity, and when to notify the physician
- Procedure for taking and monitoring pulse
- Dietary restrictions and allowances
- Weight monitoring
- Need for compliance with therapy, including taking the drug as prescribed and instructions for missed doses
- Follow-up care, including laboratory tests and physician visits

- Know that, because digoxin is excreted unchanged by the kidneys, the dosage must be reduced in patients with renal impairment
- Monitor the patient receiving I.V. infusion of inotropic drugs for worsening or new arrhythmias, hypertension, and hypotension

OTHER INOTROPIC DRUGS

Mechanism of action
- Increase myocardial contractility and decrease systemic vascular resistance and venous return, resulting in improved cardiac output

Pharmacokinetics
- Absorption: Administered I.V.
- Distribution: Distributed rapidly
- Metabolism: Conjugated pathways in the liver metabolize inamrinone
- Excretion: Excreted primarily in the urine

Drug examples
- Inamrinone lactate, milrinone (Primacor)

Indications
- Short-term management of heart failure in patients who are closely monitored and who don't respond adequately to digitalis preparations, diuretics, or vasodilators

Contraindications and precautions
- Inamrinone is contraindicated in patients who are hypersensitive to inamrinone or bisulfates or who have had an acute MI
- Milrinone is contraindicated in patients with a hypersensitivity to milrinone
- These drugs shouldn't be used in patients with severe obstructive aortic or pulmonic valvular disease; they may aggravate outflow tract obstruction in hypertrophic subaortic stenosis
- Hypokalemia should be corrected with potassium supplements before these drugs are used because of the increased risk of arrhythmias

Adverse reactions
- Because of their vasodilating effects, these drugs most commonly cause arrhythmias (ventricular) and hypotension
- These drugs also may cause thrombocytopenia, headache, nausea, vomiting, anorexia, and hypersensitivity reactions, including pericarditis, pleuritis, and ascites

Interactions
- Use of inamrinone with disopyramide may cause excessive hypotension
- Use of inamrinone with digoxin may enhance AV conduction and increase the ventricular response rate; therefore, concomitant therapy with inamrinone and digoxin is recommended for patients with atrial flutter or fibrillation

Key facts about inotropic drugs
- Increase myocardial contractility
- Decrease systemic vascular resistance
- Improve cardiac output
- Metabolized in the liver
- Excreted primarily in the uine

When to use inotropic drugs
- Heart failure

When NOT to use inotropic drugs
- Hypersensitivity to these drugs or bisulfates
- Acute MI
- Severe obstructive aortic or pulmonic valvular disease

Adverse reactions to watch for
- Arrhythmias (ventricular), hypotension, thrombocytopenia, headache, nausea, vomiting, anorexia, and hypersensitivity reactions

Key nursing actions

- Closely monitor patient's hemodynamic status.
- Monitor patient's heart rate, heart rhythm, and blood pressure frequently.
- Administer drug I.V., using an infusion pump; slow or stop infusion if patient's blood pressure drops.

Nursing responsibilities

- Closely monitor the patient's hemodynamic status, including pulmonary artery pressure and cardiac output; dosage is determined by the patient's response
- Monitor the patient's heart rate, heart rhythm, and blood pressure frequently to detect arrhythmias or hypotension
- Administer the drug I.V., using an infusion pump; slow or stop the infusion if the patient's blood pressure drops
- Monitor the patient receiving I.V. infusion of inotropic drugs for worsening or new arrhythmias, hypertension, and hypotension

ANTIARRHYTHMICS

CLASS I ANTIARRHYTHMICS

Key facts about class I antiarrhythmics

- Block sodium channels and slow conduction of electrical impulses
- Slow or normalize depolarization and shorten, normalize, or prolong repolarization
- Metabolized in the liver into several metabolites
- Excreted in the urine

Mechanism of action

- All antiarrhythmics in class I and its subclasses block sodium channels (local anesthetic effect) and slow conduction of electrical impulses
- Class IA antiarrhythmics slow depolarization and prolong repolarization
  - Disopyramide produces peripheral vasoconstriction
  - Procainamide and quinidine decrease peripheral vascular resistance
- Class IB antiarrhythmics normalize depolarization and shorten repolarization
- Class IC antiarrhythmics slow depolarization and normalize repolarization

Pharmacokinetics

- Absorption: Usually well absorbed in the GI tract after oral administration
- Distribution: Highly protein-bound
- Metabolism: Metabolized in the liver into several metabolites
- Excretion: Excreted in the urine

Drug examples

- Class I antiarrhythmics include moricizine (Ethmozine)
- Class IA antiarrhythmics include disopyramide (Norpace), procainamide (Pronestyl), and quinidine (Quinidex)
- Class IB antiarrhythmics include lidocaine (Xylocaine), mexiletine (Mexitil), phenytoin (Dilantin), and tocainide (Tonocard)
- Class IC antiarrhythmics include flecainide (Tambocor) and propafenone (Rythmol)

When to use class I antiarrhythmics

- Ventricular arrhythmias
- Ventricular ectopy
- Ventricular tachycardia

Indications

- Class I antiarrhythmics are used to treat documented life-threatening ventricular arrhythmias
- Class IA antiarrhythmics are used to treat life-threatening ventricular arrhythmias and symptomatic non-life-threatening arrhythmias
- Class IB antiarrhythmics are used to treat life-threatening ventricular arrhythmias (lidocaine) and symptomatic non-life-threatening arrhythmias

(mexiletine) and to suppress the frequency of ventricular ectopy and reduce the frequency and duration of abrupt, self-limiting ventricular tachycardia (tocainide)
- Class IC antiarrhythmics are used to treat documented life-threatening ventricular arrhythmias

Contraindications and precautions
- Antiarrhythmics are contraindicated in patients with complete atrioventricular block (from the risk of asystole) and in those hypersensitive to these or similar drugs
- Use these drugs cautiously in acute MI and heart failure

Adverse reactions
- May cause hypotension, heart failure, worsened or new arrhythmias; nausea, vomiting, and diarrhea (with oral antiarrhythmics)
- Quinidine may cause syncope, worsening AV block or asystole, hepatotoxicity, and cardiotoxicity
- Procainamide may cause a positive antinuclear antibody (ANA) test, with or without symptoms of lupus, with prolonged use
- Disopyramide may worsen heart failure or cause severe hypotension

Interactions
- Concurrent use with antihypertensives causes additive hypotension
- Concurrent use with other antiarrhythmics may cause increased toxicity
- Cimetidine increases serum levels of class I antiarrhythmics (especially disopyramide and lidocaine)
- Class I antiarrhythmics may increase serum levels of digoxin or digitoxin

Nursing responsibilities
- Before administering lidocaine, always check the label to prevent administering a form that contains epinephrine or preservatives; such solutions are used for local anesthesia only
- Know that lidocaine has a short duration of action
- Administer an I.V. bolus for ventricular arrhythmias, followed by a continuous I.V. infusion, as ordered
- Don't administer Class IA antiarrhythmics with food unless prescribed; food may affect reabsorption
- Administer mexiletine or tocainide with food or antacids to reduce GI distress
- Institute safety precautions to prevent injury
- Be aware that disopyramide has anticholinergic effects
  - Observe for urine retention, constipation, dry mouth, and blurred vision
  - Instruct the patient to follow a high-fiber diet or use a bulk laxative for constipation

When NOT to use class I antiarrhythmics
- Complete atrioventricular block
- Hypersensitivity to these drugs

Adverse reactions to watch for
- Hypotension, heart failure, worsening or new arrhythmias, nausea, vomiting, diarrhea

Key nursing actions
- Before administering lidocaine, always check label to prevent administering form containing epinephrine or preservatives.
- Administer I.V. bolus for ventricular arrhythmias, followed by continuous I.V. infusion, as ordered.
- Don't administer Class IA drugs with food unless prescribed.
- Administer mexiletine or tocainide with food or antacids.
- Institute safety precautions to prevent injury.
- Be aware that disopyramide has anticholinergic effects.

Key facts about class II antiarrhythmics

- Decrease sympathetic activity at the SA and AV nodes, decreasing automaticity and prolonging the refractory period
- Undergo extensive first-pass metabolism in the liver
- Excreted in the urine, feces, and bile

When to use class II antiarrhythmics

- Sinus tachycardia
- Atrial fibrillation or flutter
- Ventricular arrhythmias
- Hypertension

When NOT to use class II antiarrhythmics

- Persistent severe bradycardia
- Second- or third-degree heart block
- Overt cardiac failure
- Cardiogenic shock

Adverse reactions to watch for

- Dizziness, fatigue, hypotension, heart failure, bradycardia, arrhythmias, heart block, bronchospasm, GI distress

Key nursing actions

- Instruct patient to watch for signs and symptoms of fluid retention.
- Advise patient to limit fluid and salt intake to minimize fluid retention.
- Inform patient that drug should be discontinued gradually.
- Institute safety precautions to prevent injury.

CLASS II ANTIARRHYTHMICS

Mechanism of action

- Decrease sympathetic activity at the SA and AV nodes, decreasing automaticity and prolonging the refractory period

Pharmacokinetics

- Absorption: Well absorbed after oral administration
- Distribution: Acebutolol is about 26% protein-bound
- Metabolism: Undergo extensive first-pass metabolism in the liver
- Excretion: Excreted in the urine, feces, and bile

Drug examples

- Acebutolol (Sectral), esmolol (Brevibloc), propranolol (Inderal)

Indications

- These drugs are used to treat sinus tachycardia and atrial fibrillation or flutter
- Acebutolol and propranolol also are used to treat ventricular arrhythmias
- Acebutolol also is used to treat hypertension

Contraindications and precautions

- Contraindicated in patients with persistent severe bradycardia, second- and third-degree heart block, overt cardiac failure, and cardiogenic shock
- Use cautiously in patients at risk for heart failure and in those with impaired hepatic function, bronchospastic disease (including asthma), diabetes, hyperthyroidism, and peripheral vascular disease

Adverse reactions

- Dizziness, fatigue, hypotension, heart failure, bradycardia, arrhythmias, heart block, bronchospasm, GI distress

Interactions

- May increase hypotensive effects when used with alpha-adrenergic stimulants, indomethacin, NSAIDs, diuretics, phenothiazines, or calcium channel blockers

Nursing responsibilities

- Instruct the patient to watch for signs and symptoms of fluid retention, such as weight gain, peripheral edema, or shortness of breath (for specific teaching tips, see *Teaching about class II antiarrhythmics*)
- Advise the patient to limit fluid and salt intake to minimize fluid retention
- **Inform the patient that the drug should be discontinued gradually, under physician supervision, over 2 weeks**
- **Tell the patient that discontinuing the drug abruptly may exacerbate angina symptoms or precipitate MI in patients with coronary artery disease**
- Institute safety precautions to prevent injury

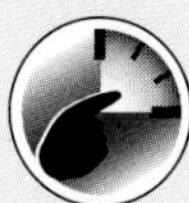

TIME-OUT FOR TEACHING

Teaching about class II antiarrhythmics

Include these topics in your teaching plan for the patient receiving a class II antiarrhythmic.

- Medication therapy regimen, including the drug's name, dose, frequency, duration, and possible adverse effects
- Signs and symptoms of possible adverse effects and when to notify the physician
- Procedure for taking and monitoring pulse
- Dietary restrictions, including fluid and sodium restrictions as appropriate
- Weight monitoring
- Safety measures
- Measures to ensure compliance with therapy
- Medical follow-up

CLASS III ANTIARRHYTHMICS

Mechanism of action

- Prolong the action potential and the absolute refractory period

Pharmacokinetics

- Absorption: Absorption is slow and variable after oral administration
- Distribution: Widely distributed in fat tissues and liver; highly protein-bound
- Metabolism: Metabolized extensively in the liver
- Excretion: Excreted in bile; amiodarone has the longest half-life of any antiarrhythmic

Drug examples

- Amiodarone (Cordarone), bretylium (Bretylol), ibutilide (Corvert), sotalol (Betapace AF)

Indications

- Recurrent ventricular fibrillation
- Unstable ventricular tachycardia
- Atrial fibrillation
- Maintenance of normal sinus rhythm in patients who have been converted from atrial fibrillation or atrial flutter (sotalol)

Contraindications and precautions

- These drugs are contraindicated in breast-feeding patients and in those with severe sinus node dysfunction or bradycardia-induced syncope
- Use amiodarone cautiously in patients with heart failure, severe hepatic dysfunction, or hypokalemia

Topics for patient discussion

- Medication therapy regimen
- Signs and symptoms of possible adverse effects and when to notify the physician
- Procedure for taking and monitoring pulse
- Dietary restrictions
- Weight monitoring
- Safety measures
- Need for compliance with therapy
- Medical follow-up

Key facts about class III antiarrhythmics

- Prolong the action potential and the absolute refractory period
- Metabolized extensively in the liver
- Excreted in bile

When to use class III antiarrhythmics

- Recurrent ventricular fibrillation
- Unstable ventricular tachycardia
- Atrial fibrillation
- Maintenance of normal sinus rhythm

When NOT to use class III antiarrhythmics

- Breast-feeding
- Severe sinus node dysfunction
- Bradycardia-induced syncope

- Use bretylium cautiously in patients with aortic stenosis or pulmonary hypertension
- Use sotalol cautiously in patients with diabetes, thyrotoxicity, or hepatic or renal impairment

Adverse reactions to watch for

- Hypotension, bradycardia, nausea, vomiting

Adverse reactions

- These drugs may cause hypotension, bradycardia, nausea, and vomiting
- Amiodarone may cause pulmonary fibrosis (with prolonged use), photosensitivity, bluish skin discoloration, corneal microdeposits, hypothyroidism, peripheral neuropathy, tremor, poor coordination, and abnormal gait
- Bretylium may cause vertigo, syncope, and dizziness
- Sotalol may cause gastric pain, heart failure, impotence, decreased libido, laryngospasm, and respiratory depression

Interactions

- Concurrent use with digoxin may increase digoxin levels and worsen arrhythmias
- Concurrent use with procainamide or quinidine may worsen hypotension
- Amiodarone also interacts with antihypertensives, warfarin, and phenytoin

Key nursing actions

- Don't administer sotalol unless patient is unresponsive to other antiarrhythmics and has a life-threatening ventricular arrhythmia
- Assess lung, thyroid, and neurologic function in patient receiving amiodarone to ensure prompt detection of adverse effects.
- After administering bretylium, keep patient supine and observe for hypotension.
- Teach patient to:
  - change position slowly if taking bretylium
  - use artificial tears and sunscreen and wear protective clothing if taking amiodarone.

Nursing responsibilities

- Assess lung, thyroid, and neurologic function in the patient receiving amiodarone to ensure prompt detection of adverse effects
- After administering bretylium, keep the patient supine and observe for hypotension
- **Don't administer sotalol unless the patient is unresponsive to other antiarrhythmics and has a life-threatening ventricular arrhythmia; monitor the patient's response carefully because the drug's proarrhythmic effects can be pronounced**
- Instruct the patient receiving bretylium to change position slowly to minimize orthostatic hypotension
- Teach the patient receiving amiodarone to use sunscreen and wear protective clothing to prevent photosensitivity reactions
- Teach the patient receiving amiodarone to use artificial tears to prevent corneal deposits

CLASS IV ANTIARRHYTHMICS (CALCIUM CHANNEL BLOCKERS)

Key facts about class IV antiarrhythmics

- Block the slow inward calcium channels, slowing conduction through the AV node
- Metabolized in the liver
- Excreted unchanged in the urine

Mechanism of action

- Block the slow inward calcium channels, slowing conduction through the AV node

Pharmacokinetics

- Absorption: Absorbed rapidly and completely from the GI tract after oral administration

- Distribution: About 90% is protein-bound
- Metabolism: Metabolized in the liver; goes through first-pass metabolism
- Excretion: Excreted in the urine as unchanged drug and active metabolites

Drug examples
- Verapamil hydrochloride (Calan, Covera-HS, Isoptin SR, Verelan)

Indications
- To treat atrial fibrillation or flutter (except when associated with accessory bypass tracts) and supraventricular tachycardias
- To manage Prinzmetal's or variant angina and unstable or chronic stable angina pectoris
- To treat hypertension

Contraindications and precautions
- Contraindicated in patients with severe left ventricular dysfunction, cardiogenic shock, second- or third-degree heart block, sick sinus syndrome (unless a functioning pacemaker is present), atrial flutter or fibrillation associated with accessory bypass tracts, severe heart failure, or severe hypotension
- **I.V. verapamil hydrochloride is contraindicated in patients receiving I.V. beta blockers and in those with ventricular tachycardia**
- Use cautiously in elderly patients and in patients with impaired hepatic or renal function or increased intracranial pressure

Adverse reactions
- Dizziness, hypotension, bradycardia, edema, constipation

Interactions
- Use with digoxin increases the risk of digoxin toxicity
- Use with beta-adrenergic blockers may increase the risk of bradycardia and heart failure
- Use with antihypertensives or nitrates causes additive hypotension

Nursing responsibilities
- Advise the patient to change position slowly to minimize orthostatic hypotension
- Encourage the patient to increase fiber intake to prevent constipation
- **If the patient is receiving I.V. verapamil hydrochloride, monitor blood pressure and ECG continuously**

MISCELLANEOUS ANTIARRHYTHMICS

Mechanism of action
- Adenosine interrupts reentrant pathways and slows conduction in the AV node
- Atropine blocks muscarinic cholinergic receptors in the SA and AV nodes and blocks the effects of the vagus nerve on cardiac conduction

Pharmacokinetics
- Absorption: Administered I.V.

When to use class IV antiarrhythmics

- Atrial fibrillation and flutter (except when associated with accessory bypass tracts)
- Supraventricular tachycardias
- Prinzmetal's or variant angina
- Unstable or chronic stable angina pectoris
- Hypertension

When NOT to use class IV antiarrhythmics

- Severe left ventricular dysfunction
- Cardiogenic shock
- Second- or third-degree heart block
- Sick sinus syndrome
- Severe heart failure
- Severe hypotension
- Atrial fibrillation and flutter associated with accessory bypass tracts

Adverse reactions to watch for

- Dizziness, hypotension, bradycardia, edema, constipation

Key nursing actions

- Advise patient to change position slowly.
- Encourage patient to increase fiber intake.
- If patient is receiving I.V. verapamil, monitor blood pressure and ECG continuously.

Key facts about adenosine and atropine

- Adenosine interrupts reentrant pathways and slows conduction in the AV node.
- Atropine blocks muscarinic cholinergic receptors in the SA and AV nodes and blocks the effects of the vagus nerve on cardiac conduction.
- Adenosine is metabolized in the tissues; atropine is metabolized by the liver.
- Atropine is excreted primarily in the urine.

When to use adenosine or atropine

- Paroxysmal supraventricular tachycardia unrelated to vagal maneuvers
- Symptomatic bradycardia and bradyarrhythmia

When NOT to use adenosine or atropine

- Second- or third-degree AV block
- Sick sinus syndrome without a pacemaker
- Atrial fibrillation, atrial flutter, and ventricular tachycardia
- Glaucoma, urine retention, or ileus

Adverse reactions to watch for

- Transient arrhythmias, dyspnea, facial flushing, hallucinations, tachycardia, dry mouth, and constipation

Key nursing actions

- Monitor heart rate, respiratory rate, blood pressure, and ECG.
- Give these drugs around the clock, as prescribed.
- Administer I.V. antiarrhythmics by infusion pump.

- Distribution: Widely distributed; adenosine's distribution is rapid
- Metabolism: Adenosine is metabolized in the tissues; atropine is metabolized by the liver
- Excretion: Excretion of adenosine is unknown; atropine is excreted in the urine, although small amounts may be excreted in the feces and in the air

Drug examples
- Adenosine (Adenocard), atropine sulfate

Indications
- Adenosine is used to treat paroxysmal supraventricular tachycardia unresponsive to vagal maneuvers
- Atropine is used to treat symptomatic sinus bradycardia and bradyarrhythmia

Contraindications and precautions
- Adenosine is contraindicated in patients with second- or third-degree AV block and sick sinus syndrome without a pacemaker, atrial fibrillation, atrial flutter, and ventricular tachycardia
- Atropine is contraindicated in patients with glaucoma, urine retention, or ileus

Adverse reactions
- Adenosine may cause transient arrhythmias, dyspnea, and facial flushing
- Atropine may cause hallucinations (with high doses), tachycardia, dry mouth, and constipation

Interactions
- Theophylline and caffeine decrease the effects of adenosine and atropine
- Dipyridamole potentiates the effects of adenosine
- Concurrent use of atropine with quinidine or tricyclic antidepressants causes additive anticholinergic effects

Nursing responsibilities
- Assess for paradoxical bradycardia when administering atropine in low doses or by slow infusion
- **Administer adenosine by rapid I.V. bolus under direct medical supervision to prevent complications; adenosine has a very short half-life**
- Monitor the patient's heart rate, respiratory rate, and blood pressure for signs of complications, such as heart failure and jugular vein distention
- Monitor the ECG for new arrhythmias or exacerbation or resolution of existing one
- Administer antiarrhythmics around the clock, as prescribed, to maintain therapeutic serum drug levels
- Know that I.V. antiarrhythmics must be administered by infusion pump for accuracy
- Teach the patient the purpose of the prescribed antiarrhythmic; emphasize the need to comply with the treatment regimen

ANTIHYPERTENSIVES

CENTRALLY ACTING ADRENERGIC INHIBITORS

Mechanism of action

- Stimulate alpha receptors in the central nervous system (CNS) to inhibit vasoconstriction and cardioacceleration, thus reducing peripheral resistance (commonly given with a diuretic)

Pharmacokinetics

- Absorption: Well absorbed from the GI tract after oral administration and after percutaneous or transdermal topical administration
- Distribution: Widely distributed
- Metabolism: Metabolized in the liver
- Excretion: Excreted in the urine and in feces

Drug examples

- Clonidine (Catapres, Catapres-TTS), guanabenz (Wytensin), guanfacine (Tenex), methyldopa and methyldopate hydrochloride (Aldomet)

Indications

- To treat moderate hypertension

Contraindications and precautions

- Contraindicated in patients with asthma, sinus bradycardia, cardiogenic shock, second- or third-degree heart block, or overt cardiac failure
- Use these drugs cautiously in pregnant or breast-feeding women and in those with severe renal or hepatic impairment

Adverse reactions

- These drugs may cause depression, drowsiness, edema, dry mouth, and impotence
- Clonidine also may cause dizziness and constipation
- Methyldopa and methyldopate hydrochloride also may cause headache, paresthesia, and sleep disturbances

Interactions

- Clonidine may decrease the effectiveness of levodopa
- Use of clonidine with beta-adrenergic-blocking agents, prazosin, or tricyclic antidepressants may block the antihypertensive effect of clonidine and cause life-threatening increases in blood pressure
- Verapamil may cause severe hypotension when given with clonidine or methyldopate hydrochloride
- Use of methyldopa with lithium increases the risk of lithium toxicity
- Use of methyldopa with MAO inhibitors may lead to excessive sympathetic stimulation
- Tricyclic antidepressants may reverse or attenuate the hypotensive effects of methyldopa

Key facts about centrally acting adrenergic inhibitors

- Stimulate alpha receptors in the CNS to inhibit vasoconstriction and cardioacceleration, thus reducing peripheral resistance
- Metabolized by the liver
- Excreted in the urine and feces

When to use centrally acting adrenergic inhibitors

- Moderate hypertension

When NOT to use centrally acting adrenergic inhibitors

- Asthma
- Sinus bradycardia
- Cardiogenic shock
- Second- or third-degree heart block
- Overt cardiac failure

Adverse reactions to watch for

- Depression, drowsiness, edema, dry mouth, impotence

Key nursing actions

- When administering clonidine or methyldopa to patient with history of mental depression, monitor him closely for worsening mental depression.
- Know that methyldopa may darken urine.
- Teach patient to:
  - take clonidine at bedtime
  - use transdermal clonidine properly, if prescribed.

Key facts about peripherally acting adrenergic inhibitors

- Reduce the effects of norepinephrine at peripheral nerve endings to decrease sympathetic vasoconstriction
- Metabolized extensively in the liver
- Excreted mostly in the bile and feces; some is excreted in the urine

When to use peripherally acting adrenergic inhibitors

- Moderate or essential hypertension

When NOT to use peripherally acting adrenergic inhibitors

- Asthma
- Sinus bradycardia
- Cardiogenic shock
- Second- or third-degree heart block
- Overt cardiac failure

Adverse reactions to watch for

- Drowsiness, edema, orthostatic hypotension, diarrhea, nasal stuffiness

- Severe increases in blood pressure may occur if methyldopa is given with nonselective beta-blockers, phenothiazines, sympathomimetics, or barbiturates

Nursing responsibilities

- When administering clonidine or methyldopa to a patient with a history of mental depression, monitor him closely for worsening mental depression
- Instruct the patient to take clonidine at bedtime to minimize orthostatic hypotension
- Teach the patient how to use transdermal clonidine, if prescribed
- Warn the patient taking methyldopa that the drug may darken urine

PERIPHERALLY ACTING ADRENERGIC INHIBITORS

Mechanism of action

- Reduce the effects of norepinephrine at peripheral nerve endings to decrease sympathetic vasoconstriction (commonly given with a diuretic)

Pharmacokinetics

- Absorption: Readily absorbed from the GI tract
- Distribution: Highly protein-bound; doxazosin appears in breast milk
- Metabolism: Extensively metabolized in the liver
- Excretion: Mostly excreted in the bile and feces; some is excreted in the urine

Drug examples

- Doxazosin (Cardura), guanadrel (Hylorel), guanethidine (Ismelin), prazosin (Minipress), reserpine (Serpasil), terazosin (Hytrin)

Indications

- To treat moderate or essential hypertension

Contraindications and precautions

- Contraindicated in patients with asthma, sinus bradycardia, cardiogenic shock, second- or third-degree heart block, or overt cardiac failure
- Use these drugs cautiously in pregnant or breast-feeding women and in those with impaired hepatic function

Adverse reactions

- These drugs may cause drowsiness, edema, orthostatic hypotension, diarrhea, and nasal stuffiness
- Guanethidine also may cause weakness, bradycardia, and ejaculation failure
- Reserpine also may cause depression, GI irritation, and impotence

Interactions

- Use of peripherally acting adrenergic inhibitors with antiarrhythmics may increase the risk of cardiac arrhythmias
- These drugs may decrease the antihypertensive effects of clonidine

- Verapamil and beta blockers may increase the acute postural hypotensive reaction when given with prazosin

Nursing responsibilities

- If the patient taking reserpine has a history of depression, monitor him closely for worsening of mental depression
- Advise the patient to take reserpine with food, milk, or water to minimize GI irritation

Key nursing actions

- If patient taking reserpine has history of mental depression, monitor him closely for worsening of depression.
- Advise patient to take reserpine with food, milk, or water.

PERIPHERAL VASODILATING DRUGS

Mechanism of action

- Exert direct action on arteries alone or on arteries and veins to decrease peripheral vascular resistance (commonly given with a beta-adrenergic blocker)

Pharmacokinetics

- Absorption: Usually administered I.V.
- Distribution: Unknown
- Metabolism: Metabolized rapidly in the tissues and red blood cells
- Excretion: Excreted in the urine

Drug examples

- Diazoxide (Hyperstat I.V.), hydralazine hydrochloride (Apresoline), minoxidil (Loniten), nitroprusside sodium (Nipride)

Indications

- These drugs are used to treat moderate to severe hypertension
- Hydralazine and minoxidil are used to treat severe and essential hypertension
- Diazoxide and nitroprusside sodium are used to treat hypertensive crisis

Contraindications and precautions

- Contraindicated in patients with asthma, sinus bradycardia, cardiogenic shock, second- or third-degree heart block, or overt cardiac failure
- Use these drugs cautiously in pregnant or breast-feeding women and in those with impaired hepatic function

Adverse reactions

- These drugs may cause fluid retention, tachycardia, orthostatic hypotension, severe hypotension (with I.V. doses), and nausea
- Minoxidil also can cause excessive hair growth

Interactions

- Antihypertensives, general anesthetics, and sildenafil may potentiate antihypertensive effects of nitroprusside
- Concurrent use of these drugs with pressor agents may increase blood pressure

Key facts about peripheral vasodilating drugs

- Exert direct action on arteries alone or on arteries and veins to decrease peripheral vascular resistance
- Metabolized rapidly in the tissues and red blood cells
- Excreted in the urine

When to use peripheral vasodilating drugs

- Moderate to severe hypertension
- Essential hypertension
- Hypertensive crisis

When NOT to use peripheral vasodilating drugs

- Asthma
- Sinus bradycardia
- Cardiogenic shock
- Second- or third-degree heart block
- Overt cardiac failure

Adverse reactions to watch for

- Fluid retention, tachycardia, orthostatic hypotension, severe hypotension (with I.V. doses), and nausea

Nursing responsibilities

- **Closely monitor the patient for fluid volume excess; monitor the patient's blood pressure every 5 minutes at the start of the infusion and at least every 15 minutes during the infusion**
- Weigh the patient daily, and record daily intake and output
- Auscultate breath sounds for crackles
- Observe for jugular vein distention and peripheral edema
- Advise the patient taking minoxidil that excessive hair growth is likely to occur 3 to 6 months after therapy begins; reassure the patient that the extra growth should disappear 1 to 6 months after therapy ends

BETA-ADRENERGIC BLOCKERS

Mechanism of action

- Compete with epinephrine for beta-adrenergic receptor sites; inhibit the response to beta-adrenergic stimulation, thereby decreasing cardiac output

Pharmacokinetics

- Absorption: Partially absorbed
- Distribution: Distributed in the tissues
- Metabolism: Minimally metabolized in the liver
- Excretion: Excreted primarily in the urine and partially in the feces

Drug examples

- Acebutolol (Sectral), atenolol (Tenormin), betaxolol (Kerlone), carteolol (Cartrol), labetalol (Normodyne, Trandate), metoprolol (Lopressor), nadolol (Corgard), penbutolol (Levatol), pindolol (Visken), propranolol (Inderal), timolol (Blocadren)

Indications

- To treat mild hypertension

Contraindications and precautions

- Contraindicated in patients with asthma, sinus bradycardia, cardiogenic shock, second- or third-degree heart block, or overt cardiac failure
- Use these drugs cautiously in pregnant or breast-feeding women and in those with impaired hepatic function

Adverse reactions

- Bradycardia, orthostatic hypotension, fatigue, nausea, vomiting

Interactions

- These drugs cause additive hypotension when used concurrently with alcohol, antihypertensives, other beta-adrenergic blockers, or calcium channel blockers
- Use of thioridazine with pindolol may prolong the QT interval and increase the risk of fatal arrhythmias

Key nursing actions

- Closely monitor patient for fluid volume excess; monitor patient's blood pressure every 5 minutes at start of infusion and at least every 15 minutes during infusion.
- Weigh patient daily, and record daily intake and output.
- Auscultate breath sounds for crackles.
- Observe for jugular vein distention and peripheral edema.

Key facts about beta-adrenergic blockers

- Compete with epinephrine for beta-adrenergic receptor sites; inhibit the response to beta-adrenergic stimulation, thereby decreasing cardiac output
- Minimally metabolized in the liver
- Excreted primarily in the urine and partially in the feces

When to use beta-adrenergic blockers

- Mild hypertension

When NOT to use beta-adrenergic blockers

- Asthma
- Sinus bradycardia
- Cardiogenic shock
- Second- or third-degree heart block
- Overt cardiac failure

Adverse reactions to watch for

- Bradycardia, orthostatic hypotension, fatigue, nausea, vomiting

Nursing responsibilities

- Warn the patient not to stop taking the drug abruptly; this can exacerbate angina or precipitate an MI
- Administer propranolol consistently with meals; food may increase absorption

Key nursing actions

- Don't discontinue drug abruptly.
- Give propranolol with food.

ANGIOTENSIN-CONVERTING ENZYME (ACE) INHIBITORS

Mechanism of action

- Block conversion of angiotensin I to angiotensin II, preventing peripheral vasoconstriction

Key facts about ACE inhibitors

- Block conversion of angiotensin I to angiotensin II, preventing peripheral vasoconstriction
- Metabolized extensively in the liver
- Excreted in the urine and feces

Pharmacokinetics

- Absorption: About 60% is absorbed from the GI tract
- Distribution: Unknown
- Metabolism: Extensively metabolized in the liver
- Excretion: Excreted in the urine and feces

Drug examples

- Benazepril (Lotensin), captopril (Capoten), enalapril (Vasotec), fosinopril (Monopril), lisinopril (Prinivil, Zestril), moexipril (Univasc), quinapril (Accupril), ramipril (Altace)

Indications

- To treat mild hypertension
- Ramipril also is used to treat heart failure after a myocardial infarction (MI) and to reduce the risk of MI, stroke, and death from cardiovascular causes

When to use ACE inhibitors

- Mild hypertension
- Heart failure after MI
- Risk of MI, stroke, and death

Contraindications and precautions

- Contraindicated in patients with asthma, sinus bradycardia, cardiogenic shock, second- or third-degree heart block, or overt cardiac failure
- Use these drugs cautiously in pregnant or breast-feeding women and in those with impaired hepatic function
- Use cautiously and at a reduced dose in patients with renal impairment

When NOT to use ACE inhibitors

- Asthma
- Sinus bradycardia
- Cardiogenic shock
- Second- or third-degree heart block
- Overt cardiac failure

Adverse reactions

- Dizziness, light-headedness, fainting, tachycardia, palpitations, rash; proteinuria (captopril)

Adverse reactions to watch for

- Dizziness, light-headedness, fainting, tachycardia, palpitations, rash, proteinuria

Interactions

- Antihypertensives, diuretics, and phenothiazines increase antihypertensive effects
- Aspirin and NSAIDs decrease the hypotensive effects
- ACE inhibitors will increase hypoglycemic effects if used with insulin and oral antidiabetics
- Concurrent use with potassium-sparing diuretics and potassium supplements should be avoided because ACE inhibitors may increase diuretic effects and increase the risk of hyperkalemia

Key nursing actions

- Administer captopril on empty stomach.
- Monitor patient taking captopril for proteinuria every 2 to 4 weeks for first 3 months.
- Teach patient to report light-headedness and avoid sudden position changes.

Key facts about calcium channel blockers

- Dilate vessels by blocking the slow channel, preventing calcium from entering the cell
- Metabolized in the liver
- Excreted in the urine

When to use calcium channel blockers

- Mild hypertension

When NOT to use calcium channel blockers

- Asthma
- Sinus bradycardia
- Cardiogenic shock
- Second- or third-degree heart block
- Overt cardiac failure

Adverse reactions to watch for

- Dizziness, AV blocks, headache, edema, flushing, nausea

Key nursing actions

- Know that nifedipine may be given sublingually.
- Warn patient not to stop drug abruptly.

Nursing responsibilities

- Administer captopril on an empty stomach, preferably 1 hour before meals, for maximum effectiveness
- Monitor the patient taking captopril for proteinuria every 2 to 4 weeks for the first 3 months of therapy to detect decreased renal function
- Tell the patient to report light-headedness, especially in the first few days of starting therapy, so dosage may be adjusted
- Advise the patient to avoid sudden position changes to minimize orthostatic hypotension

CALCIUM CHANNEL BLOCKERS

Mechanism of action

- Dilate vessels by blocking the slow channel, preventing calcium from entering the cell

Pharmacokinetics

- Absorption: Absorbed rapidly and completely from the GI tract after oral administration
- Distribution: About 90% is protein-bound
- Metabolism: Metabolized in the liver; goes through first-pass metabolism
- Excretion: Excreted in the urine as unchanged drug and active metabolites

Drug examples

- Amlodipine (Norvasc), diltiazem (Cardizem, Carizem LA), felodipine (Plendil), isradipine (DynaCirc), nicardipine (Cardene), nifedipine (Procardia), nisoldipine (Sular), verapamil (Calan, Isoptin SR)

Indications

- To treat mild hypertension

Contraindications and precautions

- Contraindicated in patients with asthma, sinus bradycardia, cardiogenic shock, second- or third-degree heart block, or overt cardiac failure
- Use these drugs cautiously in pregnant or breast-feeding women and in those with impaired hepatic function

Adverse reactions

- Dizziness, AV blocks, headache, edema, flushing, nausea

Interactions

- Increase risk of digoxin toxicity when used with digoxin
- May cause heart blocks when used with other calcium channel blockers

Nursing responsibilities

- Know that nifedipine may be given sublingually
  - The patient can puncture the end of the capsule and squeeze the liquid under the tongue
  - Some institutions vary in this policy and the patient may be asked to swallow the capsule after sublingual dosing

- Warn the patient not to stop the drug abruptly; gradually reducing the dosage under physician supervision helps prevent rebound hypertension

DIURETICS

Mechanism of action
- Inhibit sodium and chloride reabsorption, thereby increasing urine output and decreasing edema, circulating blood volume, and cardiac output

Pharmacokinetics
- See Chapter 9 for the pharmacokinetics of specific types of diuretics

Drug examples
- Chlorothiazide (Diuril), chlorthalidone (Hygroton), furosemide (Lasix), hydrochlorothiazide (Esidrix, HydroDIURIL, Oretic), indapamide (Lozol), metolazone (Diulo, Mykrox, Zaroxolyn)

Indications
- To treat mild hypertension

Contraindications and precautions
- Contraindicated in patients with asthma, sinus bradycardia, cardiogenic shock, second- or third-degree heart block, or overt cardiac failure
- Use these drugs cautiously in pregnant or breast-feeding women and in those with impaired hepatic function

Adverse reactions
- Fatigue, dizziness, orthostatic hypotension, rash, hypokalemia, hyperglycemia

Interactions
- Concurrent use with similar-acting drugs and alcohol causes additive hypotension
- Concurrent use with antidepressants, antihistamines, appetite suppressants, decongestants, NSAIDs, and sympathomimetic bronchodilators may reduce the effects of antihypertensives

Nursing responsibilities
- Monitor the patient's vital signs and assess for risk factors for hypertension
- Teach the patient about the importance of complying with therapy (for more information, see *Managing antihypertensive therapy,* page 138)
- Instruct the patient not to take a double dose after missing a dose
- Warn the patient not to stop the drug abruptly because this may cause rebound hypertension
- Teach the patient to monitor blood pressure weekly (to help determine drug effectiveness) and to watch for weight gain and peripheral edema (to detect fluid retention)
- Advise the patient to change position slowly to minimize orthostatic hypotension

Key facts about diuretics
- Inhibit sodium and chloride reabsorption
- Increase urine output
- Decrease edema, circulating blood volume, and cardiac output
- Varied metabolism and excretion

When to use diuretics
- Mild hypertension

When NOT to use diuretics
- Asthma
- Sinus bradycardia
- Cardiogenic shock
- Second- or third-degree heart block
- Overt cardiac failure

Adverse reactions to watch for
- Fatigue, dizziness, orthostatic hypotension, rash, hypokalemia, hyperglycemia

Key nursing actions
- Instruct patient not to take double dose after missing a dose.
- Warn patient not to stop drug abruptly.
- Teach patient to monitor blood pressure weekly and to watch for weight gain and peripheral edema.
- Instruct patient to avoid hot baths and showers.
- Caution patient not to consume excessive amounts of coffee, tea, or cola.

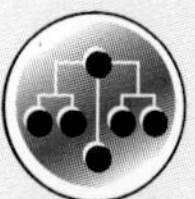

GO WITH THE FLOW

Managing antihypertensive therapy

The flowchart below is based on the approach to antihypertensive therapy endorsed by the Joint National Committee on the Detection, Evaluation, and Treatment of High Blood Pressure.

DIAGNOSIS OF HYPERTENSION SUSPECTED AND CONFIRMED

1

- Obtain baseline blood pressure readings
- Instruct patient in lifestyle modifications (weight reduction, moderate alcohol intake, regular physical activity, reduction of sodium intake, smoking cessation)

Adequate response?

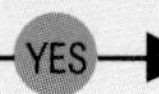

YES → Continue therapy and monitoring

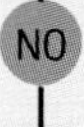

NO ↓

2

- Continue instructions for lifestyle modifications; enlist aid of family members and support groups
- Prepare patient to begin drug therapy regimen
- Anticipate use of thiazide-type diuretics, ACE inhibitor, angiotensin receptor blocker (ARB), beta-adrenergic blocker (BB), calcium channel blocker (CCB), or a combination for stage 1 hypertension in the absence of compelling indications (see below)
- Instruct patient in drug therapy regimen
- Continue monitoring blood pressure
- Assess for signs and symptoms of adverse effects
- Anticipate use of a two-drug combination (usually a thiazide-type diuretic and an ACE inhibitor, ARB, BB, or CCB) for stage 2 hypertension in the absence of compelling indications (see below)
- Anticipate use of the following drugs if the patient has any of these compelling indications: heart failure – diuretic, BB, ACE inhibitor, ARB, or aldosterone antagonist; post MI – BB, ACE inhibitor, or aldosterone antagonist; high coronary disease risk – diuretic, BB, ACE inhibitor, or CCB; diabetes – diuretic, BB, ACE inhibitor, ARB, or CCB; chronic kidney disease – ACE inhibitor or ARB; recurrent stroke prevention – diuretic or ACE inhibitor

Adequate response?

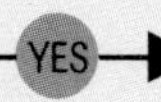

YES → Continue therapy and monitoring

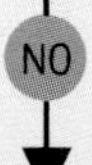

NO ↓

3

- Anticipate change in drug therapy regimen (addition of second or third antihypertensive, addition of diuretic if not already prescribed)
- Instruct patient in new drug therapy regimen; reinforce previous instructions
- Continue monitoring blood pressure
- Assess for signs and symptoms of adverse effects

Source: U.S. Department of Health and Human Services, National Institutes of Health, National Heart, Lung, and Blood Institute (2003). *The Seventh Report of the Joint National Committee on Detection, Evaluation, and Treatment of High Blood Pressure (JNC 7)*. Washington, D.C.: Government Printing Office.

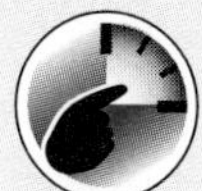

TIME-OUT FOR TEACHING

Teaching about antihypertensives

Include these topics in your teaching plan for the patient receiving an antihypertensive.

- Medication therapy regimen, including the drug's name, dose, frequency, duration, and possible adverse effects
- Signs and symptoms of possible adverse effects and when to notify the physician
- Continuation of drug even if the patient feels better
- Need for adequate drug supply and instructions for missed doses
- Dietary restrictions, including fluid and sodium restrictions as appropriate
- Weight monitoring
- Safety measures, including avoiding sudden position changes, driving, or hazardous activities until effects of drug are known, and avoiding physical exertion, especially in hot weather
- Avoidance of over-the-counter medications unless permitted by the physician
- Lifestyle modifications
- Measures to ensure compliance with therapy
- Medical follow-up

- Instruct the patient to avoid hot baths and showers, which can lead to hypotension
- Caution the patient not to consume excessive amounts of coffee, tea, or cola; these stimulants may interfere with blood pressure control and drug effectiveness
- Encourage the patient to comply with additional antihypertensive interventions, such as weight reduction, low-sodium diet, smoking cessation, regular exercise, stress management, and alcohol restrictions
- Instruct the patient to notify the physician if intolerable adverse effects occur (for specific teaching tips, see *Teaching about antihypertensives*)

Topics for patient discussion

- Therapy regimen
- Signs and symptoms of possible adverse effects and when to notify physician
- Continuation of drug even if the patient feels better
- Need for adequate drug supply
- Dietary restrictions
- Weight monitoring
- Safety measures
- Physician permission before taking over-the-counter drugs
- Lifestyle modifications
- Need for compliance with therapy
- Medical follow-up

ANTIANGINALS

NITRATES

Mechanism of action

- Produce vasodilation, decrease preload and afterload, and reduce myocardial oxygen consumption

Pharmacokinetics

- Absorption: Nitroglycerin is well absorbed in the GI tract, but it undergoes first-pass metabolism, so it's incompletely absorbed systemically
  - Completely absorbed after sublingual (S.L.) administration
  - Well absorbed after topical administration

Key facts about nitrates

- Produce vasodilation, decrease preload and afterload, and reduce myocardial oxygen consumption
- Metabolized in the liver
- Excreted in the urine

- Distribution: Widely distributed throughout the body; about 60% protein-bound
- Metabolism: Metabolized in the liver
- Excretion: Excreted in the urine

Drug examples

- Erythrityl tetranitrate (Cardilate), isosorbide dinitrate (Isordil, Sorbitrate), isosorbide mononitrate (ISMO), nitroglycerin (Nitro-Bid, Nitrodisc, Nitro-Dur, Nitrolingual, Nitrostat, Nitro-Time. Transderm-Nitro), pentaerythritol tetranitrate (Peritrate)

Indications

- These drugs are used in the treatment and prophylactic management of acute angina
- Erythrityl is used to prevent expected and chronic anginal attacks
- Pentaerythritol is used only for long-term prevention of angina
- Nitroglycerin is also administered I.V. to treat surgical hypertension

Contraindications and precautions

- Contraindicated in patients hypersensitive to nitrates and in those with early MI, severe anemia, increased intracranial pressure, angle-closure glaucoma, orthostatic hypotension, or cardiac tamponade (I.V. form)
- Use cautiously in patients with hypotension or volume depletion

Adverse reactions

- Most common adverse reaction to nitrates is headache
- May also cause dizziness, orthostatic hypotension, tachycardia, flushing, palpitations, nausea, and vomiting

Interactions

- Antihypertensives, phenothiazines, and sildenafil may increase hypotensive effects
- Use of nitrates with ergot alkaloids may precipitate angina

Nursing responsibilities

- Know that nitroglycerin is available in several forms, including I.V., S.L. tablet, sustained-release capsule, sustained-release buccal capsule, and transdermal ointment or patch
- Teach the patient about proper use and storage of nitroglycerin S.L. tablets
- Instruct the patient to sit down and take the drug at the first sign of an acute angina attack
- Teach the patient to repeat the dose if no relief occurs in 5 minutes and to seek emergency medical help if no relief occurs after taking 3 tablets in 15 minutes
- Advise the patient that S.L. tablets may be taken at the onset of activities known to cause angina, such as sexual activity
- Advise the patient to discard unused tablets and replace them with fresh ones every 3 months

When to use nitrates

- Acute angina
- Prevention of expected and chronic anginal attacks
- Long-term prevention of angina
- Surgical hypertension

When NOT to use nitrates

- Hypersensitivity to these drugs
- Early MI
- Severe anemia
- Increased intracranial pressure
- Angle-closure glaucoma
- Orthostatic hypotension
- Cardiac tamponade

Adverse reactions to watch for

- Headache, dizziness, orthostatic hypotension, tachycardia, flushing, palpitations, nausea, vomiting

Key nursing actions

- Know that nitroglycerin is available in several forms.
- Teach patient about proper use of nitroglycerin S.L. tablets.
- Teach patient to repeat dose if no relief occurs in 5 minutes and to seek emergency medical help if no relief occurs after taking 3 tablets in 15 minutes.
- Inform patient that headache is common adverse effect of nitrates and typically subsides with continued therapy.
- Advise patient to avoid alcoholic beverages.
- Know that tolerance may develop.

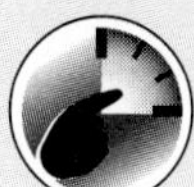

TIME-OUT FOR TEACHING

Teaching about nitrates

Include these topics in your teaching plan for the patient receiving a nitrate.

- Medication therapy regimen, including the drug's name, dose, frequency, duration, and possible adverse effects
- Forms of drug available and type prescribed
- Signs and symptoms of possible adverse effects and when to notify the physician
- Safety and emergency measures
- Application and administration techniques
- Measures to relieve common adverse effects, such as headache and orthostatic blood pressure
- Skin-care measures if topical drugs are used
- Cardiopulmonary resuscitation training
- Storage guidelines
- Dietary restrictions
- Need for compliance with therapy, including taking drug as prescribed
- Follow-up care

Topics for patient discussion

- Therapy regimen
- Forms of drug available
- Signs and symptoms of possible adverse effects and when to notify the physician
- Safety and emergency measures
- Administration techniques
- Relief of adverse effects
- Skin-care measures
- CPR training
- Storage guidelines
- Dietary restrictions
- Need for compliance with therapy
- Follow-up care

- Inform the patient that headache is a common adverse effect of nitrates and typically subsides with continued therapy; advise him to take aspirin or acetaminophen for headache relief (for specific teaching tips, see *Teaching about nitrates*)
- Teach the patient how to apply a transdermal patch or ointment, if prescribed; instruct him to remove the patch or ointment at bedtime to avoid tolerance
- Advise the patient to avoid alcoholic beverages; these can increase hypotension
- Know that tolerance may develop and a nitrate-free period of 8 to 12 hours may be prescribed

CALCIUM CHANNEL BLOCKERS

Mechanism of action

- Dilate coronary and peripheral arteries and prevent coronary vasospasm

Pharmacokinetics

- Absorption: Absorbed rapidly and completely from the GI tract after oral administration
- Distribution: About 90% is protein-bound
- Metabolism: Metabolized in the liver; goes through first-pass metabolism
- Excretion: Excreted in the urine as unchanged drug and active metabolites

Key facts about calcium channel blockers

- Dilate coronary and peripheral arteries and prevent coronary vasospasm
- Metabolized in the liver
- Excreted unchanged in the urine

When to use calcium channel blockers

- Stable and unstable angina
- Vasospastic angina

When NOT to use calcium channel blockers

- Asthma
- Sinus bradycardia
- Cardiogenic shock
- Second- or third-degree heart block
- Overt cardiac failure

Adverse reactions to watch for

- Reflex increase in heart rate, peripheral edema, constipation, dizziness, bradycardia, ventricular arrhythmias

Key nursing actions

- If patient's systolic pressure is less than 90 mm Hg or heart rate is less than 60 beats/minute, withhold dose and notify physician.
- Monitor patient for signs and symptoms of heart failure.
- Teach patient about need to continue concurrent nitrate therapy, if prescribed.

Key facts about beta-adrenergic blockers

- Reduce myocardial oxygen demands
- Minimally metabolized in the liver
- Excreted mostly in the urine and partially in the feces

Drug examples
- Bepridil (Vascor), diltiazem (Cardizem), nicardipine (Cardene), nifedipine (Procardia), verapamil (Calan, Isoptin SR)

Indications
- Stable and unstable angina, vasospastic angina (Prinzmetal's angina)
- Bepridil is used for patients who don't respond to other antianginals

Contraindications and precautions
- Contraindicated in patients with asthma, sinus bradycardia, cardiogenic shock, second- or third-degree heart block, and overt cardiac failure
- Use cautiously in pregnant or breast-feeding women and in those with impaired hepatic function

Adverse reactions
- Nifedipine may cause a reflex increase in heart rate and peripheral edema
- Diltiazem and verapamil may cause constipation, dizziness, and bradycardia
- Bepridil may cause ventricular arrhythmias

Interactions
- May increase risk of digoxin toxicity when used with digoxin
- May cause heart blocks when used with other calcium channel blockers

Nursing responsibilities
- Administer diltiazem before meals
- **If patient's systolic pressure is less than 90 mm Hg or heart rate is less than 60 beats/minute, withhold dose and notify the physician**
- Monitor the patient for signs and symptoms of heart failure, such as swelling of hands and feet and shortness of breath
- Teach the patient about the need to continue concurrent nitrate therapy, if prescribed

BETA-ADRENERGIC BLOCKERS

Mechanism of action
- Reduce myocardial oxygen demands by slowing the heart rate and decreasing the force of myocardial contractions

Pharmacokinetics
- Absorption: Partially absorbed
- Distribution: Distributed in the tissues
- Metabolism: Minimally metabolized in the liver
- Excretion: Excreted primarily in the urine and partially in the feces

Drug examples
- Atenolol (Tenormin), metoprolol (Lopressor), nadolol (Corgard), propranolol (Inderal)

Indications
- Angina pectoris

Contraindications and precautions

- Contraindicated in patients with hypotension or uncorrected hypovolemia
- Use cautiously in patients with hypoglycemia or diabetes because beta-adrenergic blockers may mask signs and symptoms of hypoglycemia
- Withdraw these drugs slowly; abrupt withdrawal may exacerbate symptoms of hyperthyroidism or cause a thyroid storm

Adverse reactions

- Flushing, headache, orthostatic hypotension

Interactions

- Produce additive hypotensive effects when used concurrently with alcohol, antihypertensives, other beta-adrenergic blockers, or calcium channel blockers

Nursing responsibilities

- Assess the location, duration, and intensity of anginal pain (signs and symptoms of angina resemble those of myocardial infarction)
- Assess the patient's vital signs regularly, and monitor the ECG for changes in heart rate or rhythm
- Monitor blood pressure and the intensity and duration of the patient's response to the drug
- Assess for factors that precipitate angina
- Teach the patient to change position slowly to minimize orthostatic hypotension
- Caution the patient to avoid hot baths or showers, which can lead to hypotension
- Warn the patient not to consume alcohol, which can lead to additive hypotension
- Observe for tolerance (tachyphylaxis)

When to use beta-adrenergic blockers

- Angina pectoris

When NOT to use beta-adrenergic blockers

- Hypotension
- Uncorrected hypovolemia

Adverse reactions to watch for

- Flushing, headache, orthostatic hypotension

Key nursing actions

- Assess location, duration, and intensity of anginal pain.
- Assess vital signs regularly and monitor ECG, blood pressure, and intensity and duration of patient's response to drug.
- Teach patient to change position slowly.
- Caution patient to avoid hot baths or showers.
- Warn patient to avoid alcohol.
- Observe for tolerance.

ANTILIPEMICS

BILE ACID SEQUESTRANTS

Mechanism of action

- Bind bile acids in the GI tract to form an insoluble complex that is excreted, thereby increasing cholesterol clearance and lowering serum low-density lipoprotein (LDL) levels

Pharmacokinetics

- Absorption: Adsorb bile from the GI tract
- Distribution: None
- Metabolism: None
- Excretion: Excreted unchanged 100% in the feces

Key facts about bile acid sequestrants

- Bind bile acids in the GI tract to form an insoluble complex that is excreted, thereby increasing cholesterol clearance and lowering serum LDL levels
- Excreted unchanged 100% in the feces

When to use bile acid sequestrants

- Hyperlipoproteinemia
- Pruritus associated with partial biliary obstruction

When NOT to use bile acid sequestrants

- Hypersensitivity to these drugs
- Complete biliary obstruction

Adverse reactions to watch for

- Constipation with fecal impaction, flatulence, nausea, heartburn

Key nursing actions

- Instruct patient to take drug before meals and at least 1 hour before or 4 to 6 hours after taking another drug.
- Monitor serum cholesterol, triglyceride, and liver enzyme levels during first 6 months.
- Instruct patient to follow recommended diet and exercise program, avoid alcohol, and stop smoking.

Key facts about HMG-CoA reductase inhibitors

- Block HMG-CoA reductase in the liver, preventing cholesterol synthesis
- Reduce serum cholesterol and LDL levels
- Metabolized extensively in the liver
- Excreted in bile

Drug examples

- Cholestyramine (Questran), colesevelam hydrochloride (WelChol), colestipol (Colestid)

Indications

- To treat hyperlipoproteinemia
- Cholestyramine also is used to relieve pruritus associated with partial biliary obstruction

Contraindications and precautions

- Contraindicated in patients hypersensitive to bile acid–sequestering resins or components of the drugs and in patients with complete biliary obstruction
- Diseases contributing to increased blood cholesterol level should be treated before starting bile acid sequestrant therapy

Adverse reactions

- The most common adverse reaction is constipation, which sometimes may be accompanied by fecal impaction, flatulence, nausea, and heartburn
- These drugs may also increase liver function test values and cause malabsorption of fat-soluble vitamins, such as vitamins A, D, E, K, and folic acid

Interactions

- Bile acid sequestrants may bind orally administered drugs and vitamins and counteract their effectiveness

Nursing responsibilities

- Instruct the patient to take the drug before meals and at least 1 hour before or 4 to 6 hours after taking another drug
- Tell the patient to mix the powder form with beverages
- Advise the patient to swallow colestipol tablets whole and not to crush, chew, or cut them
- Monitor the patient's serum cholesterol, triglyceride, and liver enzyme levels periodically during the first 6 months of therapy
- As appropriate, instruct the patient to follow his recommended diet and to restrict intake of fats, cholesterol, carbohydrates, and alcohol; to stop smoking; and to follow a recommended exercise program
- Suggest a laxative, stool softener, or increased fluid and fiber intake to prevent constipation

HMG-CoA REDUCTASE INHIBITORS

Mechanism of action

- Block 3-hydroxy-3-methylglutaryl (HMG) CoA reductase in the liver, preventing cholesterol synthesis; reduce serum cholesterol and LDL levels

Pharmacokinetics

- Absorption: Rapidly absorbed

- Distribution: More than 90% protein-bound, except for pravastatin, which is 50% protein bound
- Metabolism: Extensively metabolized by the liver; some of the metabolites exhibit pharmacologic activity
- Excretion: Excreted in bile

Drug examples

- Atorvastatin (Lipitor), fluvastatin (Lescol), lovastatin (Mevacor), pravastatin (Pravachol), simvastatin (Zocor)

Indications

- To treat hyperlipoproteinemia, hypercholesterolemia, and hypertriglyceridemia
- To reduce serum levels of LDL, cholesterol, and triglycerides
- To increase serum levels of high-density lipoproteins (HDLs)
- **Except for atorvastatin, these drugs are also used as secondary prevention of cardiovascular events**

Contraindications and precautions

- Contraindicated in patients who are hypersensitive to components of these drugs, in those with active liver disease or unexplained and persistent elevated liver function test results, and in pregnant or breast-feeding women
- Secondary causes of hyperlipidemia should be ruled out before starting therapy

Adverse reactions

- May cause headaches, insomnia, photosensitivity, blurred vision, progression of cataracts, nausea, vomiting, diarrhea, abdominal cramps, constipation, flatulence, and dyspepsia
- **May cause rhabdomyolysis, myalgia, myopathy, and hypersensitivity reactions**

Interactions

- Concurrent use of gemfibrozil and fibric acid derivatives with lovastatin may cause severe rhabdomyolysis and myopathy
- Use with cyclosporine, erythromycin, and nicotinic acid may increase the risk of rhabdomyolysis and myopathy
- Concurrent use of lovastatin and simvastatin with warfarin increases the effects of warfarin
- May increase digoxin levels

Nursing responsibilities

- **Initiate therapy with HMG-CoA reductase inhibitors only after diet therapy has proven ineffective; the patient should be on a standard cholesterol-lowering diet during therapy**
- **Give lovastatin with the evening meal; absorption is enhanced and cholesterol biosynthesis is greater in the evening**
- **Fluvastatin, pravastatin, and simvastatin are usually administered at bedtime, without regard to food**

When to use HMG-CoA reductase inhibitors

- Hyperlipoproteinemia, hypercholesterolemia, hypertriglycerideremia
- Reduction of serum levels of LDLs, cholesterol, and triglycerides
- Increase in serum levels of HDLs
- Secondary prevention of cardiovascular events

When NOT to use HMG-CoA reductase inhibitors

- Hypersensitivity to these drugs
- Active liver disease
- Elevated liver function test results
- Pregnancy
- Breast-feeding

Adverse reactions to watch for

- Headaches, insomnia, photosensitivity, blurred vision, progression of cataracts, nausea, vomiting, diarrhea, abdominal cramps, constipation, flatulence, dyspepsia, rhabdomyolysis, myalgia, myopathy, hypersensitivity reactions

Key nursing actions

- Start these drugs only after diet therapy has proven ineffective.
- Give lovastatin with the evening meal; fluvastatin, pravastatin, and simvastatin are usually administered at bedtime.
- Advise patient to avoid alcohol.
- Monitor liver function test results frequently at start of therapy and periodically thereafter.

TIME-OUT FOR TEACHING

Teaching about HMG-CoA reductase inhibitors

Include these topics in your teaching plan for the patient receiving an HMG-CoA reductase inhibitor.

- Medication therapy regimen, including the drug's name, dose, frequency, duration, and possible adverse effects
- Signs and symptoms of possible adverse effects and when to notify the physician
- Dietary modifications
- Need for compliance with therapy, including taking drug as prescribed
- Follow-up care, including laboratory tests and physician visits

- Monitor liver function tests frequently at the start of therapy and periodically thereafter
- Advise the patient to restrict alcohol intake
- Teach the patient about proper dietary management (restricting total fat and cholesterol intake), weight control, and exercise; explain their importance in controlling elevated serum lipid levels (for specific teaching tips, see *Teaching about HMG-CoA reductase inhibitors*)

MISCELLANEOUS ANTILIPEMICS

Mechanism of action

- These drugs decrease hepatic synthesis or accelerate breakdown of LDLs
- Niacin increases serum HDL levels and reduces the serum levels of LDLs, phospholipids, and very-low-density lipoproteins

Pharmacokinetics

- Absorption: Well absorbed in the GI tract
- Distribution: Peak plasma levels vary with each drug; fenofibrate is 99% protein-bound
- Metabolism: Metabolism varies with each drug
- Excretion: Excreted in the urine

Drug examples

- Clofibrate (Atromid-S), fenofibrate (Tricor), gemfibrozil (Lopid), niacin (vitamin B_3, [Nicobid, Nicolar, Nicotinex])

Indications

- As adjunct therapy to diet in patients with hypertriglyceridemia and hypercholesterolemia
- To reduce serum levels of LDL, cholesterol, and triglycerides and to increase serum levels of HDL
- Gemfibrozil is also used with diet therapy to reduce the risk of coronary heart disease

Topics for patient discussion

- Therapy regimen
- Signs and symptoms of possible adverse effects and when to notify the physician
- Dietary modifications
- Need for compliance with therapy
- Follow-up care

Key facts about antilipemics

- Decrease hepatic synthesis or accelerate breakdown of LDLs
- Increase serum HDL levels and reduce serum levels of LDLs, phospholipids, and very-low-density lipoproteins
- Metabolism varies with each drug
- Excreted in the urine

When to use antilipemics

- As adjunct in hypertriglyceridemia and hypercholesterolemia
- Reduction of LDL, cholesterol, and triglyceride levels
- Increase in HDL levels
- Reduction of coronary heart disease risk

- **Contraindications and precautions**
  - Contraindicated in patients hypersensitive to these drugs or components of these drugs
  - Also contraindicated in patients with hepatic or severe renal dysfunction, including primary biliary cirrhosis, unexplained and persistent liver function abnormalities, or preexisting gallbladder disease
  - Treatment must be discontinued if gallstones develop during therapy
- **Adverse reactions**
  - May cause diarrhea, abdominal pain, epigastric pain, nausea, vomiting, dyspepsia, pancreatitis, cholelithiasis, hyperglycemia, and hypersensitivity reactions, including severe rashes and urticaria
  - May increase liver enzyme levels
- **Interactions**
  - Use with oral anticoagulants may increase the anticoagulant effect
  - Use of clofibrate and gemfibrozil with sulfonylureas may increase hypoglycemic effects
  - Use with HMG-CoA reductase inhibitors may cause rhabdomyolysis and myopathy
  - Cyclosporine levels may increase or decrease, depending on the antilipemic used
- **Nursing responsibilities**
  - Monitor the patient's serum cholesterol, triglyceride, and liver enzyme levels periodically during the first 6 months of therapy
  - Instruct the patient to take the drug with the evening meal to enhance its effectiveness
  - As appropriate, instruct the patient to follow his recommended diet and to restrict intake of fats, cholesterol, carbohydrates, and alcohol; to stop smoking; and to follow a recommended exercise program
  - Inform the patient that abdominal pain, diarrhea, nausea, and vomiting may occur; urge the patient to notify his physician if these symptoms become pronounced or continue for a prolonged period

When NOT to use antilipemics

- Hypersensitivity to these drugs
- Hepatic or severe renal dysfunction

Adverse reactions to watch for

- Diarrhea, abdominal pain, epigastric pain, nausea, vomiting, dyspepsia, pancreatitis, cholelithiasis, hyperglycemia, hypersensitivity reactions, increased liver enzyme levels

Key nursing actions

- Monitor patient's serum cholesterol, triglyceride, and liver enzyme levels during first 6 months.
- Instruct patient to take drug with evening meal.
- Instruct patient to follow his recommended diet and exercise program, avoid alcohol, and stop smoking.
- Inform patient that abdominal pain, diarrhea, nausea, and vomiting may occur; urge him to notify physician if these symptoms become pronounced or continue for prolonged period.

NCLEX CHECKS

It's never too soon to begin your NCLEX preparation. Now that you've reviewed this chapter, carefully read each of the following questions and choose the best answer. Then compare your responses to the correct answers.

1. A 78-year-old patient is hospitalized and receives I.V. digoxin (Lanoxin). You would withhold the drug and notify the physician if the patient's:

☐ **A.** pulse rate is 54 beats/minute.
☐ **B.** history reveals liver failure.
☐ **C.** blood pressure is 72/40 mm Hg.
☐ **D.** respiratory rate is less than 14 breaths/minute.

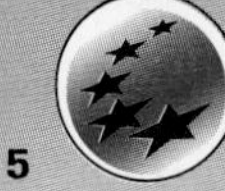

TOP 5

Items to study for your next test on drugs and the cardiovascular system

1. Indications for inotropic drugs, antiarrhythmics, antihypertensives, and antianginals
2. Mechanisms of action of cardiac drugs and antilipemics
3. Common adverse effects of cardiac drugs and antilipemics
4. Nursing responsibilities when administering a cardiac drug or an antilipemic
5. Appropriate teaching for the patient who is receiving a cardiac drug or an antilipemic

2. A patient is receiving digoxin (Lanoxin) for the treatment of atrial flutter. When you enter the room to give the medication, you find the patient is irritable and complaining of nausea and blurred vision. She is also disoriented to place and time. Your most appropriate action at this time is to:

☐ **A.** try to reorient the patient while helping her take the digoxin.
☐ **B.** return to the room later and see if the patient will take the digoxin.
☐ **C.** withhold the digoxin and notify the physician about your assessment findings.
☐ **D.** check the medication profile for possible drug interactions after giving the digoxin to the patient.

3. Which of the following statements regarding antiarrhythmics is most accurate?

☐ **A.** Antiarrhythmics act by decreasing myocardial contractility and oxygen demand.
☐ **B.** Most antiarrhythmics commonly are prescribed across the life span.
☐ **C.** Most antiarrhythmics cause new arrhythmias.
☐ **D.** Electrolyte imbalance is the most common cause of arrhythmias that require drug therapy.

4. A patient has tachycardia that hasn't responded well to propranolol (Inderal). The physician prescribes amiodarone (Cordarone). Before giving this class III antiarrhythmic, you review the patient's drug history. Which of the following drugs is most likely to interact with amiodarone?

☐ **A.** Digoxin (Lanoxin)
☐ **B.** Morphine
☐ **C.** Theophylline (Theo-Dur)
☐ **D.** Verapamil (Calan)

5. A patient with hypertension requires a selective beta-adrenergic blocker for blood pressure control. Which of the following drugs is a selective beta-adrenergic blocker?

☐ **A.** Atenolol (Tenormin)
☐ **B.** Benazepril (Lotensin)
☐ **C.** Captopril (Capoten)
☐ **D.** Clonidine hydrochloride (Catapres)

6. Which adverse reaction associated with angiotensin-converting enzyme (ACE) inhibitors is the most common and often leads to disruption of therapy?

☐ **A.** Constipation
☐ **B.** Cough
☐ **C.** Sexual dysfunction
☐ **D.** Tachycardia

7. A 60-year-old patient develops hypotension while receiving I.V. nitroglycerin (Tridil). You should:

☐ A. monitor the patient closely for signs of alcohol intoxication.
☐ B. have the patient sit up slowly to minimize hypotensive effects.
☐ C. monitor the patient for headache; then give a prescribed analgesic.
☐ D. elevate the patient's legs and retake the blood pressure before slowing the I.V. rate.

8. A patient comes to the emergency department complaining of chest pains, which started an hour ago while he was playing golf. Nitroglycerin (Nitrostat), 0.4 mg, was given sublingually stat, as prescribed. Which of the following adverse reactions would be most likely to occur?

☐ A. Hypotension
☐ B. Dizziness
☐ C. Headache
☐ D. GI distress

9. A patient is about to begin antilipemic therapy with lovastatin (Mevinolin). To enhance the drug's absorption, you should advise the patient to take the drug at what time?

☐ A. At bedtime
☐ B. Upon arising
☐ C. With the evening meal
☐ D. With morning and evening meals

10. Cholestyramine (Questran) is prescribed to a patient diagnosed with hypercholesterolemia. What information is included in the teaching plan?

☐ A. Vitamin C excretion will increase.
☐ B. Absorption of fat-soluble vitamins will be affected.
☐ C. Unlimited fats in the diet are allowed while taking this drug.
☐ D. The drug should be taken on an empty stomach.

11. The cardiologist prescribes diltiazem hydrochloride (Cardizem) 20 mg as an I.V. bolus over 2 minutes for a patient diagnosed with atrial fibrillation. The pharmacy dispenses a 5 mg/ml vial. How many milliliters (ml) should the nurse administer? ____________

12. The nurse is preparing a teaching plan for a patient who was prescribed enalapril maleate (Vasotec) for treatment of hypertension. Which of the following instructions should the nurse include in the teaching plan?

Select all that apply:

☐ A. Avoid salt substitutions.
☐ B. Light-headedness is a common adverse effect that need not be reported.
☐ C. You may experience a sore throat for the first few days of therapy.
☐ D. Report facial swelling or difficulty breathing immediately.
☐ E. Blood tests will be necessary every 3 weeks for 2 months and periodically after that.
☐ F. Don't change position suddenly; sudden changes can cause orthostatic hypotension.

ANSWERS AND RATIONALES

1. CORRECT ANSWER: A
The usual parameter for withholding digoxin is a heart rate less than 60 beats/minute. Liver failure isn't a contraindication for its use, and the drug has no effect on respirations or blood.

2. CORRECT ANSWER: C
Irritability, nausea, blurred vision, and confusion are signs and symptoms of digoxin toxicity. The digoxin dose should be withheld and the physician notified while the digoxin level is checked. You should also try to reorient the patient and prepare for possible emergency treatment pending the laboratory results. Even if the digoxin level is normal (0.5 to 2 ng/ml), patients vary greatly in response, and the dose should be withheld if the patient shows signs of toxicity. Also, the patient's medication profile should be reviewed for possible drug interactions before giving further doses of digoxin.

3. CORRECT ANSWER: C
Most antiarrhythmics can cause new arrhythmias or worsen existing ones, so the benefits need to be weighed against the risks. Only class IV antiarrhythmics decrease myocardial contractility and oxygen demand; the other classes of antiarrhythmics have different mechanisms of action. Antiarrhythmics mainly are prescribed for adults. Ischemia, not electrolyte imbalance, is the most common cause of arrhythmias.

4. CORRECT ANSWER: A
Amiodarone can interact with digoxin, increasing the serum digoxin level, thereby increasing the risk of digoxin toxicity and worsening arrhythmias. Amiodarone also may interact with other drugs, such as warfarin, procainamide, quinidine, and phenytoin. Amiodarone doesn't interact with verapamil, morphine, or theophylline.

5. CORRECT ANSWER: A
Atenolol is the only selective beta-adrenergic blocker listed. In addition to treating hypertension, atenolol is used to treat chronic stable angina and reduce cardiovascular mortality in patients with acute myocardial infarction. Benazepril also treats hypertension, but it's an angiotensin-converting enzyme inhibitor that blocks the conversion of angiotensin I to angiotensin II. Captopril may be used to treat hypertension and heart failure; although the action of captopril isn't well defined, it's thought to inhibit angiotensin-converting enzymes. Clonidine is used to treat hypertension, but it's a centrally acting alpha-adrenergic inhibitor, which inhibits the central vasomotor centers, decreasing sympathetic outflow to the heart, kidneys, and peripheral vasculature.

6. CORRECT ANSWER: B
Cough causes discontinuation of ACE inhibitor therapy in more than 10% of patients taking this class of antihypertensive because it disrupts the patient's sleep

patterns. Constipation is a common adverse reaction to calcium channel blockers and doesn't usually cause discontinuation of therapy. Sexual dysfunction is a common cause of therapy disruption when treating hypertension with antihypertensives but isn't an adverse reaction of ACE inhibitors. Tachycardia is often a reflex response that ends shortly after the start of therapy.

7. CORRECT ANSWER: D

You should position the hypotensive patient to promote venous return to the heart, such as elevating the patient's legs. If the patient's blood pressure is still hypotensive, slow the I.V. rate and call the physician. Continue to monitor the heart rate and blood pressure every 5 to 15 minutes. I.V. nitroglycerin therapy doesn't cause alcohol intoxication. Sitting the patient upright will worsen the hypotension and is contraindicated. Headaches are the most common adverse reaction to I.V. nitroglycerin and can be treated with analgesics, but treating the headache won't resolve the patient's hypotension.

8. CORRECT ANSWER: C

The most common reaction to nitrates is headache because nitrates dilate the blood vessels in the meningeal layers between the brain and the cranium. Hypotension, GI distress, and dizziness may occur, but the likelihood varies with each patient.

9. CORRECT ANSWER: C

To enhance the absorption of lovastatin, the patient should take the drug with the evening meal. The drug has a slow onset, and higher rates of cholesterol synthesis occur between midnight and 5 a.m. Antilipemics are not recommended to be taken on arising. Some are recommended to be split over two meals, which may include breakfast, but most are taken in the evening to enhance absorption for optimal effectiveness.

10. CORRECT ANSWER: B

Cholestyramine reduces the absorption of cholesterol and fat by binding with bile acids. Decreased fat absorption may lead to decreased absorption of fat-soluble vitamins, such as A, D, E, and K. Vitamin C is a water-soluble vitamin, so its excretion isn't affected by cholestyramine therapy. Cholestyramine should be mixed with fluids or pulpy fruits, not taken on an empty stomach. Cholestyramine is given with dietary restrictions.

11. CORRECT ANSWER: 4

The nurse should use the following formula to calculate drug dosages:

Dose on hand/Quantity on hand = Dose desired/X

In this example, the equation is as follows:

$$\frac{5\text{ mg}}{\text{ml}} = \frac{20\text{ mg}}{X}$$

$$5X = 20$$

$$X = 4\text{ ml}$$

12. CORRECT ANSWER: A, D, F

When teaching the patient about enalapril maleate, the nurse should tell him to avoid salt substitutions, as these products may contain potassium that can cause light-headedness and syncope. Facial swelling or difficulty breathing should be reported immediately; the drug may cause angioedema, which would require discontinuation of the drug. The patient should also be advised to change position slowly to minimize orthostatic hypotension. The nurse should tell the patient to report lightheadedness, especially in the first few days of therapy, so dosage adjustments can be made. The patient should report signs of infection, such as sore throat and fever, because the drug may decrease the white blood cell count. White blood cell and differential counts should be performed before treatment, every 2 weeks for 3 months, and periodically thereafter.

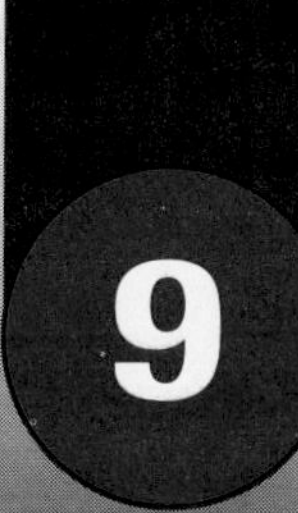

Drugs and the renal system

LEARNING OBJECTIVES

After studying this chapter, you should be able to:

- Identify medications commonly used as diuretics.
- Describe the mechanisms of action and rationales for using thiazide diuretics, loop diuretics, potassium-sparing diuretics, osmotic diuretics, and carbonic anhydrase inhibitors.
- Name the major adverse effects of each type of diuretic.
- Identify nursing responsibilities when administering each type of diuretic.
- Discuss patient teaching related to each type of diuretic.

CHAPTER OVERVIEW

Diuretics increase urine formation and promote fluid loss. These drugs are used to treat edema caused by heart failure or other drugs, to treat hypertension and glaucoma, and to prevent acute tubular necrosis. Knowing a diuretic's mechanism of action helps the nurse understand the selection of a specific diuretic. Nursing responsibilities when administering diuretics include monitoring the patient's blood pressure, fluid intake and output, daily weight, glucose and blood urea nitrogen (BUN) levels, and acid-base status. Patient teaching includes encouraging compliance, educating the patient about dietary modifications, and reminding the patient to stand up slowly and to report weight gain or edema.

A&P highlights

- The kidneys are two bean-shaped organs embedded in the dorsal part of the abdomen retroperitoneally.
- Nephrons are the structural and functional unit of the kidney.
- Each kidney contains over 1 million nephrons.
- The kidneys receive and filter a large volume of blood from the renal artery; tubular absorption and secretion convert glomerular filtrate into urine.
- Within the nephrons, glomeruli filter the blood; then the filtrate flows through the renal tubules.
- The glomerular filtration rate depends on glomerular capillary permeability, blood pressure, and effective filtration rate.
- The kidneys dispose of wastes and excess ions in the form of urine; filter blood; maintain fluid, electrolyte, and acid-base balances; produce several hormones and enzymes; convert vitamin D to a more active form; and regulate blood pressure and blood volume.

Key facts about thiazide and thiazide-like diuretics

- Increase water secretion by increasing the GFR or decreasing or inhibiting sodium reabsorption from the trubules
- Excreted primarily in the urine

ANATOMY AND PHYSIOLOGY

Anatomy

- The kidneys
  - The kidneys are two bean-shaped organs embedded in the dorsal part of the abdomen retroperitoneally
  - Kidneys have an outer region called the renal cortex, which contains blood-filtering mechanisms; a middle region called the renal medulla; and an inner region called the renal pelvis
- Nephrons
  - Nephrons are the structural and functional unit of the kidney
  - Each kidney contains over 1 million nephrons
  - Each nephron consists of a long tubule with a closed end called the glomerular capsule, or Bowman's capsule, which is divided into three portions
    - Proximal convoluted tubule
    - Loop of Henle
    - Distal convoluted tubule

Physiology

- The kidneys receive and filter a large volume of blood from the renal artery; tubular absorption and secretion convert glomerular filtrate into urine
- Within the nephrons, glomeruli filter the blood; then the filtrate flows through the renal tubules
- The tubules reabsorb and secrete various substances from the filtrate, changing its composition and concentration and ultimately producing urine
- The glomerular filtration rate (GFR) depends on glomerular capillary permeability, blood pressure, and effective filtration rate
- The cells in the kidneys also secrete renin in response to decreased blood pressure, blood volume, or plasma sodium concentration

Function of the kidneys

- Dispose of wastes and excess ions in the form of urine
- Filter blood, regulating its volume and chemical makeup
- Maintain fluid, electrolyte, and acid-base balances
- Produce several hormones and enzymes
- Convert vitamin D to a more active form
- Regulate blood pressure and blood volume by secreting renin

THIAZIDE AND THIAZIDE-LIKE DIURETICS

Mechanism of action

- Increase water excretion by either increasing the GFR or decreasing or inhibiting sodium reabsorption from the tubules

Pharmacokinetics

- Absorption: Absorbed rapidly but incompletely from the GI tract after oral administration
- Distribution: 65% to 95% protein-bound; distributed into extracellular space; crosses the placental barrier and appears in breast milk
- Metabolism: Unknown
- Excretion: Excreted primarily in the urine

Drug examples

- Chlorothiazide (Diuril), chlorthalidone (Hygroton), hydrochlorothiazide (Esidrix, HydroDIURIL, Oretic), indapamide (Lozol), metolazone (Diulo, Mykrox, Zaroxolyn)

Indications

- To treat hypertension, edema, and heart failure

Contraindications and precautions

- Contraindicated in patients sensitive to sulfonamides and in those with anuria, hepatic coma, or precoma (metolazone)
- Don't give chlorothiazide with whole blood or blood derivatives
- Give I.V. chlorothiazide only in an emergency or to adults who can't take oral medication
- Use cautiously in pregnant women and in patients with systemic lupus erythematosus or hypercholesterolemia

Adverse reactions

- May cause orthostatic hypotension, dizziness, light-headedness, headache, weakness, restlessness, insomnia, anorexia, nausea, vomiting, abdominal pain, diarrhea, constipation, impotence or reduced libido, rash, necrotizing angiitis, and photosensitivity
- May also cause hypokalemia, hyperglycemia, hyponatremia, and hypomagnesemia and other fluid and electrolyte imbalances
- May increase triglyceride and cholesterol levels

Interactions

- These drugs may decrease excretion of lithium, causing lithium toxicity
- Use with other potassium-depleting drugs and digoxin may cause additive hypokalemia, thus increasing the risk of digoxin toxicity
- Nonsteroidal anti-inflammatory drugs (NSAIDs) may reduce the antihypertensive effect of thiazide diuretics
- These drugs may produce additive hypotension when used with antihypertensives

Nursing responsibilities

- Monitor digoxin levels in patients who are receiving digoxin concurrently with thiazide and thiazide-like diuretics
- Instruct the patient to use a sunscreen and wear protective clothing to prevent photosensitivity reactions

When to use thiazide and thiazide-like diuretics

- Hypertension
- Edema
- Heart failure

When NOT to use thiazide and thiazide-like diuretics

- Hypersensitivity to sulfonamides
- Anuria
- Hepatic coma
- Precoma
- With whole blood or blood derivatives

Adverse reactions to watch for

- Orthostatic hypotension, dizziness, light-headedness, headache, weakness, restlessness, insomnia, anorexia, nausea, vomiting, abdominal pain, diarrhea, constipation, impotence or reduced libido, rash, necrotizing angiitis, photosensitivity

Key nursing actions

- Monitor digoxin levels in patients taking digoxin concurrently with these drugs.
- Monitor patient for signs and symptoms of hypokalemia.
- Give diuretic in morning or early afternoon, if possible.

- Carefully monitor the patient for signs and symptoms of hypokalemia, such as drowsiness, paresthesia, muscle cramps, and hyporeflexia
  - Administer prescribed potassium supplements
  - Advise the patient to eat foods high in potassium
- Give the diuretic in the morning or early afternoon, if possible, to prevent nocturia from disrupting the patient's sleep at night
- Keep a urinal or bedpan within reach of the patient or ensure that the bathroom is easily accessible for the patient

Key facts about loop diuretics

- Inhibit sodium and chloride reabsorption from the loop of Henle and the distal tubule
- Increase sodium and water excretion by inhibiting sodium reabsorption in the proximal tubule
- Metabolized partially or completely by the liver, except for furosemide, which is excreted primarily unchanged
- Excreted in the urine

When to use loop diuretics

- Edema associated with heart failure
- Hepatic cirrhosis
- Renal disease
- Hypertension
- Short-term management of ascites due to malignancy, idiopathic edema, or lymphedema
- Additive diuretic effects
- Cerebral edema

When NOT to use loop diuretics

- Hypersensitivity to these drugs
- Anuria
- Hepatic coma
- Severe uncorrected electrolyte depletion

LOOP DIURETICS

Mechanism of action
- Inhibit sodium and chloride reabsorption from the loop of Henle and the distal tubule
- Increase sodium and water excretion by inhibiting sodium reabsorption in the proximal tubule

Pharmacokinetics
- Absorption: Well absorbed from the GI tract
- Distribution: Rapidly distributed; extensively protein-bound
- Metabolism: Metabolized partially or completely by the liver, except for furosemide, which is excreted primarily unchanged
- Excretion: Excreted in the urine

Drug examples
- Bumetanide (Bumex), ethacrynic acid (Edecrin), furosemide (Lasix), torsemide (Demadex)

Indications
- Loop diuretics are used to treat edema associated with heart failure, hepatic cirrhosis, and renal disease, including nephrotic syndrome
- Loop diuretics also are used to treat hypertension
- Ethacrynic acid also may be used for the short-term management of ascites due to malignancy, idiopathic edema, or lymphedema
- Ethacrynic acid also is used with other diuretics for additive diuretic effects
- Furosemide may also be used with mannitol to treat cerebral edema

Contraindications and precautions
- Loop diuretics are the most potent diuretic available, producing the greatest volume of diuresis but also having the highest potential for severe adverse reactions and electrolyte depletion
- Contraindicated in patients hypersensitive to these drugs or their components, in those with anuria, hepatic coma, and in states of severe uncorrected electrolyte depletion
- Use cautiously in elderly patients, in pregnant or breast-feeding women, and in patients with hepatic cirrhosis, ascites, or systemic lupus erythematosus

Adverse reactions

- The most common adverse reactions involve fluid and electrolyte imbalances, including metabolic alkalosis, hypovolemia, hypochloremia, hypochloremic alkalosis, hyperuricemia, dehydration, hyponatremia, hypokalemia, and hypomagnesemia
- May also cause transient deafness, tinnitus, diarrhea, nausea, vomiting, abdominal pain, impaired glucose tolerance, dermatitis, paresthesia, hepatic dysfunction, photosensitivity, and orthostatic hypotension

Interactions

- These drugs may decrease excretion of lithium, causing lithium toxicity
- Use with digoxin may cause additive hypokalemia, thus increasing the risk of digoxin toxicity and arrhythmias
- Use with aminoglycosides increases the risk of ototoxicity
- Use with anticoagulants may increase anticoagulant effects
- Use with NSAIDs and probenecid may decrease the diuretic effects
- Use with thiazide diuretics causes a synergistic effect that may result in profound diuresis and serious electrolyte abnormalities

Nursing responsibilities

- Monitor serum digoxin levels in patients receiving digoxin and loop diuretics concurrently
- Instruct the patient to use a sunscreen and wear protective clothing to prevent photosensitivity reactions
- Monitor the patient for signs and symptoms of hypokalemia, such as drowsiness, paresthesia, muscle cramps, and hyporeflexia
  - Administer prescribed potassium supplements
  - Advise the patient to eat foods high in potassium
- Administer I.V. doses slowly over 1 to 2 minutes to prevent hypotension and tinnitus
- Know that bumetanide is 40 times more potent than furosemide; check the dosage with extreme care
- Be especially alert for changes in the patient's sodium and potassium levels
- When giving furosemide I.M., use the Z-track method to minimize skin irritation
- Give the diuretic in the morning or early afternoon, if possible, to prevent nocturia from disrupting the patient's sleep at night
- Keep a urinal or bedpan within reach of the patient or ensure that the bathroom is easily accessible for the patient
- Monitor the patient for signs of dehydration, such as poor skin turgor and dry mucous membranes
- Check the patient's vital signs to detect signs of hypovolemia, such as tachycardia, hypotension, and dyspnea; if signs are present, notify the physician

Adverse reactions to watch for

- Metabolic alkalosis, hypovolemia, hypochloremia, hypochloremic alkalosis, hyperuricemia, dehydration, hyponatremia, hypokalemia, hypomagnesemia, transient deafness, tinnitus, diarrhea, nausea, vomiting, abdominal pain, impaired glucose tolerance, dermatitis, paresthesia, hepatic dysfunction, photosensitivity, and orthostatic hypotension

Key nursing actions

- Monitor serum digoxin levels in patients receiving digoxin and these drugs concurrently.
- Monitor patient for signs and symptoms of hypokalemia.
- Administer I.V. doses slowly over 1 to 2 minutes.
- Know that bumetanide is 40 times more potent than furosemide.
- Be especially alert for changes in patient's sodium and potassium levels.
- Give diuretic in morning or early afternoon, if possible.
- Monitor patient for signs of dehydration.
- Check vital signs to detect signs of hypovolemia; if signs are present, notify physician.
- Accurately record fluid intake and output.
- Give diuretic with food or milk if GI upset occurs.

- **Accurately record the patient's fluid intake and output; if a large discrepancy occurs, notify the physician and expect to decrease the diuretic dosage**
- Give the diuretic with food or milk if GI upset occurs

POTASSIUM-SPARING DIURETICS

Mechanism of action
- Act at the distal tubule to cause excretion of sodium, bicarbonate, and calcium, but conserve potassium excretion
- Spironolactone acts by competing with aldosterone for receptor sites and blocks the action of aldosterone on the distal tubules

Pharmacokinetics
- Absorption: Absorbed in the GI tract
- Distribution: Unknown
- Metabolism: Metabolized by the liver, except for amiloride, which isn't metabolized
- Excretion: Excreted primarily in the urine, but also found in bile

Drug examples
- Amiloride (Midamor), spironolactone (Aldactone), triamterene (Dyrenium)

Indications
- These drugs are used primarily to conserve potassium or enhance the effects of loop or thiazide diuretics
- Spironolactone also is used to treat hyperaldosteronism, cirrhosis of the liver accompanied by edema or ascites, nephrotic syndrome, and hypokalemia
- Triamterene is used to treat idiopathic edema or edema associated with heart failure, hepatic cirrhosis, nephrotic syndrome, or steroid use, or secondary to hyperaldosteronism

Contraindications and precautions
- Contraindicated in patients who are hypersensitive to these drugs; have a serum potassium level greater than 5.5 mEq/L; are receiving antikaliuretic therapy, potassium supplementation, or another potassium-sparing diuretic; have impaired renal function; or are anuric
- Use with extreme caution in patients with diabetes, in those who have or are at risk for metabolic or respiratory acidosis or renal or hepatic impairment, and in pregnant or breast-feeding women

Adverse reactions
- **Potassium-sparing diuretics have fewer adverse reactions than other diuretics**
- May cause hyperkalemia and increased BUN level
- May cause nausea, vomiting, diarrhea, anorexia, abdominal pain, muscle cramping, headache, and dizziness

Key facts about potassium-sparing diuretics
- Act at the distal tubule to cause excretion of sodium, bicarbonate, and calcium, but conserve potassium excretion
- Metabolized by the liver
- Excreted primarily in the urine

When to use potassium-sparing diuretics
- Conservation of potassium
- Enhancement of the effects of loop or thiazide diuretics
- Hyperaldosteronism
- Cirrhosis of the liver accompanied by edema or ascites
- Nephrotic syndrome
- Hypokalemia
- Idiopathic edema or edema associated with heart failure, hepatic cirrhosis, nephrotic syndrome, or steroid use, or secondary to hyperaldosteronism

When NOT to use potassium-sparing diuretics
- Hypersensitivity to these drugs
- Serum potassium level greater than 5.5 mEq/L
- With antikaliuretic therapy, potassium supplementation, or another potassium-sparing diuretic
- Renal impairment
- Anuria

Adverse reactions to watch for
- Hyperkalemia, increased BUN level, nausea, vomiting, diarrhea, anorexia, abdominal pain, muscle cramping, headache, and dizziness

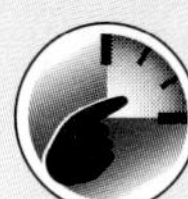

TIME-OUT FOR TEACHING

Teaching about potassium-sparing diuretics

Include these topics in your teaching plan for the patient receiving a potassium-sparing diuretic.

- Medication therapy regimen, including the drug's name, dose, frequency, duration, and possible adverse effects
- Signs and symptoms of possible adverse effects and when to notify the physician
- Signs and symptoms of hyperkalemia
- Dietary restrictions, such as alcohol
- Weight monitoring
- Intake and output
- Safety measures
- Measures to relieve minor adverse effects
- Need for compliance with therapy, including taking the drug as prescribed
- Follow-up care, including laboratory tests and physician visits

Interactions

- Giving these drugs with potassium supplements, other potassium-sparing diuretics, or angiotensin-converting enzyme inhibitors increases the risk of hyperkalemia
- **Concurrent use of spironolactone and digoxin increases the risk of digoxin toxicity**
- Salicylates decrease the effects of spironolactone

Nursing responsibilities

- **Monitor the patient for signs and symptoms of hyperkalemia, such as confusion, hyperexcitability, muscle weakness, flaccid paralysis, arrhythmias, abdominal distention, and diarrhea; notify the physician immediately if any of these symptoms occurs**
- Instruct the patient to avoid salt substitutes and potassium-rich foods, except with physician approval (for specific teaching tips, see *Teaching about potassium-sparing diuretics*)
- For maximum effectiveness, administer amiloride with food; triamterene, after meals
- Advise the patient to avoid driving or performing activities requiring mental alertness or physical dexterity because potassium-sparing diuretics may cause dizziness, headache, or visual disturbances

OSMOTIC DIURETICS

Mechanism of action

- Increase osmotic pressure of the glomerular filtrate, inhibiting reabsorption of water and electrolytes

Topics for patient discussion

- Therapy regimen
- Signs and symptoms of possible adverse effects and when to notify the physician
- Signs and symptoms of hyperkalemia
- Dietary restrictions
- Weight monitoring
- Intake and output
- Safety measures
- Measures to relieve minor adverse effects
- Need for compliance with therapy
- Follow-up care

Key nursing actions

- Monitor patient for signs and symptoms of hyperkalemia; notify physician immediately if symptoms occur.
- Instruct patient to avoid salt substitutes and potassium-rich foods, except with physician approval.
- Advise patient to avoid driving or performing activities requiring mental alertness or physical dexterity.

Key facts about osmotic diuretics

- Increase osmotic pressure of the glomerular filtrate, inhibiting reabsorption of water and electrolytes
- Create an osmotic gradient in the glomerular filtrate and the blood
- Mannitol is only slightly metabolized; the other drugs are freely filtered by the glomeruli
- Excreted primarily unchanged in the urine

- Create an osmotic gradient in the glomerular filtrate and the blood
  - In the glomerular filtrate, the gradient prevents sodium and water reabsorption
  - In the blood, the gradient allows fluid to be drawn from the intracellular into the intravascular spaces
  - The resulting increase in intravascular volume may cause fluid overload in patients with impaired kidney function

When to use osmotic diuretics

- Cerebral edema
- Reduction of intracranial and intraocular pressure
- Promotion of diuresis in acute renal failure
- Promotion of urinary excretion of toxic substances
- Interruption of acute attacks of glaucoma

Pharmacokinetics

- Absorption: Administered I.V.
- Distribution: Distributed rapidly
- Metabolism: Mannitol is only slightly metabolized; the other drugs are freely filtered by the glomeruli
- Excretion: Excreted primarily unchanged in the urine

Drug examples

- Glycerin (Osmoglyn), isosorbide (Ismotic), mannitol (Osmitrol), urea (Ureaphil)

Indications

- These drugs are used primarily to treat cerebral edema and to reduce intracranial and intraocular pressure
- Mannitol also is used to promote diuresis in acute renal failure and to promote urinary excretion of toxic substances
- Glycerin and isosorbide also may be used to interrupt acute attacks of glaucoma

When NOT to use osmotic diuretics

- Well-established anuria, severe dehydration, frank or impending acute pulmonary edema, severe cardiac decompensation, or hypersensitivity to these drugs

Contraindications and precautions

- Osmotic diuretics are contraindicated in patients with well-established anuria, severe dehydration, frank or impending acute pulmonary edema, severe cardiac decompensation, or hypersensitivity to these drugs
- Mannitol is contraindicated in patients with anuria due to severe renal disease, severe pulmonary congestion, frank pulmonary edema, active intracranial bleeding (unless during a craniotomy), severe dehydration, progressive renal damage or dysfunction after starting mannitol therapy, and progressive heart failure or pulmonary congestion after starting mannitol therapy

Adverse reactions to watch for

- Nausea, vomiting, confusion, headache, disorientation, dizziness, light-headedness, syncope, vertigo, gastric disturbances, hyponatremia, dehydration, circulatory overload, and thrombophlebitis or local irritation at the infusion site

Adverse reactions

- These drugs may cause nausea, vomiting, confusion, headache, disorientation, dizziness, light-headedness, syncope, vertigo, or gastric disturbances
- May also cause hyponatremia, dehydration, circulatory overload (from osmotic effects), and thrombophlebitis or local irritation at the infusion site
- Mannitol may cause rebound increased intracranial pressure 8 to 12 hours after diuresis; the drug also may cause chest pains, blurred vision, rhinitis, thirst, and urine retention

Interactions
- Urea may increase renal excretion of lithium, thereby decreasing the effects of lithium

Nursing responsibilities
- **Monitor the patient's vital signs, urine output, and central venous pressure for signs of circulatory overload and fluid volume depletion; assess the patient for circulatory overload when urine output is less than 30 ml/hr**
- Assess the patient's neurologic status and intracranial pressure for signs of increased intracranial pressure

CARBONIC ANHYDRASE INHIBITORS

Mechanism of action
- Inhibit the action of the enzyme carbonic anhydrase
- In the kidney, carbonic anhydrase inhibition decreases the availability of hydrogen ions, blocking sodium-hydrogen exchange mechanisms, thus increasing urinary excretion of sodium, potassium, bicarbonate, and water
- In the eye, carbonic anhydrase inhibition reduces aqueous humor production, thereby reducing intraocular pressure

Pharmacokinetics
- Absorption: Absorbed from the GI tract after oral administration; some systemic absorption occurs after ophthalmic administration
- Distribution: Distributed in tissues with high carbonic anhydrase content, such as in erythrocytes, plasma, kidneys, eyes, liver, and muscles
- Metabolism: Unknown
- Excretion: Excreted in the urine

Drug examples
- Acetazolamide (Diamox), dichlorphenamide (Daranide), methazolamide (GlaucTabs)

Indications
- To treat glaucoma
- Acetazolamide also may be used to treat epilepsy and acute mountain sickness

Contraindications and precautions
- Contraindicated in pregnant women; in patients with decreased sodium or potassium levels, marked kidney or liver disease, adrenocortical insufficiency, or severe pulmonary obstruction; and for long-term use in chronic noncongestive angle-closure glaucoma
- Carbonic anhydrase inhibitors rarely are used for diuresis in patients with drug-induced edema or heart failure because they may cause metabolic acidosis
- Use with extreme caution in patients with hepatic impairment because methazolamide may cause hepatic coma

Key nursing actions
- Monitor vital signs, urine output, and central venous pressure for signs of circulatory overload and fluid volume depletion.
- Assess neurologic status and intracranial pressure.

Key facts about carbonic anhydrase inhibitors
- Inhibit the action of the enzyme carbonic anhydrase
- In the kidney, carbonic anhydrase inhibition decreases the availability of hydrogen ions, blocking sodium-hydrogen exchange mechanisms, thus increasing urinary excretion of sodium, potassium, bicarbonate, and water
- In the eye, carbonic anhydrase inhibition reduces aqueous humor production, thereby reducing intraocular pressure
- Excreted in the urine

When to use carbonic anhydrase inhibitors
- Glaucoma
- Epilepsy
- Acute mountain sickness

When NOT to use carbonic anhydrase inhibitors
- Pregnancy
- Decreased sodium or potassium levels
- Marked kidney or liver disease
- Adrenocortical insufficiency
- Severe pulmonary obstruction
- Chronic noncongestive angle-closure glaucoma (long-term use)

- Use cautiously in patients who are allergic to sulfonamides because a cross-sensitivity reaction may occur

Adverse reactions
- May cause hypokalemia, metabolic acidosis, and other electrolyte imbalances
- May also cause fatigue, malaise, drowsiness, headache, paresthesia, urticaria, pruritus, Stevens-Johnson syndrome, and photosensitivity

Interactions
- Salicylates may cause carbonic anhydrase inhibitor toxicity, including central nervous system depression and metabolic acidosis
- Diflunisal may increase intraocular pressure when given with a carbonic anhydrase inhibitor
- Acetazolamide used concurrently with cyclosporine may increase cyclosporine levels and the risk of neurotoxicity
- Acetazolamide used concurrently with primidone may decrease serum and urine levels of primidone

Nursing responsibilities
- If GI upset occurs, give the drug with food
- Advise the patient to avoid prolonged or unprotected exposure to sunlight during drug therapy because of the risk of photosensitivity reactions

Adverse reactions to watch for

- Hypokalemia, metabolic acidosis, other electrolyte imbalances, fatigue, malaise, drowsiness, headache, paresthesia, urticaria, pruritus, Stevens-Johnson syndrome, and photosensitivity

Key nursing actions

- Give drug with food if GI upset occurs.
- Advise patient to avoid prolonged or unprotected exposure to sunlight during therapy.

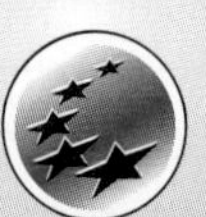

TOP 5

Items to study for your next test on drugs and the renal system

1. Medications commonly used as diuretics
2. Mechanisms of action and rationales for using thiazide diuretics, loop diuretics, potassium-sparing diuretics, osmotic diuretics, and carbonic anhydrase inhibitors
3. Major adverse effects of each type of diuretic
4. Nursing responsibilities when administering each type of diuretic
5. Patient teaching related to each type of diuretic

NCLEX CHECKS

It's never too soon to begin your NCLEX preparation. Now that you've reviewed this chapter, carefully read each of the following questions and choose the best answer. Then compare your responses to the correct answers.

1. You should observe for which electrolyte imbalance in a patient receiving furosemide (Lasix)?

☐ A. Hypercalcemia
☐ B. Hypernatremia
☐ C. Hypokalemia
☐ D. Hypophosphatemia

2. During the course of treatment for heart failure, your patient begins to complain of tinnitus. You suspect that this may be due to:

☐ A. hypokalemia.
☐ B. hypovolemia.
☐ C. insufficient diuretic use.
☐ D. excessive diuretic use.

3. A patient is taking a potassium-sparing diuretic, a drug that has weaker antihypertensive and diuretic effects than other diuretics, but preserves potassium levels in the body. Serum potassium levels should be closely monitored if the patient is also taking which drug?

- ☐ A. Cetirizine (Zyrtec)
- ☐ B. Epoprostenol (Flolan)
- ☐ C. Ibutilide (Corvert)
- ☐ D. Trandolapril (Mavik)

4. A 73-year-old man with a history of heart failure has sustained a head injury. He's receiving mannitol (Osmitrol) because he's developed cerebral edema. You should monitor the patient for which of the following conditions or symptoms?

- ☐ A. Rashes
- ☐ B. Bradycardia
- ☐ C. Disorientation
- ☐ D. Circulatory overload

5. You're instructing a patient about taking acetazolamide (Diamox) at home. Which of the following elements is most important to include in the teaching plan?

- ☐ A. The drug is safe to use and should cause few adverse reactions.
- ☐ B. Instill 2 drops into each eye every morning and before bedtime.
- ☐ C. If weakness, heart palpitations, or paresthesia occur, notify the physician.
- ☐ D. The drug may cause dim vision in low light, so night driving could be dangerous.

6. A patient comes to the facililty with acute pulmonary edema. The physician prescribes furosemide (Lasix) 80 mg I.V. b.i.d. with a 40 mg I.V. bolus. What signs and symptoms should you look for when administering the bolus?

Select all that apply:

- ☐ A. Tinnitus
- ☐ B. Dizziness
- ☐ C. Headache
- ☐ D. Abdominal pain
- ☐ E. Increased urination
- ☐ F. Fever

ANSWERS AND RATIONALES

1. CORRECT ANSWER: C

The patient's potassium level should be monitored carefully for the risk of hypokalemia. Furosemide is a loop diuretic that promotes sodium and potassium excretion. Furosemide also may cause hypocalcemia and hyponatremia because of the increased excretion of calcium and sodium in the urine. Furosemide only minimally affects phosphorus levels.

2. CORRECT ANSWER: D

Excessive diuretic use or too-rapid administration can cause tinnitus, transient deafness, and, in extreme cases, varying degrees of permanent hearing loss. The symptoms of hypokalemia typically include muscle cramps and paresthesia, not tinnitus. The symptoms of hypovolemia include light-headedness and dizziness, orthostasis, and increased thirst, not tinnitus.

3. CORRECT ANSWER: D

Trandolapril is an angiotensin-converting enzyme inhibitor, which may increase potassium levels. Trandolapril given with a potassium-sparing diuretic increases the risk of hyperkalemia. The other drugs don't increase potassium levels or cause hyperkalemia.

4. CORRECT ANSWER: D

Mannitol is an osmotic diuretic that draws fluid from the tissues into the vascular system. Because of the additional fluid in the vascular system from the cerebral edema, a patient with heart failure may develop fluid overload. Bradycardia and rashes aren't common with this drug. Mannitol may increase orientation because it decreases intracranial pressure.

5. CORRECT ANSWER: C

Acetazolamide increases urine output and can cause significant electrolyte imbalances, which may be indicated by weakness, palpitations, and paresthesia. If these occur, the patient should notify the physician because the dosage may need adjustment. Acetazolamide is safe to use, but it has many adverse reactions. It's given P.O., I.V., or I.M., but not as eyedrops. It has no miotic effects.

6. CORRECT ANSWER: A, B, D, F

Furosemide must be administered slowly over 1 to 2 minutes. Administering furosemide too quickly causes furosemide toxicity. Symptoms of toxicity include tinnitus (ringing in the ears), severe abdominal pain, dizziness, sore throat, and fever. Increased urination is the desired effect of furosemide administration. Headache is not a sign of furosemide toxicity.

Drugs and the hematologic system

LEARNING OBJECTIVES

After studying this chapter, you should be able to:

- Explain the rationale for using hematopoietics, anticoagulants, thrombolytics, and antiplatelets.
- Describe the mechanisms of action of hematopoietics, anticoagulants, thrombolytics, and antiplatelets.
- Identify laboratory tests used to monitor the patient who is receiving a hematopoietic, anticoagulant, thrombolytic, or antiplatelet drug.
- List common adverse effects of hematopoietics, anticoagulants, thrombolytics, and antiplatelet drugs.
- Identify nursing responsibilities when administering hematopoietics, anticoagulants, thrombolytics, and antiplatelet drugs.
- Discuss appropriate teaching for the patient who is receiving a hematopoietic, anticoagulant, thrombolytic, or antiplatelet drug.

CHAPTER OVERVIEW

Hematopoietic factors aid in the formation of cellular elements of blood. These drugs contribute to the production and formation of red blood cells (RBCs) in iron-deficiency anemia and megaloblastic anemia and to the production and formation of RBCs and white blood cells (WBCs) in anemia of bone marrow failure or suppression.

Anemia may result from vitamin or mineral deficiencies that impair the manufacture of RBCs; treatment focuses on replacing the deficient vitamins or minerals.

Nursing responsibilities when administering hematopoietics include monitoring the complete blood count (CBC) and differential and observing for signs and symptoms of improved energy and freedom from infection. Patient teaching focuses on rest, avoiding infection, dietary modifications, proper subcutaneous injection technique, and blood tests.

Anticoagulants and thrombolytics are used in the prophylaxis and treatment of thromboembolic disorders, such as myocardial infarction (MI), pulmonary embolism (PE), cerebrovascular accident (CVA), and deep vein thrombosis (DVT). Anticoagulants prevent clots from forming or existing clots from enlarging; thrombolytics cause clot dissolution. When used within 2 to 4 hours of the onset of MI, thrombolytics may minimize myocardial damage.

Antiplatelet drugs are used for prophylaxis of thromboembolic disorders. They're also effective in preventing new ischemic events and heart failure.

Nursing responsibilities for the administration of anticoagulants, thrombolytics, and antiplatelet drugs include verifying doses carefully, monitoring coagulation studies, implementing bleeding precautions, and checking for bruising and for occult blood in stools. Patient teaching should emphasize the need for careful compliance with the drug schedule and follow-up testing, dietary teaching, and avoiding over-the-counter vitamins or medications, unless approved by the patient's primary prescriber.

Anatomy highlights

- Blood consists of RBCs, WBCs, and platelets that are in a viscous fluid called plasma.
- RBCs are the most numerous elements in the blood.
- WBCs are classified as granulocytes (neutrophils, eosinophils, and basophils) and agranulocytes (lymphocytes and monocytes).
- Platelets resemble small plates and are anucleated cells about one-third the size of RBCs.
- Plasma accounts for about 55% of the total blood volume and consists of albumin, globulins, and fibrinogen.

ANATOMY AND PHYSIOLOGY

Anatomy

- Blood
  - Blood is made up of RBCs (or erythrocytes), WBCs, and platelets (or thrombocytes) that are in a viscous fluid called plasma
  - RBCs are the most numerous elements in the blood
  - WBCs are less numerous than RBCs and are classified as granulocytes (neutrophils, eosinophils, and basophils) and agranulocytes (lymphocytes and monocytes)
  - Platelets resemble small plates and are anucleated cells about one-third the size of RBCs; they are formed from large multinucleated cells called megakaryocytes in the bone marrow
- Plasma
  - Plasma accounts for about 55% of the total blood volume
  - It consists of albumin, globulins, and fibrinogen

Physiology

- RBC production is called erythropoiesis; it occurs in the bone marrow of certain bones and is regulated by the oxygen content of the arterial blood
- RBC maturation and function require hemoglobin
- Iron forms an essential part of hemoglobin
- Small amounts of iron circulate in the plasma with the iron-binding transport protein, transferrin

- Transferrin transports iron from the intestinal tract (where iron is absorbed) and from mononuclear phagocytes (where iron is recovered from RBC breakdown) to the bone marrow, liver, and spleen (where extra iron is stored as ferritin and hemosiderin)
- WBCs mature in the bone marrow, circulate in the blood, and enter the tissues
- WBCs participate in the inflammatory and immune responses, either by phagocytosis (the process by which WBCs ingest and digest solid substances, such as other cells, bacteria, necrotic tissues, and foreign particles) or by releasing chemicals in response to foreign antigens or bacteria that enter the body
- Platelets, coagulation factors (such as clotting activators and fibrin), RBCs, and other blood components help blood to clot, which stops bleeding
- After a bleeding blood vessel has healed and the clot is no longer needed, it must be lysed (dissolved), which is done by fibrinolysis
- Coagulation inhibitors and anticoagulants that retard clotting counterbalance coagulation factors and mechanisms and prevent excessive (disseminated) intravascular coagulation
  - Antithrombin in plasma inhibits thrombin formation
  - Heparin, which exists in basophils and mast cells, has anticoagulant properties
  - Prostaglandin derivatives inhibit platelet aggregation and phospholipid release that initiate coagulation
- The fibrinolytic system is a clot-dissolving system that's activated simultaneously with the coagulation mechanism
  - It restricts clotting to a limited area, thereby preventing excessive intravascular coagulation
  - It activates plasmin, a proteolytic (protein-digesting) enzyme, which breaks down the fibrin strands in a clot

Function of blood and plasma

- Blood
  - Blood delivers oxygen to body cells from the lungs and delivers nutrients to body cells from the GI tract
  - It transports carbon dioxide to the lungs and nitrogenous wastes to the kidneys for elimination
  - It transports hormones from endocrine glands to their target tissues
  - It maintains body temperature by absorbing and distributing body heat
  - It maintains acid-base balance
    - Blood proteins and other solutes act as buffers to prevent sudden changes in blood pH
    - Blood also stores bicarbonate atoms (an important component of the blood-buffer system needed to maintain normal blood pH)
  - It maintains adequate fluid volume; salts (such as sodium chloride) and proteins (such as albumin) in the blood prevent excessive fluid loss
  - It helps prevent blood loss through hemostasis, a mechanism that involves a vascular spasm, platelet formation, and coagulation

Physiology highlights

- RBC production is called erythropoiesis.
- WBCs mature in the bone marrow, circulate in the blood, and enter the tissues.
- WBCs participate in the inflammatory and immune responses.
- Platelets, coagulation factors, RBCs, and other blood components help blood to clot.
- After a bleeding blood vessel has healed and the clot is no longer needed, it must be lysed.
- Coagulation inhibitors and anticoagulants that retard clotting counterbalance coagulation factors and mechanisms and prevent excessive intravascular coagulation.
- The fibrinolytic system is a clot-dissolving system that's activated simultaneously with the coagulation mechanism.

Function highlights

- Blood:
  - delivers oxygen and nutrients to body cells
  - transports carbon dioxide to lungs and nitrogenous wastes to kidneys for elimination
  - transports hormones from endocrine glands to target tissues
  - maintains body temperature
  - maintains acid-base balance
  - stores bicarbonate atoms
  - maintains adequate fluid volume
  - helps prevent blood loss through hemostasis.

Plasma:
- helps maintain colloid osmotic pressure of blood
- transports enzymes, hormones, vitamins, and other substances
- plays a major role in blood coagulation.

- It helps prevent infection through the action of antibodies, complement proteins, and WBCs
- Plasma
  - Albumin is essential in maintaining the colloid osmotic pressure of the blood, which plays a major role in regulating fluid flow between the capillaries and interstitial tissues
  - Globulins transport enzymes, hormones, vitamins and other substances; gamma globulins act as antibodies, defending the body against infection
  - Fibrinogen plays a major role in blood coagulation; it's converted to fibrin (a protein that forms a meshlike network across a wound) when the blood coagulates

HEMATOPOIETICS

IRON PRODUCTS

Mechanism of action

- Supplement and replace depleted iron stores in the bone marrow to assist in erythropoiesis (RBC production)

Pharmacokinetics

- Absorption: Iron is absorbed primarily in the duodenum and upper jejunum
  - Iron absorption depends partially on the body stores of iron; when the body stores are low, iron absorption increases; when the body stores are high, iron absorption decreases
  - The lymphatic system absorbs the parenteral forms; food will decrease absorption
- Distribution: Iron is transported by the blood and bound to transferrin, its carrier plasma-protein
- Metabolism: Occurs in a closed system where most of the iron that's broken down is reused by the body
- Excretion: Iron is excreted in the urine, feces, and sweat and through intestinal cell sloughing; it appears in breast milk

Drug examples

- Ferrous fumarate (Femiron, Feostat, Ircon, Hemocyte), ferrous gluconate (Fergon), ferrous sulfate (Feosol, Fer-In-Sol, Fer-Gen-Sol, Feratab, Mol-Iron, Fer-Iron, Fero-Gradumet Filmtabs), iron dextran (InFeD, DexFerrum), iron sucrose (Venofer), sodium ferric gluconate (Ferrlecit)

Indications

- To prevent and treat iron deficiency and iron deficiency anemias
- As a dietary supplement for iron

Contraindications and precautions

- Contraindicated in patients with hemochromatosis, hemosiderosis, hemolytic anemias, or hypersensitivity to the drug, tartrazine, or sulfites

Key facts about iron products

- Supplement and replace depleted iron stores in the bone marrow to assist in erythropoiesis
- Metabolism occurs in a closed system where most of the iron that's broken down is reused by the body
- Excreted in the urine, feces, and sweat and through intestinal cell sloughing; appear in breast milk

When to use iron products

- Iron deficiency
- Iron deficiency anemias
- As dietary iron supplement

When NOT to use iron products

- Hypersensitivity to these products, tartrazine, or sulfites
- Hemochromatosis
- Hemosiderosis
- Hemolytic anemias

- Not intended for long-term use in patients with normal iron stores

Adverse reactions

- Oral iron preparations may cause nausea, vomiting, constipation, dark stools, diarrhea, and GI distress
- Parenteral iron preparations may cause nausea, vomiting, headache, staining at the I.M. injection site, localized phlebitis at the I.V. injection site, and anaphylaxis
- Liquid iron preparations may temporarily stain teeth
- Iron sucrose injection also may cause heart failure, sepsis, and mild to moderate hypersensitivity reactions (wheezing, dyspnea, hypotension, rash, pruritus)

Interactions

- Antacids, cimetidine, and tetracyclines decrease absorption of oral iron preparations
- Ascorbic acid and chloramphenicol increase absorption of oral iron preparations
- Iron may decrease the absorption or effect of levodopa, levothyroxine, methyldopa, penicillamine, and quinolones

Nursing responsibilities

- Administer drugs according to the prescribed route
  - For oral administration
    - Administer between meals
    - If GI distress occurs, administer with meals
    - Administer tablets with juice or water, but not with milk or antacids; orange juice or ascorbic acid promotes iron absorption
    - Dilute liquid iron preparations and administer with a straw to avoid staining teeth
  - For I.M. administration
    - Use the Z-track technique, which prevents leakage and staining into subcutaneous tissues
  - For I.V. administration
    - Check institutional policy before administering I.V.; some institutions don't permit the infusion method because its safety is controversial
    - Use the I.V. route in these situations
      - Insufficient muscle mass for deep I.M. injection
      - Impaired absorption from muscle caused by stasis or edema
      - Possibility of uncontrolled I.M. bleeding from trauma (as may occur in hemophilia)
      - Massive and prolonged parenteral therapy (as may be necessary in cases of chronic substantial blood loss)
    - Before I.V. administration, give an initial test dose to rule out hypersensitivity
    - On completion of I.V. iron dextran infusion, flush the vein with 10 ml of 0.9% sodium chloride solution
    - Tell the patient to rest for 15 to 30 minutes after I.V. administration

Adverse reactions to watch for

- Nausea, vomiting, constipation, dark stools, diarrhea, GI distress, headache, staining at I.M. injection site, localized phlebitis at I.V. injection site, anaphylaxis, temporary staining of teeth

Key nursing actions

- Administer drugs according to prescribed route.
- Monitor patient's CBC count, hemoglobin, and plasma iron level.
- Check for constipation.
- Caution parents to be alert for iron poisoning in children.
- Know that signs and symptoms of iron poisoning include nausea, vomiting, diarrhea, and GI bleeding, which can lead to shock, coma, and death.
- Teach patient to:
  - continue regular dosing schedule after missing dose; caution against doubling dose
  - drink at least 2 L of fluid daily (unless contraindicated) and to exercise regularly
  - avoid antacids, coffee, tea, dairy products, eggs, and whole-grain breads for 1 hour before and 2 hours after taking oral iron preparations
  - be aware that iron preparations may turn stools dark green or black.

Topics for patient discussion

- Therapy regimen
- Available forms and proper administration method
- Signs and symptoms of possible adverse effects and when to notify the physician
- Dietary allowances
- Changes in stool color
- Measures to relieve minor adverse effects
- Need for compliance with therapy
- Follow-up care

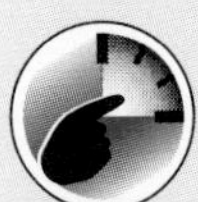

TIME-OUT FOR TEACHING

Teaching about iron products

Include these topics in your teaching plan for the patient receiving an iron product.

- Medication therapy regimen, including the drug's name, dose, frequency, duration, and possible adverse effects
- Available forms and proper administration method
- Signs and symptoms of possible adverse effects and when to notify the physician
- Dietary allowances, including the need for high-iron foods
- Changes in stool color
- Measures to relieve minor adverse effects such as constipation
- Need for compliance with therapy, including taking the drug as prescribed
- Follow-up care, including laboratory tests and physician visits

- Monitor the patient's CBC, hemoglobin, and plasma iron level
- Check for constipation
  - Record the color, amount, and consistency of stool
  - Teach dietary measures for preventing constipation (for specific teaching tips, see *Teaching about iron products*)
- Tell the patient to continue the regular dosing schedule after missing a dose; caution against doubling the dose
- **Caution parents to be aware of iron poisoning in children and to contact their pediatrician or local poison control center immediately**
  - **Signs and symptoms of iron poisoning can occur within minutes to hours after swallowing tablets**
  - **They include nausea, vomiting, diarrhea, and GI bleeding, which can lead to shock, coma, and death**
- Instruct the patient to drink at least 2 L (64 ounces) of fluid daily (unless contraindicated), to increase fiber intake, and to exercise regularly to prevent constipation
- **Advise the patient to avoid antacids, coffee, tea, dairy products, eggs, and whole-grain breads for 1 hour before and 2 hours after taking oral iron preparations; these substances may interfere with absorption**
- Inform the patient that iron preparations may turn stools dark green or black

Key facts about vitamins

- Replace depleted vitamin stores
- Vitamin B_{12}, folic acid, and leucovorin are metabolized and stored in the liver
- Vitamin B_{12} is excreted in the urine but some is excreted in the bile and then reabsorbed in the ileum; also excreted in breast milk
- Folic acid and leucovorin are excreted in the urine and feces; some excreted in breast milk

VITAMINS

Mechanism of action

- Replace depleted vitamin stores

Pharmacokinetics

- Absorption

  - Vitamin B_{12}: Absorbed by simple diffusion, but depends on intrinsic factor, which is secreted by the parietal cells of the gastric mucosa and which regulates the amount of vitamin B_{12} absorbed; therefore, the parenteral form usually is used
  - Hydroxocobalamin (vitamin B_{12}; crystalline): Absorbed more slowly from the injection site than cyanocobalamin
  - Folic acid and leucovorin: Undergo hydrolysis in the GI tract before being completely absorbed
- Distribution
  - Vitamin B_{12}: Protein-bound and distributed in the tissues
  - Folic acid and leucovorin: Distributed rapid to all body tissues
- Metabolism: Vitamin B_{12}, folic acid, and leucovorin are metabolized and stored in the liver
- Excretion
  - Vitamin B_{12}: Excreted in the urine but some is excreted in the bile and then reabsorbed in the ileum; also excreted in breast milk
  - Folic acid and leucovorin: Excreted in the urine and feces; some excreted in breast milk

Drug examples

- Cyanocobalamin (Nascobal), hydroxocobalamin, vitamin B_{12} (Betalin 12, Big Shot B-12); folic acid or vitamin B_9 (Folvite); leucovorin calcium (folinic acid, citrovorum factor)

Indications

- Cyanocobalamin is used to treat vitamin B_{12} deficiency (also known as megaloblastic anemia)
  - The oral form is *not* used to treat pernicious anemia
  - The nasal and parenteral (hydroxocobalamin) forms are used to treat vitamin B_{12} deficiency as seen with pernicious anemia
- Folic acid and parenteral leucovorin are used to treat megaloblastic anemia due to folic acid deficiency
- Oral and parenteral forms of leucovorin also are used to treat toxicity associated with methotrexate therapy

Contraindications and precautions

- Cyanocobalamin is contraindicated in patients hypersensitive to these vitamins or cobalt
- Folic acid and leucovorin are contraindicated in patients with pernicious anemia and other megaloblastic anemias caused by vitamin B_{12} deficiency

Adverse reactions

- Cyanocobalamin may cause headache, infection, nausea, mild diarrhea, asthenia, paresthesia, itching, and rash
- Folic acid may cause an allergic reaction or allergic bronchospasm

Interactions

- Folic acid may increase the metabolism or counteract the effects of anticonvulsants, causing a subtherapeutic phenytoin level and increasing the risk of seizures

When to use vitamins

- Vitamin B_{12} deficiency
- Megaloblastic anemia due to folic acid deficiency
- Toxicity associated with methotrexate therapy

When NOT to use vitamins

- Hypersensitivity to these vitamins or cobalt
- Pernicious anemia, other megaloblastic anemias caused by vitamin B_{12} deficiency

Adverse reactions to watch for

- Headache, infection, nausea, mild diarrhea, asthenia, paresthesia, itching, rash, allergic reaction or allergic bronchospasm

- Alcohol, aspirin, neomycin, and colchicine may reduce absorption of cyanocobalamin, impairing the vitamin's effectiveness
- Aspirin, hormonal contraceptives, methotrexate, and sulfasalazine may decrease folate levels
- Concurrent use of leucovorin with fluorouracil (5-FU) may increase 5-FU toxicity

Nursing responsibilities

- **Inform patients with pernicious anemia that they will require monthly injections of vitamin B12 for the rest of their lives; failure to do so will result in return of the anemia and in the development of incapacitating and irreversible damage to the nerves of the spinal cord**
- **Take seizure precautions in a patient receiving large doses of folic acid while on anticonvulsant therapy**
- Encourage the patient to eat foods rich in vitamin B_{12}, such as meat, seafood, eggs, legumes, and liver
- Monitor laboratory test results, such as hematocrit and reticulocyte counts, to determine the effectiveness of therapy
- Check folate levels in a patient who is receiving more than 10 mcg daily of vitamin B_{12}; the hematologic results may seem normal but may mask a folate deficiency, which could be the actual cause of megaloblastic anemia
- Monitor the patient's potassium level during the first 48 hours of treatment, particularly if the patient has addisonian pernicious anemia or megaloblastic anemia

Key nursing actions

- Inform patients with pernicious anemia that they will require monthly injections of vitamin B_{12} for the rest of their lives.
- Take seizure precautions in a patient receiving large doses of folic acid while on anticonvulsant therapy.
- Encourage patient to eat foods rich in vitamin B_{12}.
- Monitor lab test results, such as hematocrit and reticulocyte counts.
- Check folate levels in patient receiving more than 10 mcg daily of vitamin B_{12}.
- Monitor potassium level during first 48 hours of treatment, particularly if patient has addisonian pernicious anemia or megaloblastic anemia.

BIOLOGIC RESPONSE MODIFIERS

Mechanism of action

- Stimulate RBC production in the bone marrow by boosting the production of erythropoietin

Key facts about biologic response modifiers

- Stimulate RBC production in the bone marrow by boosting the production of erythropoietin

Pharmacokinetics

- Absorption: Absorption is slow and rate limiting with S.C. administration; darbepoetin alfa has a threefold longer terminal half-life than epoetin alfa when given by I.V. or S.C. route
- Distribution: Distribution of darbepoetin alfa is confined to the vascular space
- Metabolism: Unknown
- Excretion: Unknown

Drug examples

- Darbepoetin alfa (Aranesp), epoetin alfa (Epogen, Procrit)

Indications

- Darbepoetin alfa is used to treat anemia associated with chronic renal failure, whether or not the patient is on dialysis
- Epoetin alfa is used to treat anemia associated with end-stage renal disease, chemotherapy, or zidovudine therapy

When to use biologic response modifiers

- Anemia associated with chronic renal failure, end-stage renal disease, chemotherapy, or zidovusine therapy
- Decrease in need for perioperative blood transfusions

- Epoetin alfa is used to decrease the need for perioperative blood transfusions in surgery patients

Contraindications and precautions

- These drugs are contraindicated in patients with uncontrolled hypertension or hypersensitivity to the drugs or their components, such as mammalian-derived products or human albumin
- Epoetin alfa isn't intended for patients with chronic renal disease who have severe anemia or for HIV-infected patients or cancer patients with anemia that's caused by other factors, such as iron or folate deficiencies, hemolysis, or GI bleeding that should be managed appropriately
- Use darbepoetin alfa with extreme caution in patients with underlying hematologic disease, such as hemolytic anemia, sickle cell anemia, thalassemia, or porphyria, because safety hasn't been established
- Use these drugs with extreme caution in pregnant and breast-feeding women

Adverse reactions

- These drugs may cause hypertension, seizures, iron deficiency, increased risk of thrombotic events (including MI, stroke, or transient ischemic attack), or hypersensitivity and allergic reactions
- The most common adverse reactions for darbepoetin alfa are vascular access thrombosis, heart failure, sepsis, cardiac arrhythmias, infection, hypertension, hypotension, myalgia, headache, and diarrhea

Interactions

- None reported

Nursing responsibilities

- Monitor hemoglobin and hematocrit frequently, especially early in therapy, to evaluate the drug's effectiveness
  - A rapid rise in hematocrit value is associated with seizures and hypertension
  - Adequate iron, folic acid, and vitamin B_{12} stores must be present for erythropoiesis
- Institute seizure precautions and closely monitor the patient's neurologic status
- Frequently monitor the patient's blood pressure for signs of hypertension
- Teach the patient or family the proper technique for S.C. injection

COLONY-STIMULATING FACTOR

Mechanism of action

- Stimulates production of granulocytes and macrophages in the bone marrow by binding to specific cell surface receptors

Pharmacokinetics

- Unknown

When NOT to use biologic response modifiers

- Hypersensitivity to these drugs
- Uncontrolled hypertension

Adverse reactions to watch for

- Hypertension, seizures, iron deficiency, increased risk of thrombotic events, and hypersensitivity and allergic reactions

Key nursing actions

- Monitor hemoglobin and hematocrit frequently, especially early in therapy.
- Institute seizure precautions and closely monitor patient's neurologic status.
- Frequently monitor patient's blood pressure for signs of hypertension.
- Teach proper technique for S.C. injection.

Key facts about colony-stimulating factor

- Stimulates production of granulocytes and macrophages in the bone marrow by binding to specific cell surface receptors

When to use colony-stimulating factor

- Aplastic anemia secondary to chemotherapy
- Acceleration of bone marrow recovery in malignant lymphoma and Hodgkin's disease
- Failed bone marrow transplant
- Increase of WBCs during zidovudine therapy

When NOT to use colony-stimulating factor

- Hypersensitivity to these drugs
- Excessive leukemic myeloid blasts in the bone marrow or peripheral blood
- Simultaneous administration of cytotoxic chemotherapy or radiotherapy
- Within 24 hours before or after chemotherapy or radiotherapy

Adverse reactions to watch for

- Respiratory symptoms, supraventricular arrhythmias, bone pain, arthralgia, myalgia, anorexia, nausea, vomiting, diarrhea, stomatitis, fluid retention, and hypersensitivity reactions

Key nursing actions

- Monitor WBC count.
- Discontinue drug when absolute neutrophil count is 10,000 for filgrastim and 20,000 for sargramostim.
- Teach proper technique for S.C. injection.
- Teach importance of maintaining nutritionally balanced diet and complying with therapy.

Drug examples

- Filgrastim (Neupogen), pegfilgrastim (Neulasta), sargramostim (Leukine)

Indications

- To treat aplastic anemia secondary to chemotherapy
- To accelerate bone marrow recovery in malignant lymphoma and Hodgkin's disease
- To treat delayed or failed bone marrow transplant
- To increase WBCs in patients taking zidovudine

Contraindications and precautions

- Filgrastim and pegfilgrastim are contraindicated in patients with hypersensitivity to *Escherichia coli*–derived proteins or to other components of the drugs
- Sargramostim is contraindicated in patients with excessive leukemic myeloid blasts in the bone marrow or peripheral blood (10% or more) or hypersensitivity to the drug or its components, in patients receiving simultaneous administration of cytotoxic chemotherapy or radiotherapy, and within 24 hours before or after chemotherapy or radiotherapy

Adverse reactions

- May cause respiratory symptoms, supraventricular arrhythmias, bone pain, arthralgia, myalgia, anorexia, nausea, vomiting, diarrhea, stomatitis, fluid retention, and hypersensitivity reactions

Interactions

- Concurrent use with lithium may potentiate the release of neutrophils
- Lithium, corticosteroids, and other drugs may potentiate the myeloproliferative effects of sargramostim

Nursing responsibilities

- Monitor the patient's WBC count
- Monitor the patient for signs and symptoms of infection
- Discontinue the drug when the absolute neutrophil count is 10,000 for filgrastim and 20,000 for sargramostim
- Know that pegfilgrastim is longer acting than filgrastim
- Instruct the patient or family in the proper technique for S.C. injection
- Teach the patient about the importance of maintaining a nutritionally balanced diet and complying with the therapeutic regimen

ANTICOAGULANTS

Mechanism of action

- Prevent extension and formation of clots by inhibiting factors in the clotting cascade

Pharmacokinetics

- Absorption: Heparin is administered I.V. or S.C.
- Distribution: Distribution varies after S.C. administration
- Metabolism: Heparin is metabolized by the liver
- Excretion: Excreted in the urine

Drug examples

- Argatroban, bivalirudin (Angiomax), dalteparin sodium (Fragmin), enoxaparin sodium (Lovenox), fondaparinux sodium (Arixtra), heparin sodium, lepirudin (Refludan), tinzaparin sodium (Innohep), warfarin sodium (Coumadin)

Indications

- To prevent and treat thromboembolic disorders (such as DVT, PE, and atrial fibrillation with embolization) and ischemic complications
- Bivalirudin also is used with aspirin in patients with unstable angina undergoing percutaneous transluminal coronary angioplasty (PTCA)

Contraindications and precautions

- Contraindicated in patients with underlying coagulation disorders, ulcer disease, recent surgery, cancer, or active bleeding
- Also contraindicated in patients with severe thrombocytopenia, uncontrolled bleeding, or hypersensitivity to the drugs or their components
- Enoxaparin sodium isn't recommended in patients with prosthetic heart valves; these patients are at a higher risk for thromboembolism

Adverse reactions

- May cause hyperlipidemia, thrombocytopenia (with heparin), hemorrhages, and spinal or epidural hematoma (with indwelling catheters)
- May cause fever, pain at the injection site, nausea, constipation, and insomnia

Interactions

- Androgens, chloral hydrate, chloramphenicol, metronidazole, quinidine, sulfonamides, thrombolytics, and valproic acid increase the risk of bleeding and enhance the effects of warfarin
- Alcohol, barbiturates, estrogen-containing hormonal contraceptives, and foods high in vitamin K increase the risk of clotting and may decrease the effects of warfarin
- Concurrent use with other drugs that affect platelet function (such as aspirin, dextran, dipyridamole, and NSAIDs) increases the risk of bleeding

Nursing responsibilities

- Don't give heparin by I.M. route
- Minimize venipunctures and injections; apply pressure to all puncture sites to prevent bleeding
- Know that heparin is given initially because of its rapid action; the patient may then be started on warfarin, which takes several days to reach a therapeutic level
- Once therapeutic levels are reached, heparin will be discontinued and the patient will be maintained on warfarin
- Know that heparin directly affects partial thromboplastin time (PTT) and warfarin directly affects prothrombin time (PT) and international normalized ratio (INR)

Key facts about anticoagulants

- Prevent extension and formation of clots by inhibiting factors in the clotting cascade
- Heparin is metabolized by the liver
- Excreted in the urine

When to use anticoagulants

- Thromboembolic disorders
- Ischemic complications
- Unstable angina in PTCA

When NOT to use anticoagulants

- Hypersensitivity to these drugs
- Underlying coagulation disorders
- Ulcer disease
- Recent surgery
- Cancer
- Active bleeding
- Severe thrombocytopenia
- Uncontrolled bleeding

Adverse reactions to watch for

- Hyperlipidemia, thrombocytopenia, hemorrhages, spinal or epidural hematoma, fever, pain at injection site, nausea, constipation, and insomnia

GO WITH THE FLOW

Monitoring heparin therapy

When monitoring a patient who is receiving heparin, the nurse plays a key role in ensuring maximum effectiveness while minimizing possible adverse effects. Use the flowchart below to initiate therapy and monitor the patient's response.

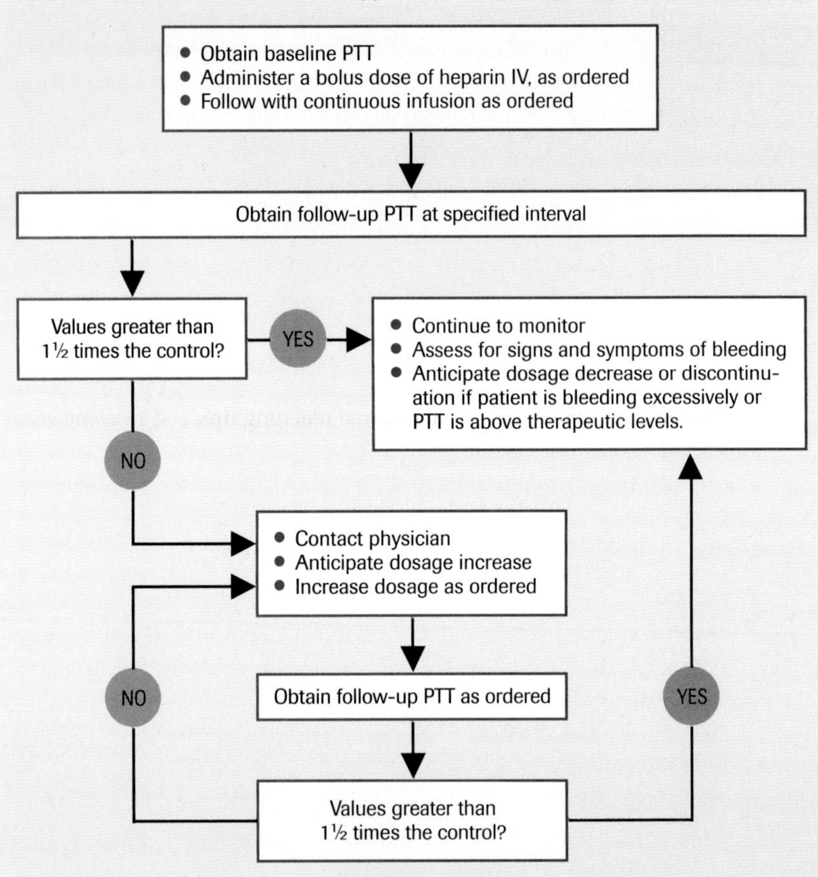

Key nursing actions

- Don't give heparin by I.M. route.
- Minimize venipunctures and injections; apply pressure to all puncture sites.
- Inject S.C. heparin and enoxaparin into abdomen; don't aspirate or rub injection site and rotate injection sites.
- Assess for signs and symptoms of bleeding; instruct patient to report bleeding immediately.
- Monitor hemoglobin and clotting factor and platelet levels.
- Caution patients not to increase dietary vitamin K or drastically and suddenly change diet.
- Teach patient to:
  - inform physician and dentist of therapy regimen before undergoing any medical treatments
  - be aware of importance of routine lab tests to monitor coagulation times
  - carry ID describing disease and drug regimen
  - not take drugs or vitamins, including over-the-counter or herbal products, without medical approval.

- Monitor activated partial thromboplastin time (aPTT) in the patient taking argatroban
- Enoxaparin usually doesn't significantly affect INR, PT, PTT, or platelet function (for more information, see *Monitoring heparin therapy*)
- Inject S.C. heparin and enoxaparin into the abdomen; don't aspirate or rub the injection site and rotate injection sites
- Know that protamine sulfate is the antidote for heparin
- Know that phytonadione (vitamin K1) is the antidote for warfarin
- Assess for signs and symptoms of bleeding and instruct the patient to report signs and symptoms of bleeding immediately

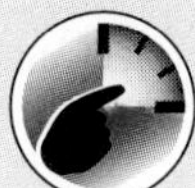

TIME-OUT FOR TEACHING

Teaching about anticoagulants

Include these topics in your teaching plan for the patient receiving an anticoagulant.

- Medication therapy regimen, including the drug's name, dose, frequency, duration, and possible adverse effects
- Signs and symptoms of possible adverse effects and when to notify the physician
- Subcutaneous administration technique if indicated
- Safety measures and bleeding precautions
- Avoidance of over-the-counter products unless permitted by the physician
- Need for compliance with therapy, including taking the drug as prescribed
- Follow-up care, including laboratory tests and physician visits

- Monitor hemoglobin and clotting factor and platelet levels
- Instruct the patient to use a soft toothbrush and an electric razor to prevent trauma and bleeding (for additional teaching tips, see *Teaching about anticoagulants*)
- Instruct the patient to inform the physician and dentist of the medication regimen before undergoing any medical treatments
- **Caution patients not to increase dietary vitamin K or drastically and suddenly change their diet; doing either of these can impair warfarin's effectiveness**
- Teach the patient about the importance of routine laboratory tests to monitor coagulation times
- Instruct the patient to carry identification describing the disease and drug regimen
- Instruct the patient not to take any drugs or vitamins, including over-the-counter or herbal preparations, unless directed by a medical professional

Topics for patient discussion

- Therapy regimen
- Signs and symptoms of possible adverse effects and when to notify the physician
- Subcutaneous administration technique, if indicated
- Safety measures and bleeding precautions
- Avoidance of over-the-counter products unless permitted by the physician
- Need for compliance with therapy
- Follow-up care

THROMBOLYTICS

Mechanism of action

- Activate plasminogen, leading to its conversion to plasmin (a substance that degrades clots)

Pharmacokinetics

- Absorption: Administered I.V.
- Distribution: Distributed immediately throughout the circulation
- Metabolism: Varies with each drug; may be metabolized by the liver or in plasma
- Excretion: Varies with each drug

Key facts about thrombolytics

- Activate plasminogen, leading to its conversion to plasmin
- Metabolism varies with each drug; may be metabolized by the liver or in plasma
- Excretion varies with each drug

When to use thrombolytics

- Lysis of thrombi
- Massive pulmonary emboli, DVT, acute ischemic stroke, and acute MI
- Clearing of arterial catheters and arteriovenous cannuli
- Reduction of mortality in severe sepsis associated with acute organ dysfunction and a high risk of death

When NOT to use thrombolytics

- Recent streptococcal infection
- Active internal bleeding
- Recent stroke
- Underlying coagulation disorders
- Ulcer disease
- Recent surgery
- Cancer
- Uncontrolled hypertension

Adverse reactions to watch for

- Bleeding, arrhythmias, hypersensitivity reactions, urticaria, fever, and hemorrhage

Key nursing actions

- Assess for signs and symptoms of bleeding; tell patient to report bleeding immediately.
- Ensure that aminocaproic acid is readily available.
- Minimize venipunctures, injections, and other invasive procedures; apply pressure to puncture sites to prevent bleeding.
- Keep typed and crossmatched blood on hand to administer in case of hemorrhage.

Drug examples

- Alteplase (tissue plasminogen activator [Activase]), drotrecogin alfa (activated) (Xigris), reteplase (Retavase), streptokinase (Streptase), tenecteplase (TNKase), urokinase (Abbokinase)

Indications

- These drugs are used to produce lysis of thrombi and may be used to treat massive pulmonary emboli, acute ischemic stroke, and acute MI
- These drugs also are used to treat DVT and to clear arterial catheters and arteriovenous cannuli
- Drotrecogin alfa is used to reduce mortality in patients with severe sepsis associated with acute organ dysfunction and a high risk of death

Contraindications and precautions

- Contraindicated in patients with recent streptococcal infection (streptokinase), active internal bleeding, recent stroke, underlying coagulation disorders, ulcer disease, recent surgery, cancer, or uncontrolled hypertension
- Streptokinase isn't indicated for arterial embolism originating from the left side of the heart because of the risk of new embolic phenomena, such as cerebral embolism

Adverse reactions

- The most common adverse reactions are bleeding and arrhythmias
- May also cause hypersensitivity reactions, urticaria, fever, and hemorrhage

Interactions

- May increase risk of bleeding when used concurrently with other drugs that affect platelet function (such as aspirin, dextran, dipyridamole, and NSAIDs)
- Aminocaproic acid inhibits streptokinase and can be used to reverse its fibrinolytic effects

Nursing responsibilities

- Know that thrombolytics should be administered only when the patient's hematologic function and clinical response can be monitored
- When administering an anticoagulant or thrombolytic, assess the patient for signs and symptoms of bleeding, monitor coagulation values, and implement appropriate safety measures to prevent bleeding
- Ensure that aminocaproic acid (Amicar), the antidote for thrombolytic overdose, is readily available
- Minimize venipunctures, injections, and other invasive procedures to decrease the risk of bleeding; apply pressure to all puncture sites to prevent bleeding
- Monitor hemoglobin and clotting factor and platelet levels
- Assess for signs and symptoms of bleeding and instruct the patient to report signs and symptoms of bleeding immediately
- Frequently monitor the patient's vital signs for indications of bleeding or hypotension; check peripheral pulses to ensure adequate circulation to the extremities

- Keep typed and crossmatched blood on hand to administer in case of hemorrhage

ANTIPLATELET DRUGS

Mechanism of action

- Interfere with platelet aggregation in different drug-specific and dose-specific ways, preventing thromboembolic events

Pharmacokinetics

- Absorption: Absorption varies with each drug
- Distribution: Usually distributed quickly and widely throughout the body; highly protein-bound
- Metabolism: Metabolized in the liver
- Excretion: Depending on the form, may be excreted in the bile, the urine, or the feces

Drug examples

- Aspirin, cilostazol (Pletal), clopidogrel (Plavix), dipyridamole (Persantine), ticlopidine (Ticlid)

Indications

- These drugs are used as prophylaxis for thromboembolic events and intermittent claudication
- Aspirin is used in patients with previous MI or unstable angina to reduce the risk of death from these conditions and in men to reduce the risk of transient ischemic attacks
- Cilostazol is used to reduce the symptoms of intermittent claudication
- Clopidogrel is used to reduce a cardiovascular event and mortality in patients with a recent MI, recent stroke, established peripheral arterial disease, or acute coronary syndrome
- Ticlopidine is a second-line drug used to prevent stroke in high-risk individuals

Contraindications and precautions

- Contraindicated in patients with active bleeding, thrombocytopenia, severe liver impairment, underlying coagulation disorders, ulcer disease, recent surgery, or cancer

Adverse reactions

- May cause bleeding, pancytopenia, neutropenia or agranulocytosis (ticlopidine), hemorrhage, or thrombotic thrombocytopenic purpura
- May also cause dizziness, diarrhea, abnormal stools, headache, infection, rash, nausea, or pain at the injection site

Interactions

- May increase the risk of bleeding when used with other drugs that affect platelet function (such as aspirin, dextran, dipyridamole, and NSAIDs)

Key facts about antiplatelet drugs

- Interfere with platelet aggregation in different drug-specific and dose-specific ways, preventing thromboembolic events
- Metabolized in the liver
- Depending on the form, may be excreted in the bile, the urine, or the feces

When to use antiplatelet drugs

- As prophylaxis for thromboembolic events and intermittent claudication

When NOT to use antiplatelet drugs

- Active bleeding
- Thrombocytopenia
- Severe liver impairment
- Underlying coagulation disorders
- Ulcer disease
- Recent surgery
- Cancer

Adverse reactions to watch for

- Bleeding, pancytopenia, neutropenia or agranulocytosis, hemorrhage, thrombotic thrombocytopenic purpura, dizziness, diarrhea, abnormal stools, headache, infection, rash, nausea, and pain at injection site

Key nursing actions

- Monitor patient for bruising or bleeding.
- Assess for signs and symptoms of bleeding; tell patient to report bleeding immediately.
- Monitor hemoglobin and clotting factor and platelet levels.
- Minimize venipunctures and injections; apply pressure to all puncture sites to prevent bleeding.

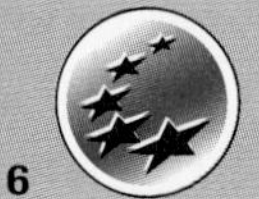

TOP 6

Items to study before your next test on drugs and the hematologic system

1. Rationale for using hematopoietics, anticoagulants, thrombolytics, and antiplatelets
2. Mechanisms of action of hematopoietics, anticoagulants, thrombolytics, and antiplatelets
3. Laboratory tests used to monitor the patient who is receiving a hematopoietic, anticoagulant, thrombolytic, or antiplatelet drug
4. Common adverse effects of hematopoietics, anticoagulants, thrombolytics, and antiplatelet drugs
5. Nursing responsibilities when administering hematopoietics, anticoagulants, thrombolytics, and antiplatelet drugs
6. Appropriate teaching for the patient who is receiving a hematopoietic, anticoagulant, thrombolytic, or antiplatelet drug

Nursing responsibilities

- Monitor the patient for bruising or bleeding
- Assess for signs and symptoms of bleeding and instruct the patient to report signs and symptoms of bleeding immediately
- Monitor hemoglobin and clotting factor and platelet levels
- Minimize venipunctures and injections; apply pressure to all puncture sites to prevent bleeding

NCLEX CHECKS

It's never too soon to begin your NCLEX preparation. Now that you've reviewed this chapter, carefully read each of the following questions and choose the best answer. Then compare your responses to the correct answers.

1. A patient on a weight-reduction diet has been diagnosed with iron deficiency anemia. When teaching the patient about hematinics, what should he understand about the pharmacokinetics of these agents?

☐ A. Hematinics are absorbed through the liver and kidneys.
☐ B. Different routes of administration provide peak drug levels at about the same time.
☐ C. Iron deficiency anemia is correctable with oral administration of an iron preparation.
☐ D. Normal hemoglobin levels and body iron stores are restored after 1 month of therapy.

2. What agent would you use to treat anemia related to renal disease?

☐ A. Cyanocobalamin
☐ B. Epoetin alfa
☐ C. Ferrous sulfate
☐ D. Folic acid

3. A 21-year-old female college student takes birth control pills and is a heavy smoker. She develops a thrombus in her leg, is admitted to the hospital, and is started on heparin. Which of the following actions is the most important?

☐ A. Keep her on strict bed rest.
☐ B. Limit her smoking to one pack a day.
☐ C. Give her aspirin for headaches and joint stiffness.
☐ D. Have her walk after 4 hours to prevent pneumonia and joint stiffness.

4. While hospitalized, a patient is receiving heparin, which the physician ordered to be continued while starting warfarin sodium (Coumadin) therapy. Which of the following rationales explains why these two drugs are given together?

☐ A. Heparin activates warfarin.
☐ B. Heparin hastens warfarin's onset of action.
☐ C. Warfarin and heparin have an antagonistic effect.
☐ D. Warfarin's therapeutic effects don't start until clotting factors are depleted.

5. Your patient is allergic to salicylates. He is prescribed an antiplatelet drug as a prophylactic against stroke. What drug would you expect to administer?

☐ **A.** dipyridamole (Persantine)
☐ **B.** folic acid
☐ **C.** ticlopidine (Ticlid)
☐ **D.** warfarin sodium (Coumadin)

6. A patient is admitted to the emergency department with an acute inferior wall myocardial infarction (MI). After receiving oxygen, I.V. nitroglycerin, and I.V. morphine, the patient still feels pain. The physician orders streptokinase (Streptase), 140,000 IU, by intracoronary infusion. Which condition would contraindicate the use of streptokinase?

☐ **A.** Age 60 or older
☐ **B.** History of MI
☐ **C.** Acute pulmonary thromboembolism
☐ **D.** Cerebrovascular accident (CVA) in the past 2 months

7. A 75-year-old patient is admitted to the hospital with anemia secondary to end-stage renal disease. His hemoglobin on admission to the emergency department is 10.2 g/dl. The physician prescribes epoetin alfa (Epogen) 100 units/kg I.V. 3 times/week. The patient, on admission, weighed 150 lbs. How many units will you administer? ________

ANSWERS AND RATIONALES

1. CORRECT ANSWER: C

Iron deficiency anemia, which is commonly caused by inadequate dietary intake of iron, is correctable with oral iron preparations, such as ferrous fumarate, ferrous gluconate, or ferrous sulfate. It usually takes 6 months of iron therapy to restore normal hemoglobin levels and create iron stores in the body. Peak levels differ according to the route of administration and absorption factors. Drug levels may peak in 4 weeks with oral administration and within 4 to 8 weeks with I.V. and I.M. administration. Oral hematinics are absorbed primarily from the duodenum and upper jejunum mucosal cell membranes; hematinics administered by injection are absorbed by the lymphatic system or transported by the bloodstream to be stored in the liver.

2. CORRECT ANSWER: B

Epoetin alfa imitates erythropoietin, which is necessary for the stimulation of red blood cell (RBC) production, and which may correct normocytic anemia related to renal disease. This agent also has been used to stimulate RBC production before surgery when transfusions are refused. Clinical response normally takes 2 to 6 weeks. Cyanocobalamin, vitamin B_{12}, is used to treat pernicious anemia. Ferrous sulfate is used to prevent and treat iron deficiency anemia. Folic acid is used to treat megaloblastic anemia related to folic acid deficiency.

3. CORRECT ANSWER: A

A patient with a thrombus needs to be on strict bed rest to prevent dislodgment of the clot, which could migrate to the pulmonary system and result in a pulmonary embolus. Smoking constricts blood vessels and may contribute to clot formation, so it should be avoided entirely. Aspirin potentiates the effects of anticoagulants and should be avoided while the patient is receiving heparin. The patient should be instructed not to walk because bed rest is needed to prevent dislodgment of the clot.

4. CORRECT ANSWER: D

Therapeutic anticoagulation with warfarin or other oral anticoagulants may not be achieved for 3 to 5 days after initiation of therapy. This is the amount of time it takes for oral anticoagulants to deplete the blood of clotting factors. Heparin administration provides continued anticoagulation during this transition to oral anticoagulation therapy. Heparin accelerates the interaction between thrombin and antithrombin III, but it doesn't activate or hasten the onset of the effects of warfarin. Heparin doesn't antagonize the effects of warfarin.

5. CORRECT ANSWER: C

For patients with salicylate (aspirin) sensitivity, ticlopidine is used most often as a preventive antiplatelet drug against stroke. Dipyridamole's status as an antiplatelet drug is questionable because research has shown mixed results. Folic acid and warfarin aren't antiplatelet drugs.

6. CORRECT ANSWER: D

Streptokinase is contraindicated when a patient has had a CVA within the past 2 months, is undergoing intracranial or intraspinal surgery, or has active internal bleeding, intracranial neoplasm, severe uncontrolled hypertension, or drug hypersensitivity because bleeding is an adverse reaction of this drug. Acute pulmonary thromboembolism and a history of an acute MI aren't contraindications to streptokinase therapy. Streptokinase is to be used with caution in patients older than age 75. There's no age-related caution for patients age 75 and younger.

7. CORRECT ANSWER: 6,800

To start, first convert the patient's weight from lb into kg.

Use the following equation (2.2 lb = 1 kg):

$$2.2 \text{ lb}/1 \text{ kg} = 150 \text{ lb}/x \text{ kg}$$

$$2.2x = 150$$

$$x = 68.1 \text{ kg}$$

Then, determine the number of units:

$$100 \text{ units}/1 \text{ kg} = x \text{ units}/68 \text{ kg}$$

$$x = 6{,}800 \text{ units}$$

Drugs and the endocrine system

LEARNING OBJECTIVES

After studying this chapter, you should be able to:

- Describe the mechanisms of action for pituitary, thyroid, and parathyroid drugs; insulin; and oral hypoglycemics.
- Discuss the rationale for using pituitary, thyroid, and parathyroid drugs; insulin; and oral hypoglycemics.
- Name major adverse effects of pituitary, thyroid, and parathyroid drugs.
- Identify nursing responsibilities when administering pituitary, thyroid, and parathyroid drugs; insulin; and oral hypoglycemics.
- Discuss patient teaching related to insulin and oral hypoglycemics.
- Identify the purpose, mechanism of action, adverse reactions, and nursing considerations of antihypercalcemic drugs.

CHAPTER OVERVIEW

Pituitary hormones and thyroid and parathyroid drugs are used to replace or inhibit hormones in states of deficiency or excess. Pituitary hormones, secreted by the anterior and posterior pituitary gland, are used as hormone replacement. Thyroid drugs replace endogenous thyroid hormone in deficiency states, and antithyroid drugs treat hypersecretion and decrease the size and vascularity of the thyroid gland before surgery. Parathyroid drugs regulate calcium imbalances, which usually result from underlying pathology. Nursing responsibilities include monitoring related laboratory and X-ray studies and observing for adverse effects. Patient teaching focuses on the importance of adhering to the prescribed regimen and keeping follow-up appointments.

Antidiabetics are used to control hyperglycemia secondary to diabetes mellitus, stress responses, total parenteral nutrition, hyperkalemia, medications, and other disorders. Type 1 diabetes is controlled with injectable insulin and diet therapy. Insulin may be derived from pork or human (produced by recombinant deoxyribonucleic acid technology) sources. Type 2 diabetes is managed with diet therapy and an oral hypoglycemic, and possibly insulin, as needed. Oral hypoglycemics stimulate beta cells of the pancreas to release insulin, enhance insulin receptor sites, potentiate insulin's action, or delay absorption of dietary carbohydrates in the intestine. Nursing responsibilities include recognizing and treating symptoms of hypoglycemia and hyperglycemia, monitoring blood glucose and glycosylated hemoglobin levels, and teaching proper timing and techniques for drug administration and nutrition.

A&P highlights

- The endocrine system includes the pituitary gland, thyroid gland, parathyroid glands, adrenal glands, and the islets of Langerhans (in the pancreas).
- These endocrine glands release various hormones:
  - Anterior pituitary gland secretes GH, TSH, ACTH, FSH, LH, and prolactin.
  - Posterior pituitary gland secretes oxytocin and ADH.
  - Thyroid gland secretes T_3, T_4, and thyrocalcitonin.
  - Parathyroid glands secrete PTH.
  - Adrenal cortex secretes glucocorticoids, mineralocorticoids, and sex hormones.
  - Adrenal medulla secretes epinephrine and norepinephrine.
  - Islets of Langerhans secrete glucagon, insulin, and somatostatin.

ANATOMY AND PHYSIOLOGY

Anatomy

- The endocrine system consists of the endocrine glands, which are ductless glands located throughout the body, and other structures
  - The major endocrine glands are the pituitary, thyroid, parathyroid, and adrenal glands, the islets of Langerhans (in the pancreas), the ovaries, and the testes (For more detailed information on the ovaries and the testes, see chapter 15)
  - The other structures, such as the pineal and thymus glands, are considered minor glands
- The pituitary gland, also known as the master gland, is located at the base of the brain and has two main lobes—the anterior lobe and the posterior lobe
- The thyroid gland, one of the largest endocrine glands, is located in the lower anterior portion of the neck
- Four small parathyroid glands are located in the posterior surface of the thyroid gland; these pea-sized glands are the smallest endocrine glands
- The adrenal glands are located on top of each kidney and consist of the adrenal cortex and the adrenal medulla
  - The adrenal cortex forms the bulk of the adrenal gland
  - The adrenal medulla forms the inner part of the adrenal gland
  - The adrenal cortex and the adrenal medulla function as separate endocrine glands
- The pancreas lies horizontally in the left upper quadrant of the abdomen and has millions of cell clusters known as the islets of Langerhans scattered throughout; each islet is composed of six different cells that secrete different hormones

Physiology

- Endocrine glands release hormones directly into the blood or the lymph

- Hormones are chemical substances that regulate the activities of specific organs
- Once secreted into the bloodstream, hormones travel to their target tissue and act by altering the metabolism of the specific cells in the target tissue

- The pituitary gland receives chemical and nervous stimulation from the hypothalamus
  - The hypothalamus activates, controls, and integrates various endocrine functions
  - The hypothalamus releases hormones that are stored in the anterior and posterior pituitary glands
  - The release of these hormones is controlled by a negative feedback mechanism, whereby further hormone output is suppressed when there is an elevated level of hormone or hormone-regulated substance in the body
  - The anterior pituitary gland secretes growth hormone (GH), thyroid-stimulating hormone (TSH), adrenocorticotropic hormone (ACTH), follicle-stimulating hormone (FSH), luteinizing hormone (LH), and prolactin
  - The posterior pituitary gland secretes oxytocin and antidiuretic hormone (ADH)
- The thyroid gland secretes triiodothyronine (T_3) and thyroxine (T_4), which regulate the metabolic rate, and thyrocalcitonin, which helps control calcium metabolism
- All four parathyroid glands secrete parathyroid hormone (PTH), the principal regulator of calcium metabolism
- The adrenal cortex secretes glucocorticoids, mineralocorticoids, and sex hormones; the adrenal medulla secretes epinephrine and norepinephrine
- The islets of Langerhans contain alpha cells, which secrete glucagon; beta cells, which secrete insulin; and delta cells, which secrete somatostatin

Function

- The endocrine system and nervous system control all body functions through hormones
- The anterior pituitary gland secretes GH, TSH, ACTH, FSH, LH, and prolactin
  - GH stimulates bone and muscle growth
  - TSH stimulates the thyroid gland to release thyroid hormone
  - ACTH stimulates the adrenal cortex to release glucocorticoid
  - FSH stimulates ovarian follicle maturation and production in women and sperm production in men
  - LH stimulates ovulation and ovarian production of progesterone and testicular production of testosterone in males
  - Prolactin stimulates the breasts to produce milk
- The posterior pituitary gland secretes oxytocin and ADH
  - Oxytocin stimulates contraction of the pregnant uterus

Functions of the anterior pituitary gland

- GH: stimulates bone and muscle growth
- TSH: causes the release of thyroid hormone
- ACTH: causes the release of glucocorticoid
- FSH: stimulates ovarian production and sperm production
- LH: stimulates ovulation and stimulates the breasts to produce milk

Functions of the posterior pituitary gland

- Oxytocin: stimulates uterine contraction
- ADH: causes cells to be more permeable to water

– ADH causes the cells of the renal and collecting tubules to be more permeable to water, thus altering urine concentration

- The thyroid gland secretes T_3, T_4, and thyrocalcitonin
  - T_3 and T_4 control the rate of metabolism, which is necessary for normal growth and development and for the development and maturation of the nervous system
  - Thyrocalcitonin maintains the blood calcium level by inhibiting calcium release from bone (thereby lowering the blood calcium level)
- The four parathyroid glands secrete PTH
  - PTH helps regulate calcium metabolism by adjusting the rate at which the kidneys remove calcium and magnesium ions from the urine
  - PTH raises the blood calcium level
- The adrenal cortex secretes glucocorticoids, mineralocorticoids, and sex hormones
  - Glucocorticoids raise the blood glucose level by decreasing glucose metabolism and promoting glucose formation from protein and fat (also known as gluconeogenesis)
  - Mineralocorticoids regulate electrolyte and water balance by promoting sodium absorption and potassium excretion by the renal tubules
  - Sex hormones are responsible for the sex drive in men and women
- The adrenal medulla secretes norepinephrine and epinephrine
  - Norepinephrine and epinephrine cause widespread physiologic effects in response to stress, also known as the fight-or-flight response
  - They increase heart rate and cardiac output and cause vasoconstriction
  - They also increase the blood glucose level and the responsiveness of the nervous system
- The islets of Langerhans secrete glucagon, insulin, and somatostatin
  - Glucagon, secreted by the alpha cells in the islets of Langerhans, increases the blood glucose level in response to hypoglycemia
  - Insulin, secreted by the beta cells in response to blood glucose elevation, controls carbohydrate metabolism and increases the use of glucose as a source of energy, thereby decreasing blood glucose levels
  - Somatostatin, secreted by the delta cells, inhibits insulin and glucagon secretion and suppresses growth hormone, resulting in decreased blood glucose levels; somatostatin also inhibits glucose absorption from the GI tract

GROWTH HORMONES

Mechanism of action

- These drugs are therapeutically equivalent to and simulate the action of endogenous growth hormones; they interact with specific plasma membrane receptors to stimulate linear growth and increase the number and size of muscle cells to stimulate skeletal growth
- Growth hormones decrease carbohydrate metabolism by decreasing insulin sensitivity in children with hypopituitarism

Functions of the thyroid gland

- T_3 and T_4: control the rate of metabolism
- Thyrocalcitonin: maintains blood calcium level

Functions of PTH in the parathyroid glands

- Helps regulate calcium metabolism
- Raises the blood calcium level

Functions of the adrenal cortex

- Glucocorticoids: raise the blood glucose level
- Mineralocorticoids: regulate electrolyte and water balance
- Sex hormones: responsible for the sex drive

Functions of norepinephrine and epinephrine in the adrenal medulla

- Cause physiologic effects in response to stress
- Increase heart rate, cardiac output
- Cause vasoconstriction
- Increase blood glucose level

Functions of the islets of Langerhans

- Glucagon: increases blood glucose level
- Insulin: controls carbohydrate metabolism and increases glucose use
- Somatostatin: inhibits insulin and glucagon secretion; suppresses growth hormone

- Growth hormones increase protein metabolism by retaining nitrogen and increasing cellular protein synthesis
- Growth hormones reduce body fat stores, increase lipid mobilization, and increase plasma fatty acids to increase lipid metabolism and decrease mean cholesterol levels
- Growth hormones stimulate the synthesis of chondroitin sulfate and collagen and the urinary excretion of hydroxyproline to cause connective tissue metabolism

Pharmacokinetics

- Absorption: Levels peak in 7.5 hours; bioavailability is 75% after subcutaneous injection and 63% after I.M. administration
- Distribution: Drugs localize to highly perfused organs, particularly the liver and kidneys
- Metabolism: Metabolized by the liver and the kidneys
- Excretion: Excreted in the urine and feces

Drug examples

- Somatrem (Protropin), somatropin (Genotropin, Humatrope, Norditropin, Nutropin, Nutropin AQ, Nutropin Depot, Saizen, Serostim)

Indications

- Except for Serostim, growth hormones are used to treat growth failure due to lack of adequate endogenous growth hormones
- Nutropin and Nutropin AQ also are used to treat growth failure in children with chronic renal failure
- Serostim only is used to treat cachexia or wasting due to AIDS
- Humatrope, Nutropin, and Nutropin AQ are used for the long-term treatment of short stature associated with Turner syndrome
- Humatrope is used to treat somatropin deficiency syndrome
- Genotropin is used to treat growth failure in patients with Prader-Willi syndrome and in those born small for gestational age who don't achieve catch-up growth by age 2

Contraindications and precautions

- Contraindicated in patients with closed epiphyses or with evidence of intracranial tumors or active neoplasia
- Some of these drugs contain benzyl alcohol, which is contraindicated in neonates and in patients hypersensitive to it
- Humatrope is contraindicated in patients with an allergy to m-cresol or glycerin
- Use cautiously in breast-feeding women and in patients with diabetes or glucose tolerance

Adverse reactions

- These drugs may cause malignant transformation of skin lesions, clipped capital femoral epiphysis or avascular necrosis of the femoral head, gynecomastia, and intracranial hypertension with visual changes, headache, nausea, or vomiting
- These drugs may cause leukemia in children

Key facts about growth hormones

- Therapeutically equivalent to and simulate the action of endogenous growth hormones
- Stimulate linear growth and increase the number and size of muscle cells
- Decrease carbohydrate metabolism; increase protein metabolism
- Reduce body fat, increase lipid mobilization, and decrease mean cholesterol levels
- Metabolized by liver and kidneys
- Excreted in urine and feces

When to use growth hormones

- Growth failure; short stature
- Cachexia or wasting
- Somatropin deficiency syndrome

When NOT to use growth hormones

- Closed epiphyses, intracranial tumors, or active neoplasia
- Drug allergies
- Neonates

Adverse reactions to watch for

- Malignant transformation of skin lesions, clipped capital femoral epiphysis or avascular necrosis of femoral head, gynecomastia, intracranial hypertension, leukemia, swelling, musculoskeletal discomfort, carpal tunnel syndrome, pain at injection site, mild and transient edema, glucose intolerance, headache, weakness, localized muscle pain, antibodies to growth hormones, increased growth of preexisting nevi, and pancreatitis

Key nursing actions

- Monitor thyroid function tests regularly.
- Rotate injection sites.
- Monitor for intracranial hypertension.

Key facts about antidiuretic hormones

- Enhance reabsorption of water in kidneys
- Promote vasoconstriction; decrease hepatic blood flow
- Metabolized by liver and kidneys (vasopressin)
- Excreted unchanged in urine (vasopressin)

- Serostim also may cause swelling, musculoskeletal discomfort, and carpal tunnel syndrome
- Somatropin also may cause pain at injection site, mild and transient edema, glucose intolerance, headache, weakness, localized muscle pain, and antibodies to growth hormones
- Nutropin AQ also may cause mild and transient peripheral edema, increased growth of preexisting nevi, and pancreatitis

Interactions

- These drugs may cause epiphyseal closure when used with androgens, estrogens, or thyroid hormones
- These drugs diminish the growth rate when given with glucocorticoids

Nursing responsibilities

- Monitor serum and urine glucose levels regularly to prevent glucose intolerance
- Monitor thyroid function tests regularly
- Know that injection of growth hormones may cause pain and swelling; therefore, rotate injection sites to decrease these effects
- Teach the patient self-injection techniques, if appropriate
- Stress the importance of regular blood and urine glucose monitoring to detect adverse effects
- Recommend annual bone age determinations for children receiving growth hormone
- Monitor the patient for intracranial hypertension by performing a funduscopic examination periodically

ANTIDIURETIC HORMONES

Mechanism of action

- These drugs enhance reabsorption of water in the kidneys and smooth muscle contraction (vasoconstriction), promoting an antidiuretic effect and regulating fluid balance
- Vasopressin also promotes vasoconstriction and decreases hepatic blood flow
- Desmopressin has a greater antidiuretic response than vasopressin; response time following I.V. administration is about 10 times greater than that following intranasal administration

Pharmacokinetics

- Absorption
  - Intranasal desmopressin is absorbed in the nasal mucosa
  - Oral desmopressin is only minimally absorbed in the GI tract: bioavailability is 5% compared with that of intranasal administration and 0.16% compared with that of I.V. administration
  - Vasopressin's duration of action is 2 to 8 hours following I.M. or S.C. injection

- Distribution
  - Unknown for desmopressin, except that it appears in breast milk
  - Vasopressin is distributed throughout the extracellular fluid
- Metabolism
  - Unknown for desmopressin
  - Vasopressin is metabolized in the liver and the kidneys
- Excretion
  - Unknown for desmopressin
  - Vasopressin is excreted unchanged in the urine

Drug examples

- Desmopressin (DDAVP, Stimate), vasopressin (Pitressin)

Indications

- These drugs are used to treat diabetes insipidus
- Desmopressin also is used to treat nocturnal enuresis (nighttime bedwetting) and to control bleeding in hemophilia A and mild to moderate von Willebrand's disease (type I) with factor VIII levels greater than 5%
- Vasopressin also is used to prevent and treat postoperative abdominal distention and to dispel interfering gas shadows in abdominal roentgenography

Contraindications and precautions

- Desmopressin is contraindicated in patients with type IIB, or platelet-type, pseudo von Willebrand's disease
- Vasopressin is contraindicated in patients with anaphylaxis or hypersensitivity to the drug or its components and in patients with chronic nephritis with nitrogen retention
- Use vasopressin with extreme caution in patients with vascular disease (especially coronary artery disease), epilepsy, migraines, asthma, heart failure, or states in which a rapid increase in extracellular water may result in further compromise, and in pregnant or breast-feeding women

Adverse reactions

- These drugs may cause water intoxication, hyponatremia, abdominal cramps, nausea, nasal congestion or changes (with nasal administration), facial flushing, hypertension, chest pain, headache, epistaxis, sore throat, cough, and injection site redness, swelling, or burning

Interactions

- Alcohol, demeclocycline, epinephrine, heparin, and lithium reduce antidiuretic hormone activity when used with these drugs
- Carbamazepine, chlorpropamide, clofibrate, fludrocortisone, tricyclic antidepressants, and urea increase antidiuretic hormone activity when used with these drugs

Nursing responsibilities

- Frequently monitor the patient's fluid intake and output and urine osmolality
- Teach the patient how to use the intranasal drug form, if prescribed

When to use antidiuretic hormones

- Diabetes insipidus
- Nocturnal enuresis
- Bleeding in hemophilia A
- Mild to moderate von Willebrand's disease
- Postoperative abdominal distention

When NOT to use antidiuretic hormones

- Type IIB or pseudo von Willebrand's disease
- Anaphylaxis or hypersensitivity to the drug

Adverse reactions to watch for

- Water intoxication, hyponatremia, abdominal cramps, nausea, nasal congestion, facial flushing, hypertension, chest pain, headache, epistaxis, sore throat, cough, and injection site redness, swelling, or burning

- Instruct the patient to consult the physician if rhinitis or nasal congestion occurs because these conditions may decrease the effects of intranasal therapy
- Caution the patient to abstain from alcohol to prevent adverse drug interactions and dehydration
- Teach the patient to self-administer and alternate injection sites to prevent tissue damage, if appropriate
- **Warn patients, especially children and elderly patients, to ingest only enough fluid to satisfy thirst to decrease the risk of water intoxication and hyponatremia; early signs of water intoxication include drowsiness and listlessness, and headaches precede coma and convulsions**

Key nursing actions

- Monitor fluid intake and output and urine osmolality frequently.
- Warn patients to ingest only enough fluid to satisfy thirst to decrease risk or water intoxication and hyponatremia.

THYROID HORMONES

Mechanism of action

- These drugs control the metabolic rate of tissues and accelerate heat production and oxygen consumption
- Synthetic thyroid hormones have the same physiologic effects as natural hormones; they result in T_3 activity and are used to replace hormonal deficits or suppress excessive hormone production

Key facts about thyroid hormones

- Control metabolic rate of tissues
- Accelerate heat production and oxygen consumption
- Result in T_3 activity
- Used to replace hormonal deficits or suppress excessive hormone production
- Metabolized in liver and other tissues
- Excreted in bile and urine

Pharmacokinetics

- Absorption: Absorbed from the GI tract; fasting increases absorption
- Distribution: Drug is over 99% protein-bound
- Metabolism: Metabolized in the liver and other tissues
- Excretion: Excreted in the bile and urine

Drug examples

- Levothyroxine sodium (T_4 [Levothroid, Levoxine, Levoxyl, Synthroid, Thyro-Tabs, Unithroid]), liothyronine sodium (T_3 [Cytomel], Triostat), liotrix (Thyrolar), thyroid USP (desiccated [Armour Thyroid], S-P-T)

Indications

- As thyroid hormone replacement in primary or secondary hypothyroidism (including cretinism, myxedema, and nontoxic goiter) and in hypothyroidism caused by functional deficiency, primary atrophy, partial or total absence of thyroid gland, or effects of surgery, radiation, or drugs
- Also used to treat or prevent goiters by suppressing secretion of TSH from the pituitary gland
- May be used with antithyroid drugs to treat thyrotoxicosis, to prevent goitrogenesis and hypothyroidism, and to prevent thyrotoxicosis during pregnancy

When to use thyroid hormones

- Primary or secondary hypothyroidism
- Goiters
- Thyrotoxicosis

Contraindications and precautions

- Thyroid hormones are contraindicated in patients with an acute myocardial infarction or thyrotoxicosis uncomplicated by hypothyroidism; if hypothyroidism is a complication, thyroid hormones may be used judiciously

- Contraindicated when hypothyroidism and hypoadrenalism (Addison's disease) coexist, unless the treatment of hypoadrenalism with adrenocortical steroids precedes the initiation of thyroid therapy
- Use thyroid hormones cautiously in patients with heart disease, hypertension, diabetes mellitus or insipidus, myxedema, or adrenal insufficiency
- Thyroid hormones aren't intended to be used as primary or adjunctive therapy in a weight control program

Adverse reactions

- Prolonged and excessive use may cause signs and symptoms of hyperthyroidism or may aggravate existing hyperthyroidism
- May cause tachycardia, arrhythmias, palpitations, nervousness, sweating, heat intolerance, insomnia, weight loss, and headache, which are symptoms of overdosage
- May decrease bone density with long-term use in pre- and postmenopausal women
- May cause partial hair loss in children in the first few months of therapy; however, hair loss is usually temporary

Interactions

- Thyroid hormones increase the effects of oral anticoagulants
- Colestipol and cholestyramine decrease the effects of thyroid hormones and may cause hypothyroidism
- Thyroid hormones may impair the effects of beta blockers and digoxin
- Thyroid hormones may increase theophylline levels
- Estrogen decreases the effects of thyroid hormones

Nursing responsibilities

- **Administer thyroid hormones in the morning to prevent insomnia**
- Teach the patient to take the drug 1 hour before meals or 2 hours after meals to improve drug absorption
- Because colestipol and cholestyramine decrease the effects of thyroid hormones, give these drugs at least 4 hours apart
- Monitor the patient's pulse rate and evaluate results of thyroid function studies
- **Caution the patient not to change medication brands because potency differs among brands**
- Teach the patient about the importance of complying with therapy
- **Tell the patient to notify the prescriber if headache, nervousness, diarrhea, excessive sweating, heat intolerance, chest pain, increased pulse rate, palpitations (symptoms of hyperthyroidism), or other unusual events occur**

ANTITHYROID DRUGS

Mechanism of action

- Iodine
  - Iodine is circulated into the thyroid gland as iodide

When NOT to use thyroid hormones

- Acute MI or thyrotoxicosis
- Coexistence of hypothyroidism and hypoadrenalism, unless treatment of hypoadrenalism with adrenocortical steroids precedes initiation of thyroid therapy

Adverse reactions to watch for

- Hyperthyroidism, tachycardia, arrhythmias, palpitations, nervousness, sweating, heat intolerance, insomnia, weight loss, headache, decreased bone density, partial hair loss

Key nursing actions

- Administer thyroid hormones in the morning to prevent insomnia.
- Caution patient not to change medication brands.
- Instruct patient to notify prescriber if headache, nervousness, diarrhea, or other unusual events occur.

Key facts about antithyroid drugs

- Iodine is circulated into the thyroid glands as iodide; iodide helps yield thyroid hormones; large doses of iodide can inhibit T_3 and T_4 synthesis
- PTU and methimazole inhibit synthesis of thyroid hormones; don't inactivate existing T_3 or T_4
- Sodium iodide I 131 limits thyroid hormone secretion; facilitates reuptake of drug to cancerous thyroid tissue
- Metabolized rapidly into conjugate and minor metabolites (PTU)
- Excreted in urine

When to use antithyroid drugs

- Hyperthyroidism
- Thyroid blocking
- Thyroid carcinoma

When NOT to use antithyroid drugs

- Pregnancy and breast-feeding
- Hypersensitivity to iodides

  - Iodide oxidation helps yield thyroid hormones
  - Large doses of iodide can inhibit T_3 and T_4 synthesis
- Propylthiouracil (PTU) and methimazole
  - These drugs inhibit the synthesis of thyroid hormones
  - They don't inactivate existing T_4 or T_3 or interfere with exogenous thyroid hormones
  - PTU partially inhibits the conversion of T_4 to T_3
- Sodium iodide I 131
  - It limits thyroid hormone secretion by destroying thyroid tissue
  - Because thyroid tissue has an affinity to radioactive iodine, it facilitates the reuptake of the drug to cancerous thyroid tissue that has metastasized

Pharmacokinetics

- Absorption: Absorbed in the GI tract
- Distribution: Crosses the placental barrier and appears in breast milk; PTU is highly protein-bound, but methimazole isn't
- Metabolism: Unknown, but PTU is metabolized rapidly into its conjugate and minor metabolites and requires frequent administration
- Excretion: Excreted in the urine

Drug examples

- Iodine (Strong Iodine Solution, USP [Lugol's solution], Thyro-Block), methimazole (Tapazole), PTU, sodium iodide I 131 (Iodotope, Sodium Iodide I 131 Therapeutic)

Indications

- Antithyroid drugs are used to treat hyperthyroidism (Graves' disease)
- PTU also is used when a thyroidectomy is contraindicated or not advisable
- Iodine is used adjunctively with an antithyroid drug in hyperthyroid patients to decrease hyperthyroidism and reduce thyroid friability before surgery and to treat thyrotoxic crisis or neonatal thyrotoxicosis
- Iodine may also be used for thyroid blocking in a radiation emergency
- Sodium iodine I 131 also may be used palliatively in selected cases of thyroid carcinoma

Contraindications and precautions

- Iodine is contraindicated in pregnant women and in patients hypersensitive to iodides
- PTU and methimazole are contraindicated in pregnant and breast-feeding women
- Sodium iodide I 131 is contraindicated in women who are or intend to become pregnant, or who are breast-feeding, and in patients who are younger than age 30 or who have preexisting vomiting and diarrhea

Adverse reactions

- Iodine may cause hypothyroidism, diarrhea, hypersensitivity, and iodism (characterized by vomiting, abdominal pain, metallic taste, rash, and sore salivary glands)

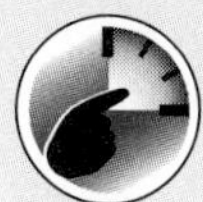

TIME-OUT FOR TEACHING

Teaching about thyroid hormones

Include these topics in your teaching plan for the patient receiving a thyroid hormone.

- Medication regimen, including the drug's name, dosage, frequency, duration, and possible adverse effects
- Signs and symptoms to discuss with the physician, including those relating to adverse effects and thyroid hormone deficiency or excess (including toxicity)
- Consistency regarding time of administration and brand used
- Possible dietary restrictions, such as foods containing iodine
- Avoidance of other products containing iodine
- Compliance with therapy, including taking the drug as prescribed
- Follow-up care, including laboratory tests and physician visits

Topics for patient discussion

- Therapy regimen
- Signs and symptoms
- Dietary restrictions

- Methimazole and PTU may cause nausea, vomiting, agranulocytosis, and rash
- Sodium iodide I 131 may cause bone marrow depression, acute leukemia, anemia, radiation sickness, chest pains, tachycardia, itching, neck tenderness or swelling, sore throat, cough, and temporary thinning of the hair

Adverse reactions to watch for

- Hypothyroidism, diarrhea, hypersensitivity, iodism, nausea, vomiting, agranulocytosis, rash, bone marrow depression, acute leukemia, anemia, radiation sickness, chest pains, tachycardia, itching, neck tenderness or swelling, sore throat, cough, and temporary thinning of the hair

Interactions

- Iodine use with lithium may cause hypothyroidism
- PTU and methimazole may enhance the effects of anticoagulants
- Recent intake of stable forms of iodine, thyroid hormone, or antithyroid drug affects the uptake of sodium iodide I 131

Nursing responsibilities

- Give the drug at regular intervals (usually every 8 hours), unless directed otherwise by the physician
- **Administer the drug at a consistent time 1 hour before or 2 hours after meals because food may affect drug absorption**
- Dilute strong iodine solution with water or fruit juice to improve taste
- Monitor the patient's serum thyroid levels and thyroid function test results
- Assess the patient for signs and symptoms of overdose (hypothyroidism) or under dose (thyrotoxicosis)
- Advise the patient to consult the physician before eating iodized salt and iodine-rich foods (for additional teaching tips, see *Teaching about thyroid hormones*)
- Teach the patient to avoid aspirin and drugs containing iodine
- Teach the patient about the importance of complying with therapy and undergoing routine follow-up evaluation
- Advise caregivers that children receiving growth hormone should have annual bone age determinations

Key nursing actions

- Administer drug at a consistent time 1 hour before or 2 hours after meals.
- Assess for signs and symptoms of overdose or under dose.
- Advise caregiver that children receiving growth hormone should have annual bone age determinations.

PARATHYROID AND ANTIHYPERCALCEMIC DRUGS

Key facts about parathyroid and antihypercalcemic drugs

- Parathyroid drugs: increase serum calcium level; metabolized in liver and kidneys; excreted in feces
- Antihypercalcemic drugs: reduce serum calcium level; not metabolized; excreted in urine

When to use parathyroid and antihypercalcemic drugs

- Parathyroid drugs: hypocalcemia, hypoparathyroidism, pseudohypoparathyroidism, osteoporosis
- Antihypercalcemic drugs: hypercalcemia, Paget's disease, osteoporosis, heterotopic ossification following total hip replacement or spinal cord injury, hypercalcemia of malignancy, metastases of breast cancer, osteolytic lesions of multiple myeloma

When NOT to use parathyroid and antihypercalcemic drugs

- Parathyroid drugs: hypercalcemia, vitamin D toxicity
- Antihypercalcemic drugs: hypersensitivity to bisphosphonates, hypocalcemia, abnormalities of the esophagus that delay gastric emptying, inability to stand or sit upright for 30 minutes, clinically overt osteomalacia, severe renal impairment

Mechanism of action

- Parathyroid drugs increase the serum calcium level, causing a corresponding decrease in the serum phosphate level
- Antihypercalcemic drugs reduce the serum calcium level by reducing bone resorption, increasing GI absorption of calcium, and interfering with renal calcium clearance

Pharmacokinetics

- Absorption
  - Parathyroid drugs are readily absorbed in the GI tract after oral administration
  - Absorption by bone of antihypercalcemic drugs is rapid; food reduces the bioavailability of antihypercalcemic drugs
- Distribution
  - Parathyroid drugs are distributed widely and are protein-bound
  - Distribution of antihypercalcemic drugs varies
- Metabolism
  - Parathyroid drugs are metabolized in the liver and kidneys
  - Antihypercalcemic drugs aren't metabolized
- Excretion
  - Parathyroid drugs are excreted primarily in the feces
  - Antihypercalcemic drugs are excreted in the urine

Drug examples

- Parathyroid drugs: calcitriol (Calcijex, Rocaltrol), calcium carbonate (Os-Cal), calcium citrate, calcium chloride, calcium gluconate, calcium lactate
- Antihypercalcemic drugs: alendronate sodium (Fosamax), calcitonin (salmon [Calcimar]), etidronate disodium (Didronel), gallium nitrate (Ganite), pamidronate disodium (Aredia), risedronate sodium (Actonel), teriparatide (Furteo), tiludronate disodium (Skelid), zoledronic acid (Zometa)

Indications

- Parathyroid drugs are used to treat hypocalcemia, hypoparathyroidism, and pseudohypoparathyroidism and to prevent and treat osteoporosis
- Antihypercalcemic drugs are used to treat hypercalcemia, Paget's disease, osteoporosis, heterotopic ossification following total hip replacement or spinal cord injury, hypercalcemia of malignancy, metastases of breast cancer, and osteolytic lesions of multiple myeloma

Contraindications and precautions

- Parathyroid drugs are contraindicated in patients with hypercalcemia or vitamin D toxicity
- Use parathyroid drugs cautiously in patients with renal failure

- Antihypercalcemic drugs are contraindicated in patients with hypersensitivity to bisphosphonates or other components of the drugs and in those with hypocalcemia, abnormalities of the esophagus that delay gastric emptying, inability to stand or sit upright for at least 30 minutes, clinically overt osteomalacia, or severe renal impairment
- Use antihypercalcemic drugs cautiously in patients with asthma or upper GI problems and in pregnant or breast-feeding women (except zoledronic acid, which is contraindicated)

Adverse reactions to watch for

- Hypercalcemia and hypocalcemia

Adverse reactions

- **Parathyroid drugs may cause hypercalcemia (characterized by nausea, vomiting, anorexia, polyuria, polydipsia, constipation, arrhythmias, calculi, and lethargy)**
- **Antihypercalcemic drugs may cause hypocalcemia (marked by nausea, vomiting, facial flushing, tetany, positive Trousseau's sign, and positive Chvostek's sign)**

Interactions

- Use of parathyroid and antihypercalcemic drugs with magnesium-containing antacids may cause hypermagnesemia
- Use of calcium salts with cardiac glycosides increases the risk of digitalis toxicity
- Oral calcium salts reduce absorption of tetracyclines
- Aminoglycosides may potentiate antihypercalcemic effects

Key nursing actions

- Instruct patient to take antihypercalcemic drugs on an empty stomach with 6 to 8 ounces of water either 2 hours before or after meals or 30 minutes before the first food of the day.
- Teach patient to avoid excessive consumption of spinach, whole grains, and rhubarb and to maintain adequate intake of calcium and vitamin D.

Nursing responsibilities

- **Tell the patient to take antihypercalcemic drugs on an empty stomach with 6 to 8 ounces of water either 2 hours before or after meals or 30 minutes before the first food of the day**
- Monitor the patient's serum electrolyte levels to prevent imbalances
- Assess the patient for hypocalcemia and hypercalcemia
- **Teach the patient receiving an oral calcium drug to avoid excessive consumption of spinach, whole grains, and rhubarb and to maintain adequate intake of calcium and vitamin D**

ANTIDIABETICS (INSULIN AND ORAL HYPOGLYCEMICS)

INSULIN

Key facts about insulin

- Reduces serum glucose level
- Metabolized in kidneys and liver
- Filtered by renal glomeruli; undergoes some tubular resorption

Mechanism of action

- Reduces the serum glucose level by increasing glucose transport into cells and promoting glucose conversion to glycogen

Pharmacokinetics

- Absorption: Given parenterally because it's destroyed in the GI tract
- Distribution: Distributed widely throughout the body
- Metabolism: Metabolized in the liver and kidneys

Comparing types of insulin

The following chart compares rapid-acting, intermediate-acting, and long-acting insulins. Onset of action, peak concentration levels, and duration of action are based on subcutaneous administration. Only regular insulin can be administered intravenously.

	GENERIC NAME	TRADE NAME	ONSET (HOURS)	PEAK (HOURS)	DURATION (HOURS)
Rapid-acting	Insulin injection (regular)	Humulin R Novolin R Regular Iletin II Velosulin BR	½ to 1	Unknown	8 to 12
	Lispro insulin solution	Humalog	¼	½ to 1½	6 to 8
	Insulin aspart solution	NovoLog	¼	1 to 3	3 to 5
Intermediate-acting	Isophane insulin suspension (NPH)	Novolin N Humulin N NPH Iletin II	1 to 1½	4 to 12	24
	Insulin zinc suspension (lente)	Humulin L Lente Iletin II	1 to 2½	7 to 15	24
Long-acting	Insulin glargine solution	Lantus	1.1	5	24
	Extended insulin zinc suspension (ultralente)	Humulin U	4 to 8	10 to 30	36

Duration of insulin

- Insulin injection: 8 to 12 hours
- Lispro insulin solution: 6 to 8 hours
- Insulin aspart solution: 3 to 5 hours
- Isophane insulin suspension: 24 hours
- Insulin zinc suspension: 24 hours
- Insulin glargine solution: 24 hours
- Extended insulin zinc suspension: 36 hours

- Excretion: Filtered by the renal glomeruli; undergoes some tubular resorption

Drug examples

- Rapid-acting insulins include prompt insulin aspart (NovoLog), lispro (Humalog), and regular insulin (Humulin R, Novolin R, Regular Iletin II, Velosulin BR)
- Intermediate-acting insulins include isophane insulin suspension (NPH [Humulin N, Novolin N]) and insulin zinc suspension (lente [Humulin L, Lente Iletin II)
- Long-acting insulins include extended insulin zinc suspension (ultralente [Humulin U, Ultralente Insulin]) and glargine (Lantus) (for more information, see *Comparing types of insulin*)
- Mixed insulins include 30% regular insulin and 70% NPH insulin (Humulin 70/30, Novolin 70/30), 50% lispro protamine and 50% insulin lispro

(Humalog Mix 50/50, Humalog Mix 75/25), 50% regular insulin and 50% NPH insulin (Humulin 50/50)

Indications

- Insulin is indicated for type 1 (insulin-dependent) and type 2 (non-insulin-dependent) diabetes mellitus that's unresponsive to dietary measures and oral hypoglycemics

Contraindications and precautions

- Insulin is contraindicated in persons with known hypersensitivity

Adverse reactions

- Hypoglycemia, rebound hyperglycemia (Somogyi effect), lipodystrophy, lipoatrophy, skin reactions at injection site (warmth, stinging, swelling)

Interactions

- Insulin causes a disulfiram-like reaction (abdominal cramps, nausea, vomiting, flushing, headache, hypoglycemia) when used with alcohol
- Use of antidiabetics with beta-adrenergic blockers may mask signs and symptoms of hypoglycemia
- Use of insulin with corticosteroids, sympathomimetics, thiazide diuretics, or thyroid preparations may cause hyperglycemia, necessitating an increase in the insulin dosage
- Alcohol, anabolic steroids, anticoagulants, chloramphenicol, clofibrate, guanethidine, isoniazid, monoamine oxidase (MAO) inhibitors, niacin, phenothiazines, salicylates, sulfonamides, and tetracyclines may cause hypoglycemia, possibly requiring a decreased insulin dosage

Nursing responsibilities

- **Know that only regular insulin can be administered I.V., if needed in an emergency**
- **When administering mixed insulin, draw regular insulin into the syringe first to avoid contaminating the clear regular insulin vial with the cloudy, longer-acting insulin mixture**
- **Don't shake the insulin vial; instead, roll it between the hands**
- Teach the patient how to inject insulin, rotate injection sites, and dispose of used syringes
- Keep in mind that some patients may be allergic to certain types of insulin
- **Schedule snacks to coincide with insulin's peak action, when hypoglycemia is most likely to occur; know that the patient receiving more than one type of insulin may be at risk for hypoglycemia several times daily**
- Monitor the patient's blood glucose levels
- Assess the patient for signs and symptoms of hypoglycemia or hyperglycemia
- Periodically monitor the glycosylated hemoglobin level, which reflects the degree of glycemic control for the previous 2 to 3 months
- **Know that stress, fever, trauma, infection, and surgery may increase insulin requirements**

When to use insulin

- Type 1 and type 2 diabetes mellitus

When NOT to use insulin

- Hypersensitivity

Adverse reactions to watch for

- Hypoglycemia, rebound hyperglycemia, lipodystrophy, lipoatrophy, skin reactions at injection site

Key nursing actions

- Know that only regular insulin can be administered I.V., if needed in an emergency.
- When administering mixed insulin, draw regular insulin into the syringe first to avoid contaminating the clear regular insulin vial with the cloudy, longer-acting insulin mixture.
- Don't shake the insulin vial; instead, roll it between hands.
- Schedule snacks to coincide with insulin's peak action.

- **Know that I.V. glucose or glucagon may be necessary in severe hypoglycemia**
- Inform the patient that antidiabetics control but don't cure diabetes; emphasize the need for lifelong therapy
- Teach the patient to follow the recommended diabetic diet and to use the exchange system when planning meals
- Emphasize the importance of regular exercise, daily foot inspection, sick-day rules, and alcohol restriction
- Instruct the patient to contact the physician if unable to eat, such as from illness; inadequate intake increases the risk of hypoglycemia
- Teach the patient how to recognize signs and symptoms of hypoglycemia and hyperglycemia and what to do if these occur
- Instruct the patient to carry sugar or a glucose-raising substance, such as hard candy or glucose tablets, and identification describing the disease and drug regimen in case of hypoglycemic reaction
- Refrigerate insulin

ORAL HYPOGLYCEMICS

Key facts about oral hypoglycemics

- Stimulate the pancreas to produce more insulin and decrease the serum glucose level
- Acarbose delays absorption of carbohydrates
- Metabolized by liver or localized to GI tract
- Excreted in urine

When to use oral hypoglycemics

- Type 2 diabetes mellitus unresponsive to dietary measures and exercise

Mechanism of action

- Oral hypoglycemics stimulate the pancreas to produce more insulin and increase the sensitivity of peripheral receptors to insulin, ultimately decreasing the serum glucose level
- Acarbose delays absorption of carbohydrates

Pharmacokinetics

- Absorption: Well absorbed in the GI tract
- Distribution: Varies widely with each form of the drug
- Metabolism: Either metabolized by the liver or localized to the GI tract, depending on the drug
- Excretion: Excreted in the urine

Drug examples

- Alpha-glucoside inhibitors: acarbose (Precose), miglitol (Glyset)
- Biguanides: metformin hydrochloride (Glucophage, Glucophage XL)
- Combination: glyburide/metformin hydrochloride (Glucovance), rosiglitazone maleate/metformin hydrochloride (Avandamet), glipizide/metformin hydrochloride (Metaglip)
- Meglitinides: repaglinide (Prandin), nateglinide (Starlix)
- Sulfonylureas: acetohexamide (Dymelor), chlorpropamide (Diabinese), glimepiride (Amaryl), glipizide (Glucotrol, Glucotrol XL), glyburide (DiaBeta, Micronase), tolazamide (Tolinase), tolbutamide (Orinase)
- Thiazolidinediones: rosiglitazone maleate (Avandia), pioglitazone hydrochloride (Actos)

Indications

- Type 2 diabetes mellitus unresponsive to dietary measures and exercise

Contraindications and precautions

- These drugs are contraindicated in patients with type 1 diabetes mellitus
- Alpha-glucoside inhibitors are contraindicated in patients with cirrhosis or other conditions that may deteriorate because of increased intestinal gas formation
- Meglitinides are contraindicated in patients with liver cirrhosis or intestinal diseases; use cautiously in patients with liver impairment
- Metformin is contraindicated in patients with renal or hepatic insufficiency or alcoholism
- Sulfonylurea hypoglycemics are contraindicated in patients who are allergic to sulfa drugs
- Thiazolidinediones are contraindicated in patients with liver cirrhosis or heart failure: use cautiously in patients with liver impairment, edema, or heart failure
- Use these drugs cautiously in pregnant and breast-feeding women

Adverse reactions

- Hypoglycemia, nausea, vomiting, heartburn, dizziness, drowsiness, headache, photosensitivity reactions (sulfonylureas), lactic acidosis (metformin), flatulence and diarrhea (alpha-glucoside inhibitors), upper respiratory tract infections (meglitinides), edema, heart failure

Interactions

- Concurrent use of antidiabetics with beta-adrenergic blockers may mask signs and symptoms of hypoglycemia
- Anabolic steroids, anticoagulants, chloramphenicol, MAO inhibitors, salicylates, and sulfonamides may cause hypoglycemia (necessitating a reduced insulin dosage) and may increase the hypoglycemic effects of oral hypoglycemics

Nursing responsibilities

- **Tell the patient to take alpha-glucoside inhibitors with the first bite of food and to take meglitinides within 30 minutes of each meal**
- Instruct the patient to contact the physician if unable to eat; inadequate intake increases the risk of hypoglycemia
- Instruct the patient taking a sulfonylurea to use sunscreen and protective clothing to prevent photosensitivity reactions (for additional teaching tips, see *Teaching about sulfonylureas,* page 200)
- Assess the patient for signs and symptoms of hypoglycemia or hyperglycemia
- Advise the patient to consult the physician before adjusting the dosage of an oral hypoglycemic
- Teach the patient how to recognize signs and symptoms of hypoglycemia and hyperglycemia
- Provide information about recommended dietary measures, exercise, foot care, and sick-day rules
- Teach the patient to follow the recommended diabetic diet and to use the exchange system when planning meals

When NOT to use oral hypoglycemics

- Type 1 diabetes mellitus
- Cirrhosis
- Intestinal disease
- Renal or hepatic insufficiency or alcoholism
- Allergies to sulfa drugs
- Heart failure

Adverse reactions to watch for

- Hypoglycemia, nausea, vomiting, heartburn, dizziness, drowsiness, headache, photosensitivity reactions, lactic acidosis, flatulence and diarrhea, upper respiratory tract infections, edema, and heart failure

Key nursing actions

- Instruct patient to take alpha-glucoside inhibitors with the first bite of food and to take meglitinides within 30 minutes of each meal.
- Assess the patient for signs and symptoms of hypoglycemia or hyperglycemia.
- Provide information about recommended dietary measures, exercise, foot care, and sick-day rules.

Topics for patient discussion

- Therapy regimen
- Signs and symptoms
- Blood glucose monitoring

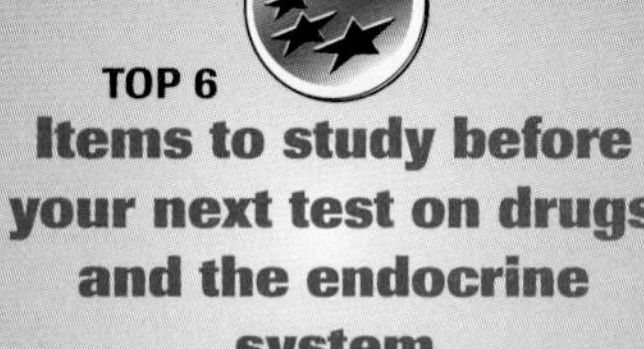

TOP 6

Items to study before your next test on drugs and the endocrine system

1. The mechanisms of action for pituitary, thyroid, and parathyroid drugs; insulin; and oral hypoglycemics
2. The rationale for using pituitary, thyroid, and parathyroid drugs; insulin; and oral hypoglycemics
3. Major adverse effects of pituitary, thyroid, and parathyroid drugs
4. Nursing responsibilities when administering pituitary, thyroid, and parathyroid drugs; insulin; and oral hypoglycemics
5. Patient teaching related to insulin and oral hypoglycemics
6. Purpose, mechanism of action, adverse reactions, and nursing considerations of antihypercalcemic drugs

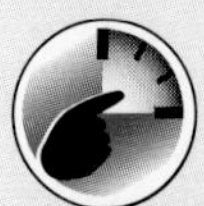

TIME-OUT FOR TEACHING

Teaching about sulfonylureas

Include the following topics in your teaching plan for the patient receiving a sulfonylurea.

- Medication regimen, including the drug's name, dosage, frequency, duration, and possible adverse effects
- Signs and symptoms to discuss with the physician, including hypoglycemia and hyperglycemia, and measures to correct them
- Blood glucose monitoring
- Avoidance of alcohol
- Medical alert identification
- Measures to deal with sun exposure
- Follow-up care, including laboratory tests and physician visits

- Emphasize the importance of regular exercise, daily foot inspection, sick-day rules, and alcohol restriction
- Know that stress, fever, trauma, infection, and surgery may increase insulin requirements or necessitate switching from an oral hypoglycemic to insulin
- Inform the patient that antidiabetics control but don't cure diabetes; emphasize the need for lifelong therapy
- Instruct the patient to carry sugar and identification describing the disease and drug regimen in case of hypoglycemic reaction

NCLEX CHECKS

It's never too soon to begin your NCLEX preparation. Now that you've reviewed this chapter, carefully read each of the following questions and choose the best answer. Then compare your responses to the correct answers.

1. A patient diagnosed with hypothyroidism is prescribed levothyroxine (Synthroid). Which laboratory test must be closely monitored to evaluate the effectiveness of the drug therapy?

☐ **A.** $CD4^+$
☐ **B.** Hemoglobin A_{1c}
☐ **C.** Prothrombin time
☐ **D.** Thyroxine (T_4)

2. You're treating a child with primary nocturnal enuresis. Which of the following pituitary agents is indicated for children with this disorder?

☐ **A.** Corticotropin
☐ **B.** Cosyntropin (Cortrosyn)
☐ **C.** Desmopressin (DDAVP)
☐ **D.** Somatropin (Humatrope)

3. A patient diagnosed with hypoparathyroidism is prescribed the vitamin D analogue calcitriol, 0.25 mcg P.O. daily. You explain to the patient that calcitriol increases the plasma level of calcium by which of the following actions?

- ☐ A. Reduces bone resorption
- ☐ B. Decreases osteoclastic activity
- ☐ C. Increases GI absorption and bone resorption of calcium
- ☐ D. Stimulates the parathyroid gland to secrete parathyroid hormone

4. What type of insulin and route of administration should you use in a medical emergency?

- ☐ A. NPH insulin I.M.
- ☐ B. NPH insulin S.C.
- ☐ C. Regular insulin I.V.
- ☐ D. Regular insulin S.C.

5. A physician orders glipizide (Glucotrol) for a patient with type 2 diabetes mellitus. Instruct the patient to take the drug:

- ☐ A. with meals.
- ☐ B. after meals.
- ☐ C. 30 minutes before bedtime.
- ☐ D. 30 minutes before breakfast.

6. A patient is admitted with a diagnosis of diabetic ketoacidosis. An insulin drip is initiated with 50 U of insulin in 100 ml of normal saline solution. The I.V. is being infused via an infusion pump and the pump is currently set at 10 ml/hour. The nurse determines that the patient is receiving how many units of insulin each hour?

____

7. A patient who suffered a brain injury after falling off a ladder has recently developed syndrome of inappropriate antidiuretic hormone (SIADH). What findings indicate that the treatment he's receiving for SIADH is effective?

Select all that apply:

- ☐ A. Decrease in body weight
- ☐ B. Rise in blood pressure and drop in heart rate
- ☐ C. Absence of wheezes in the lungs
- ☐ D. Increase in urine output
- ☐ E. Decrease in urine osmolarity

ANSWERS AND RATIONALES

1. CORRECT ANSWER: D

Monitor T_4 levels, which indicate thyroid function, to evaluate the effectiveness of levothyroxine therapy. $CD4^+$ cell count is used to evaluate the progression of human immunodeficiency virus infection. Hemoglobin A_{1c} is used to measure a patient's glucose levels over a 4-month period. Prothrombin time is used to measure clotting times for patients taking oral anticoagulants.

2. CORRECT ANSWER: C

It's believed that children with primary nocturnal enuresis have insufficient antidiuretic hormone, so desmopressin is indicated. Cosyntropin and corticotropin stimulate the adrenal glands and won't help with enuresis. Somatropin is used for growth failure.

3. CORRECT ANSWER: C

Calcitriol increases GI absorption and bone resorption of calcium and decreases renal calcium clearance, thereby increasing serum calcium level. It isn't known to reduce bone resorption, stimulate the parathyroid gland to secrete parathyroid hormone, or decrease osteoclastic activity.

4. CORRECT ANSWER: C

In a medical emergency, speed and onset of action are important. The I.V. route is the fastest route to action, and only regular insulin may be given by this route. Although regular insulin is fast acting, the S.C. route isn't the fastest route to correct glycemic problems. If the goal is prolonged action, then NPH insulin given S.C. would be the drug of choice. NPH insulin is never given I.M.

5. CORRECT ANSWER: D

Glipizide is well absorbed; onset of action may be as soon as 30 minutes after intake, peaking within 2 to 3 hours. Taking the drug 30 minutes before breakfast ensures effectiveness at the first meal and throughout the day. Taking the drug with or after meals doesn't ensure effectiveness. Taking the drug before bedtime could result in nighttime hypoglycemia.

6. CORRECT ANSWER: 5

To determine the number of insulin units the patient is receiving per hour, the nurse must first determine the number of units in each ml of fluid (50 U ÷ 100 ml = 0.5 U/ml). Next, she multiplies the units/ml by the rate of ml/hour (0.5 units × 10 ml/hr = 5 U).

7. CORRECT ANSWER: A, D, E

SIADH is an abnormality involving an abundance of diuretic hormone. The predominant feature is water retention with oliguria, edema, and weight gain. Successful treatment should result in weight reduction, increased urine output, and decreased urine concentration (urine osmolarity).

Drugs and the immune system

LEARNING OBJECTIVES

After studying this chapter, you should be able to:

- Describe the mechanism of action of corticosteroids, immunosuppressants, antibacterials, antifungals, anthelmintics, antivirals, and antituberculotics.
- Describe the general characteristics of penicillins, cephalosporins, aminoglycosides, tetracyclines, fluoroquinolones, and urinary tract antiseptics.
- Identify indications for corticosteroids, immunosuppressants, antibacterials, antifungals, anthelmintics, antivirals, and antituberculotics.
- List common adverse effects of corticosteroids, immunosuppressants, the various classes of antibacterials, antifungals, anthelmintics, antivirals, and antituberculotics.
- Identify nursing responsibilities when administering corticosteroids, immunosuppressants, antibacterials, antifungals, anthelmintics, antivirals, and antituberculotics.
- Discuss appropriate teaching for the patient who is receiving a corticosteroid, an immunosuppressant, an antibacterial, an antifungal, an antiviral, or an antituberculotic.
- Identify precautions that may help prevent infection in the immunosuppressed patient.
- Discuss appropriate teaching for patients and families infected with helminths.

CHAPTER OVERVIEW

Corticosteroids comprise two subgroups: glucocorticoids and mineralocorticoids. Glucocorticoids are used to decrease inflammation and immune response in a variety of disorders. Mineralocorticoids cause reabsorption of sodium and water in the nephron and are used as replacement therapy in adrenocortical insufficiency. Immunosuppressants are used to prevent transplanted organ rejection and to treat certain autoimmune disorders, such as systemic lupus erythematosus and idiopathic thrombocytopenic purpura. Because of the risk of infection in patients taking steroids and immunosuppressants, the patient and nurse must observe carefully for masked signs of infection. Other nursing responsibilities include monitoring fluid and electrolyte balance and renal function studies. Patient teaching focuses on signs and symptoms of infection, exacerbation of illness, or transplant rejection and on the importance of strict and lifelong compliance with drug therapy.

Antibacterial drugs, including penicillins, cephalosporins, aminoglycosides, tetracyclines, fluoroquinolones, miscellaneous anti-infectives, and urinary tract antiseptics, are used to treat systemic microbial infections. Each class of drug kills (bactericidal) or inhibits (bacteriostatic) the growth of susceptible organisms. Before therapy begins, specimens for culture and sensitivity tests should be obtained. Nursing responsibilities focus on around-the-clock administration, monitoring the patient for possible allergic reaction, assessment of peak and trough levels of specific drugs, and evaluation of drug effectiveness. Patient teaching focuses on proper drug administration, compliance with therapy, and necessary follow-up care.

Antifungals are used to treat fungal infections, including candidiasis, tinea, histoplasmosis, and aspergillosis. Infections may be local or systemic; systemic infections are more difficult to treat. Nursing responsibilities focus on providing physiologic support and preventing or minimizing adverse effects. Patient teaching centers on proper cleaning of the infected area and prevention of the infection from spreading.

Anthelmintics are used to treat parasitic worms of the intestinal tract and other organs. Nursing responsibilities and patient teaching focus on preventing the condition and reducing the risk of transmission. When one member of a family is diagnosed with helminths, all family members should be tested. The nurse should assess the patient for dehydration and the need for fluid and electrolyte replacement secondary to diarrhea.

Antivirals are used to treat such common viral infections as herpes simplex I and II, genital herpes, herpes zoster varicella, certain influenza viruses, and human immunodeficiency virus (HIV). Replicating viruses invade the human cell and interfere with cellular metabolism, making them difficult to treat. Nursing responsibilities include preventing transmission of the virus and helping the patient understand that zidovudine and didanosine are palliative measures, not cures, for acquired immunodeficiency syndrome (AIDS).

Antituberculotics are used to treat tuberculosis (TB), an infection of the lung and other organs caused by *Mycobacterium tuberculosis*. Treatment for TB or for exposure to TB lasts 6 months to 2 years, making compliance difficult and contributing to the prevalence of resistant TB. The nurse plays a major role in encouraging compliance, monitoring liver function studies, and observing for adverse effects.

ANATOMY AND PHYSIOLOGY

Anatomy

- The lymphatic system consists of lymphocyte-containing (lymphoid) tissues, lymph, and a network of lymphatic vessels
- Lymph tissues are concentrated in the lymph nodes, spleen, thymus, tonsils, adenoids, appendix, and Peyer's patches in the intestines

Physiology

- Lymph carries foreign substances that have entered the tissue fluids to the lymph nodes, where lymphocytes act on them
- Lymphatic vessels collect lymph and return it to the circulation
- Beginning from the tiny lymphatic capillaries, lymph flows through progressively larger vessels until it reaches the subclavian vein
- Lymphocytes are a type of white blood cell (WBC) that develop from stem cells in the bone marrow and then differentiate into lymphocyte precursor cells
- The precursor cells develop into two types of lymphocytes—T lymphocytes and B lymphocytes—both of which perform specific immune functions
- T lymphocytes and B lymphocytes mature and continuously recirculate between the blood and the various lymphatic tissues and organs
- Two mechanisms—nonspecific resistance and acquired immunity—protect the body against microorganisms and other potentially harmful substances
  - Nonspecific resistance is a group of general protective mechanisms that function without prior exposure to harmful agents to ward off a wide range of pathogens
    - These mechanisms include the skin and mucous membranes, antimicrobial substances, phagocytosis, inflammation, and fever
    - Resistance refers to the body's ability to fend off disease; susceptibility refers to a lack of resistance
  - Acquired immunity consists of specific immune responses provided by the lymphatic system and directed against specific organisms or toxins
    - These responses usually require previous exposure to a foreign substance
    - They cause antibody formation (humoral immunity) or lymphatic activation (cell-mediated immunity)

Function

- The lymphatic system functions as a second circulatory system
  - Lymphatic vessels drain excess fluid from interstitial spaces and return it to the blood

A&P highlights

- The lymphatic system consists of lymphoid tissues, lymph, and a network of lymphatic vessels.
- Lymph carries foreign substances to the lymph nodes.
- Lymphatic vessels collect lymph and return it to circulation.
- Lymphocytes are white blood cells that develop from stem cells in the bone marrow.
- There are two types of lymphocytes: T lymphocytes and B lymphocytes. Each performs specific immune functions.
- Two mechanisms – nonspecific resistance and acquired immunity – protect the body against microorganisms and other potentially harmful substances.
  - Nonspecific resistance is a group of general protective mechanisms, such as skin, mucous membranes, antimicrobial substances, and inflammation, that ward off pathogens to which the body has not previously been exposed.
  - Acquired immunity consists of specific immune responses (antibody formation or lymphatic activation) directed against specific organisms or toxins to which the body most likely has already been exposed.

- Lymphatic vessels absorb fats from the GI tract and transport them to the bloodstream
- The lymphatic system also has immune functions
- B lymphocytes have distinct initial and ultimate immune functions
  - Initially, B lymphocytes synthesize antibodies (called *surface immunoglobulin*) that rise to the surface of the lymphocyte, where they function as B-cell receptors
  - When mature, B lymphocytes produce humoral immunity
    - Their plasma cells secrete antibodies
    - Their memory cells become plasma cells during subsequent exposure to an antigen
- T lymphocytes also have initial and ultimate immune functions
  - Initially, T lymphocytes seek, recognize, and attach to antigens that fit their surface receptors
  - Later, they produce cell-mediated immunity
- The lymphatic system also provides acquired immunity
  - Cell-mediated immunity, which relies on sensitized T lymphocytes, is the main defense against viruses, fungi, parasites, and some bacteria
  - It also eliminates abnormal cells that may arise during cell division, which can develop into tumors if not destroyed
  - **Cell-mediated immunity causes organ transplant rejection**
  - Humoral immunity, which relies on B-lymphocyte function, provides the major defense against many bacteria and bacterial toxins by producing immunoglobulin antibodies and an allergic response to the antigen

Functions of B lymphocytes

- Synthesize antibodies that function as B-cell receptors on the surface of the lymphocyte
- Produce humoral immunity (main defense against bacteria and bacterial toxins)
- Secrete antibodies

Functions of T lymphocytes

- Seek, recognize, and attach to antigens that fit their surface receptors
- Produce cell-mediated immunity (main defense against viruses, fungi, parasites, and some bacteria)

CORTICOSTEROIDS (ADRENOCORTICOIDS)

Mechanism of action

- Glucocorticoids (normally secreted by the adrenal cortex) produce various metabolic effects, suppress inflammation, and alter the normal immune response; they also promote sodium and water retention and potassium excretion
- Mineralocorticoids (normally secreted by the adrenal cortex) enhance reabsorption of sodium and chloride and promote excretion of potassium and hydrogen from the renal tubules, thereby helping to maintain fluid and electrolyte balance

Key facts about corticosteroids

- Also called *adrenocorticoids*
- Two types: glucocorticoids and mineralocorticoids
  - Glucocorticoids: produce various metabolic effects, suppress inflammation, alter normal immune response, and promote sodium and water retention and potassium excretion
  - Mineralocorticoids: enhance reabsorption of sodium and chloride and promote excretion of potassium and hydrogen (to help maintain fluid and electrolyte balance)
- Metabolized in the liver
- Excreted in urine

Pharmacokinetics

- Absorption: Readily absorbed from the GI tract
- Distribution: Reversibly bound to corticosteroid-binding globulin (CBG) and corticosteroid-binding albumin (CBA)
- Metabolism: Metabolized in the liver
- Excretion: Excreted in the urine

Drug examples

- Glucocorticoids: betamethasone (Celestone), cortisone (Cortone), dexamethasone (Decadron, Hexadrol), hydrocortisone (Cortef, Hydrocortone,

Solu-Cortef), methylprednisolone (Depo-Medrol, Medrol, Solu-Medrol), prednisolone (Delta-Cortef, Prelone), prednisone (Deltasone, Orasone), triamcinolone (Aristocort, Azmacort, Kenacort, Kenalog)
- Mineralocorticoids: fludrocortisone (Florinef)

Indications
- Glucocorticoids
  - These drugs are used as replacement therapy for adrenocortical insufficiency
  - They also are used to treat neoplastic diseases, septic shock, autoimmune diseases, cerebral edema, and inflammation of the joints, GI tract, respiratory tract, and skin
- Mineralocorticoids are used as replacement therapy in primary or secondary adrenal insufficiency

Contraindications and precautions
- Use glucocorticoids with extreme caution in patients with serious infection because they may mask signs and symptoms of infection
- Use mineralocorticoids with caution in patients with cardiovascular disease and hypertension

Adverse reactions
- Glucocorticoids may cause muscle wasting, osteoporosis, growth retardation (in children), peptic ulcer, increased serum glucose level, hypertension, convulsions, mood swings, cataracts, glaucoma, fragile skin, hirsutism, increased appetite and altered fat distribution
  - They may also mask signs and symptoms of infection
  - They are more likely to cause adverse effects when given in doses above normal body levels for nonendocrine disorders than when given as replacement therapy
- Mineralocorticoids may cause sodium and fluid retention, hypokalemia, euphoria, depression, hyperglycemia, acute adrenal insufficiency after abrupt withdrawal, redistribution of fat, insomnia, hirsutism, and GI distress or ulcers

Interactions
- Concurrent use with drugs that induce hypokalemia (such as potassium-depleting diuretics) causes additive hypokalemia
- Concurrent use with insulin or oral hypoglycemics may increase blood glucose levels, thereby increasing insulin or oral hypoglycemic requirements
- Phenobarbital, phenytoin, and rifampin may enhance the metabolism of glucocorticoids, decreasing the latter's effects
- Hormonal contraceptives may block the metabolism of glucocorticoids

Nursing responsibilities
- **Administer daily doses in the morning to mimic the body's normal pattern of cortisol secretion**
- Assess the patient for symptomatic improvement and adverse effects

When to use corticosteroids
- Replacement therapy for adrenocortical insufficiency
- Neoplastic diseases
- Septic shock
- Autoimmune diseases
- Cerebral edema
- Inflammation of the joints, GI tract, respiratory tract, or skin

When NOT to use corticosteroids
- Serious infection

Adverse reactions to watch for
- Muscle wasting, osteoporosis, growth retardation, peptic ulcer, increased serum glucose level, hypertension, convulsions, mood swings, cataracts, glaucoma, fragile skin, hirsutism, increased appetite, altered fat distribution, sodium and fluid retention, hypokalemia, euphoria, depression, hyperglycemia, acute adrenal insufficiency after abrupt withdrawal, redistribution of fat, insomnia, hirsutism, GI distress or ulcers

Topics for patient discussion

- Medication regimen, including guidelines for missed doses
- Signs and symptoms to discuss with the physician
- Avoidance of abrupt drug discontinuation
- Avoidance of alcohol, cigarettes, caffeine, and aspirin-containing products
- Possible mood alterations
- Dietary restrictions and allowances
- Follow-up care

Key nursing actions

- Administer daily doses in the morning.
- Assess patient for symptomatic improvement and adverse effects.
- Administer additional doses during periods of stress or infection, as ordered.
- Monitor regularly for weight changes and fluid and electrolyte imbalances.
- Instruct the patient to consult with physician before receiving vaccinations.

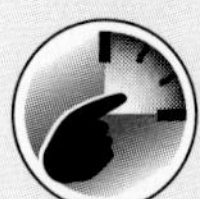

TIME-OUT FOR TEACHING

Teaching about glucocorticoids

Include these topics in your teaching plan for the patient receiving a glucocorticoid.

- Medication regimen, including the drug's name, dosage, frequency, duration, and possible adverse effects
- Signs and symptoms to discuss with the physician
- Avoidance of abrupt drug discontinuation
- Consistent dosing
- Guidelines for missed doses
- Avoidance of alcohol, cigarettes, caffeine, and aspirin-containing products
- Possible mood alterations
- Dietary restrictions and allowances
- Follow-up care, including physician visits

- Know that the patient may need additional doses during periods of stress or infection
- Monitor the patient regularly for weight changes and fluid and electrolyte imbalances, especially hypokalemia; promote increased intake of high-potassium foods to prevent hypokalemia
- Monitor the patient taking a mineralocorticoid for signs of fluid retention by weighing the patient daily, assessing lung sounds, and checking for peripheral edema
- Warn the patient not to stop the drug abruptly because this may cause life-threatening adrenal insufficiency
- Instruct the patient to consult the physician before receiving vaccinations
- Teach the patient to avoid such foods as fresh fruit and raw vegetables because they tend to have higher levels of bacteria than cooked foods, thereby increasing the risk of infection in an already immunosuppressed patient
- Teach the patient about the importance of complying with therapy (for additional teaching tips, see *Teaching about glucocorticoids*)
- Teach the patient to carry identification describing the disease and drug regimen

IMMUNOSUPPRESSANTS

Mechanism of action

- Azathioprine suppresses cell-mediated immunity and alters antibody formation
- Basiliximab and daclizumab are monoclonal antibodies that inhibit the activation of lymphocytes
- Cyclosporine and sirolimus inhibit proliferation and function of T lymphocytes

- Muromonab-CD3 reacts with the T_3 complex, blocking T-cell function
- Mycophenolate mofetil inhibits the proliferation of T lymphocytes and B lymphocytes, inhibits the recruitment of leukocytes to the sites of inflammation, and suppresses antibody formation by B lymphocytes
- Prednisone inhibits macrophage formation and hinders migration of macrophages and leukocytes to inflamed areas
- Tacrolimus inhibits T-lymphocyte activation

Pharmacokinetics

- Absorption: Varies widely with each drug
- Distribution: Varies widely with each drug
- Metabolism: Metabolized in the liver
- Excretion: Excreted in the urine and feces

Drug examples

- Antilymphocyte globulin, antilymphocyte serum, antithymocyte globulin (Atgam), azathioprine (Imuran), basiliximab (Simulect), cyclosporine (Sandimmune, Neoral), daclizumab (Zenapax), muromonab-CD3 (Orthoclone OKT3), mycophenolate mofetil (CellCept), prednisone (Deltasone), sirolimus (Rapamune), tacrolimus (Prograf)

Indications

- Antithymocyte globulin, antilymphocyte globulin, and antilymphocyte serum are used in organ or bone marrow transplant to reduce circulating T lymphocytes without affecting other immune cells
- Azathioprine is used to prevent rejection of renal transplants and may be prescribed for rheumatoid arthritis (with cyclophosphamide or methotrexate) in patients who don't respond to conventional therapy
- Basiliximab, daclizumab, and sirolimus are used to prevent rejection of kidney transplants
- Muromonab-CD3, mycophenolate mofetil, and cyclosporine are used to prevent rejection of renal, hepatic, and cardiac transplants (usually combined with glucocorticoids)
- Prednisone is used for its anti-inflammatory or immunosuppressive actions
- Tacrolimus is used to prevent rejection of liver or kidney transplants

Contraindications and precautions

- Mycophenolate mofetil (I.V. form) is contraindicated in patients with a hypersensitivity to polysorbate 80 (Tween)
- Use mycophenolate cautiously in patients with GI disorders or bone marrow depression
- Tacrolimus is contraindicated in patients with a hypersensitivity to castor oil derivatives (I.V. form)
- Use tacrolimus cautiously in patients with impaired liver or kidney function or lymphomas
- Use azathioprine cautiously in patients with bone marrow depression, infection, or cancer

Key facts about immunosuppressants

- Azathioprine: suppresses cell-mediated immunity and alters antibody formation
- Basiliximab and daclizumab: inhibit activation of lymphocytes
- Cyclosporine and sirolimus: inhibit proliferation and function of T lymphocytes
- Muromonab-CD3: blocks T-cell function
- Mycophenolate mofetil: inhibits proliferation of T and B lymphocytes, inhibits recruitment of leukocytes to sites of inflammation, and suppresses B lymphocyte antibody formation
- Prednisone: inhibits macrophage formation and hinders migration of macrophages and leukocytes to inflamed areas
- Tacrolimus: inhibits T-lymphocyte activation
- Metabolized in the liver
- Excreted in urine and feces

When to use immunosuppressants

- Organ or bone marrow transplant
- Rheumatoid arthritis

When NOT to use immunosuppressants

- Hypersensitivity polysorbate 80
- GI disorders
- Bone marrow depression, infection, or cancer
- Hypersensitivity to castor oil derivatives
- Impaired liver or kidney function
- Lymphomas
- Pregnancy or breast-feeding
- Hyperlipidemia

- Use all immunosuppressants cautiously in pregnant and breast-feeding women and in patients with bone marrow depression, infection, or cancer
- Use sirolimus cautiously in patients with hyperlipidemia or impaired liver or kidney function

Adverse reactions

- These drugs may cause peptic ulcer, edema, altered fat distribution, increased serum glucose levels, mood swings, hirsutism, fragile skin, nausea, vomiting, diarrhea, anorexia, anemia, leukopenia, thrombocytopenia, hepatotoxicity
- Azathioprine also may cause fever and chills
- Basiliximab and daclizumab also may cause the formation of antibodies, anaphylaxis, GI disorders, renal impairment, respiratory depression, flulike symptoms, and electrolyte changes
- Cyclosporine also may cause gingival hyperplasia, hypertension, infection, nephrotoxicity, and tremor
- Mycophenolate mofetil also may cause dyspnea, electrolyte changes, and GI disorders
- Sirolimus and tacrolimus may cause neurotoxicity, nephrotoxicity, GI disorders, CNS effects (such as insomnia, headache, depression), weight gain, electrolyte imbalance, flulike symptoms, tremor, and respiratory effects

Adverse reactions to watch for

- Peptic ulcer, edema, altered fat distribution, increased serum glucose levels, mood swings, hirsutism, fragile skin, nausea, vomiting, diarrhea, anorexia, anemia, leukopenia, thrombocytopenia, hepatotoxicity, fever and chills, antibody formation, anaphylaxis, GI disorders, renal impairment, respiratory effects, flulike symptoms, electrolyte changes, gingival hyperplasia, hypertension, infection, nephrotoxicity, tremor, dyspnea, neurotoxicity, CNS effects, weight gain

Interactions

- Allopurinol increases the risk of toxicity from azathioprine
- Concurrent use of cyclosporine with other nephrotoxic drugs causes additive nephrotoxicity
- Cimetidine and ketoconazole increase the risk of toxicity from cyclosporine
- Phenobarbital, phenytoin, rifampin, and co-trimoxazole (sulfamethoxazole-trimethoprim) I.V. decrease the effects of cyclosporine
- Sirolimus may interact with many drugs, possibly increasing the risk of nephrotoxicity and neurotoxicity; may increase cholesterol and triglyceride levels
- Tacrolimus may interact with many drugs, possibly increasing the risk of nephrotoxicity and neurotoxicity; may alter glucose and potassium levels

Nursing responsibilities

- **When administering a monoclonal antibody (basiliximab or daclizumab), monitor the patient for anaphylaxis**
- **When giving sirolimus or tacrolimus, monitor the patient for signs of rejection, nephrotoxicity, or neurotoxicity**
- **When administering cyclosporine, monitor the serum drug level to prevent toxicity; teach the patient to maintain proper oral hygiene to prevent gingival hyperplasia**
- **Know that Sandimmune and Neoral are NOT interchangeable**
- After organ transplantation, protect the patient from visitors and staff with infections; as indicated, maintain isolation precautions

Key nursing actions

- Monitor for adverse effects, toxicity, and signs and symptoms of infection.
- Maintain isolation precautions, as indicated.
- Monitor fluid intake and output.
- Instruct patient to report unusual bleeding or signs and symptoms of infection or transplant rejection.
- Urge the patient to use contraception to prevent pregnancy.
- Teach the patient to avoid flowers, plants, fresh fruit, and raw vegetables because they increase the risk of infection.
- Teach the patient about the importance of lifelong compliance with immunosuppressive therapy to prevent organ rejection.

- Assess the patient for signs and symptoms of infection, such as fever, tachycardia, malaise, redness, and inflammation
- **Monitor the patient's fluid intake and output during immunosuppressive therapy to prevent nephrotoxicity; know that decreased urine output may lead to azathioprine toxicity**
- Instruct the patient to report immediately any signs and symptoms of infection, unusual bleeding, or transplant rejection (fever, graft tenderness, decreased urine output, and edema)
- Inform the patient about potential teratogenic effects of these drugs during pregnancy and urge the patient to use contraception
- **Teach the patient to avoid flowers and plants and such foods as fresh fruit and raw vegetables because they tend to have higher levels of bacteria than cooked foods, thereby increasing the risk of infection in an already immunosuppressed patient**
- Teach the patient about the importance of lifelong compliance with immunosuppressive therapy to prevent organ transplant rejection

ANTIBACTERIAL DRUGS

PENICILLINS

Mechanism of action

- Penicillins usually are bactericidal, inhibiting synthesis of the bacterial cell wall and causing rapid cell lysis
- Penicillins are most effective against fast-growing susceptible bacteria

Pharmacokinetics

- Absorption: Varies widely for oral form; absorption is slow after I.M. administration
- Distribution: Highly bound to albumin and widely distributed
- Metabolism: Partially metabolized in the liver
- Excretion: Most penicillins are excreted in the urine; nafcillin undergoes extrahepatic circulation and is excreted in the bile

Drug examples

- Aminopenicillins: amoxicillin (Amoxil), amoxicillin/clavulanate (Augmentin, Augmentin XR), ampicillin (Principen), and ampicillin/sulbactam (Unasyn)
- Extended-spectrum penicillins: carbenicillin (Geocillin), piperacillin (Pipracil), piperacillin/tazobactam sodium (Zosyn), ticarcillin (Ticar), and ticarcillin/clavulanate (Timentin)
- Natural penicillins: procaine penicillin G, penicillin G potassium (Pfizerpen), and penicillin V (Pen-Vee K)
- Penicillinase-resistant penicillins: dicloxacillin (Dynapen), nafcillin, and oxacillin

Indications

- Penicillins are used to treat infection by gram-positive cocci and bacilli and some gram-negative cocci; they also are effective against some anaerobes

Key facts about penicillins

- Usually bactericidal
- Most effective against fast-growing susceptible bacteria
- Partially metabolized in the liver
- Mostly excreted in urine

When to use penicillins

- Gram-positive cocci and bacilli infections
- Some gram-negative cocci infections
- Some anaerobe infections
- Enterococcal infections
- Gram-negative bacteria infections
- Gonorrhea
- Staphylococci infections

When NOT to use penicillins

- Allergy to penicillin or cephalosporin
- Allergy to caine-type local anesthetics

Adverse reactions to watch for

- Nausea, vomiting, diarrhea, epigastric distress, rash, allergic reaction, pain at I.M. injection site, phlebitis at I.V. infusion site, resistant bacterial and fungal superinfections

Key nursing actions

- Obtain an allergy history.
- Obtain appropriate specimens for culture and sensitivity.
- Watch for signs and symptoms of an allergic reaction; if any occur, discontinue the drug and notify the physician.
- Instruct the patient to avoid taking oral penicillin with acidic juices or carbonated beverages.
- Assess for signs and symptoms of superinfection.

- Aminopenicillins are active against many organisms and have special use in treating enterococcal infections
- Extended-spectrum penicillins have increased activity against gram-negative bacteria
- Natural penicillins are the drugs of choice for treating gonorrhea
- Penicillinase-resistant penicillins are used mainly to treat infections caused by staphylococci that synthesize the enzyme penicillinase

Contraindications and precautions

- Penicillins are contraindicated in patients who are allergic to any penicillin or cephalosporin; the patient may have up to a 10% cross-sensitivity to other penicillins in this group
- Procaine penicillin G is contraindicated in patients who are allergic to caine-type local anesthetics

Adverse reactions

- Nausea, vomiting, diarrhea, epigastric distress, rash, allergic reaction, pain at the I.M. injection site, phlebitis at the I.V. infusion site, resistant bacterial and fungal superinfections (with broad-spectrum drugs)

Interactions

- Penicillins may decrease the effectiveness of aminoglycosides
- Use of penicillins with a hormonal contraceptive increases the risk of breakthrough bleeding and may diminish the efficacy of the contraceptive
- Use of extended-spectrum penicillins with other penicillins may inhibit platelet aggregation and potentiate bleeding
- Probenecid decreases renal excretion of penicillin, thereby increasing penicillin levels and enhancing penicillin's effectiveness
- Use of penicillins with clavulanate or sulbactam enhances resistance against bacteria that produce beta-lactamase (an enzyme that inactivates penicillin)
- Tetracyclines may decrease the bactericidal effects of penicillins

Nursing responsibilities

- **Before administering a penicillin, obtain the patient's allergy history**
- **Know that an allergic reaction to penicillin may occur even in a patient who has no history of an allergic reaction**
- Obtain appropriate specimens for culture and sensitivity before initiating drug therapy (however, the first dose may be given pending results)
- After administering a penicillin, observe for signs and symptoms of an allergic reaction; if these occur, discontinue the drug and notify the physician
- **Instruct the patient to avoid taking oral penicillin with acidic juices or carbonated beverages because they may reduce drug absorption**
- **Assess the patient, especially if elderly or debilitated, for signs and symptoms of superinfection, particularly if the patient is on prolonged therapy**
- Instruct the woman taking hormonal contraceptives to use an alternative contraceptive method (barrier method) during the entire course of penicillin therapy

- Instruct the patient to notify the physician if he notes signs of superinfection, such as black, furry overgrowth on the tongue, loose or foul-smelling stools, and (in women) vaginal itching or discharge
- Teach the patient about the importance of complying with therapy and completing the full therapeutic course, even if feeling better; inadequate dosage or premature discontinuation of therapy may exacerbate the infection and lead to resistant organisms

CEPHALOSPORINS

Mechanism of action

- Cephalosporins are chemically and pharmacologically similar to penicillins
- These drugs are bactericidal and kill or inhibit many gram-positive and gram-negative bacteria, and some anaerobic bacteria
- These drugs don't kill fungi or viruses

Pharmacokinetics

- Absorption: Oral absorption of cephalosporins varies widely; many are given I.V.
- Distribution: Distributed widely to most tissues and fluids
  - Third- and fourth- generation cephalosporins penetrate the blood-brain barrier and appear in cerebrospinal fluid (CSF)
  - All cephalosporins cross the placental barrier
- Metabolism: Varies widely; some drugs are metabolized extensively and some aren't metabolized at all
- Excretion
  - Excreted primarily in the urine
  - Some drugs appear in breast milk
  - May be removed by hemodialysis

Drug examples

- First-generation cephalosporins: cefadroxil (Duricef), cefazolin sodium (Ancef), cephalexin monohydrate (Keflex, Keftab), cephapirin (Cefadyl), and cephradine (Velosef)
- Second-generation cephalosporins: cefaclor (Ceclor, Ceclor CD), cefotetan (Cefotan), cefoxitin (Mefoxin), cefprozil (Cefzil), cefuroxime (Ceftin), and loracarbef (Lorabid)
- Third-generation cephalosporins: cefdinir (Omnicef), cefditoren pivoxil (Spectracef), cefoperazone (Cefobid), cefotaxime (Claforan), cefpodoxime proxetil (Vantin), ceftazidime (Fortaz, Tazicef, Tazidime), ceftibuten (Cedax), ceftizoxime (Cefizox), and ceftriaxone (Rocephin)
- Fourth-generation cephalosporin: cefepime hydrochloride (Maxipime)

Indications

- Cephalosporins are active against infections caused by gram-positive and gram-negative bacteria

Key facts about cephalosporins

- Chemically and pharmacologically similar to penicillins
- Bactericidal (not antifungal or antiviral)
- Metabolism varies by drug
- Excreted primarily in urine

When to use cephalosporins

- Gram-positive and gram-negative bacterial infections
- Gram-positive and gram-negative cocci infections
- Certain gram-negative bacilli infections

When NOT to use cephalosporins

- Allergy to penicillin
- Pregnancy or breast-feeding
- History of GI disease, particularly colitis

Adverse reactions to watch for

- Nausea, vomiting, diarrhea, rash, anaphylaxis, pain at I.M. injection site, phlebitis at I.V. infusion site, pseudomembranous colitis

Key nursing actions

- Before administering a cephalosporin, obtain an allergy history.
- After administering a cephalosporin, observe for signs and symptoms of an allergic reaction; discontinue the drug and notify the physician if any occur.

Key facts about aminoglycosides

- Bactericidal
- Exact mechanism unknown
- Not metabolized
- Excreted unchanged in urine

- First-generation cephalosporins are active against infections caused by most gram-positive cocci and certain gram-negative bacilli
- Each subsequent cephalosporin generation has increased activity against gram-negative organisms and reduced activity against gram-positive organisms

Contraindications and precautions

- Use cephalosporins cautiously in patients who are allergic to penicillins to prevent cross-sensitivity
- Use cephalosporins cautiously in pregnant or breast-feeding women and in those with a history of GI disease, particularly colitis

Adverse reactions

- Nausea, vomiting, diarrhea, rash, anaphylaxis, pain at I.M. injection site, phlebitis at I.V. infusion site, pseudomembranous colitis

Interactions

- If cephalosporins must be administered with aminoglycosides, they should be given in separate sites to prevent inactivation
- Probenecid decreases excretion of cephalosporins, increasing cephalosporin levels
- Use of cefotetan or cefoperazone with alcohol may cause a disulfiram-like reaction (flushing, headache, tachycardia)

Nursing responsibilities

- **Before administering a cephalosporin, obtain the patient's allergy history**
- **Know that an allergic reaction to a cephalosporin may occur even in a patient with no history of an allergic reaction**
- After administering a cephalosporin, observe for signs and symptoms of an allergic reaction; discontinue the drug and notify the physician if these occur

AMINOGLYCOSIDES

Mechanism of action

- Aminoglycosides are bactericidal
- The exact mechanism of action is not clear, but they are thought to bind to ribosomal subunits, inhibiting bacterial protein synthesis

Pharmacokinetics

- Absorption: Oral absorption is poor; most of these drugs are given parenterally
- Distribution: Widely distributed into extracellular fluid; minimal CSF penetration
- Metabolism: Most are not metabolized
- Excretion: Excreted unchanged in the urine; neomycin is excreted in the feces after oral administration

Drug examples

- Amikacin (Amikin), gentamicin (Garamycin), kanamycin (Kantrex), neomycin (Mycifradin), streptomycin, tobramycin (Nebcin)

Indications

- These drugs are used to treat infections caused by aerobic gram-negative bacilli and some gram-positive bacteria
- Used to treat septicemia; postoperative pulmonary, intra-abdominal, and serious recurrent urinary tract infections; infections of the bones, skin, soft tissues, and joints; and ammonia-forming bacteria in the GI tract of patients with hepatic encephalopathy
- Aminoglycosides may be used with other antibacterials to treat serious staphylococcal infections, serious *Pseudomonas aeruginosa* infections, enterococcal infections, nosocomial pneumonia, tuberculosis, pelvic inflammatory disease, and serious *Klebsiella* infections

Contraindications and precautions

- Contraindicated in pregnant or breast-feeding women
- Use cautiously in patients with renal failure or neuromuscular disease and in elderly or debilitated patients

Adverse reactions

- **The most serious complications are vestibular and cochlear ototoxicity, nephrotoxicity, and neurotoxicity (as evidenced by paresthesia, respiratory depression, and neuromuscular weakness); ototoxicity and nephrotoxicity are reversible only if detected early and if the drug is discontinued immediately**
- The most common adverse reactions are nausea, vomiting, and diarrhea
- Aminoglycosides may also cause hypersensitivity reactions, hemolytic anemia, transient neutropenia, leukopenia, thrombocytopenia, elevated liver enzyme levels; and vein irritation, phlebitis, and sterile abscess (with I.V. form)

Interactions

- Use with another aminoglycoside or with loop diuretics may cause additive ototoxicity
- Inactivation occurs when aminoglycosides are mixed with penicillins
- Administration with cephalosporins in the same site may cause inactivation
- Use with certain inhalation anesthetics or neuromuscular blockers may cause respiratory paralysis

Nursing responsibilities

- **Before starting drug therapy and during therapy, assess eighth cranial nerve function to detect vertigo and hearing loss (which usually involves high frequencies); permanent damage may occur without immediate intervention**
- **Monitor renal function for evidence of nephrotoxicity**

When to use aminoglycosides

- Aerobic gram-negative bacilli and some gram-positive bacterial infections
- Septicemia
- Postoperative pulmonary, intra-abdominal, and serious recurrent urinary tract infections
- Infections of the bones, skin, soft tissues, and joints
- Ammonia-forming bacterial infections in the GI tract
- Staphylococcal infections
- Serious *Pseudomonas aeruginosa* infections
- Enterococcal infections
- Nosocomial pneumonia
- Tuberculosis
- Pelvic inflammatory disease
- Serious *Klebsiella* infections

When NOT to use aminoglycosides

- Pregnancy
- Breast-feeding

Adverse reactions to watch for

- Vestibular and cochlear ototoxicity, nephrotoxicity, and neurotoxicity; nausea; vomiting; diarrhea; hypersensitivity reactions; hemolytic anemia; transient neutropenia; leukopenia; thrombocytopenia; elevated liver enzyme levels; vein irritation, phlebitis, and sterile abscess

Key nursing actions

- Assess eighth cranial nerve function to detect vertigo and hearing loss.
- Monitor renal function for evidence of nephrotoxicity.
- Promote fluid intake of 1,500 to 2,000 ml/day.
- Monitor peak and trough levels to evaluate drug effectiveness and prevent toxicity.

- Make sure patient is well hydrated during drug therapy; promote a fluid intake of 1,500 to 2,000 ml/day to maintain adequate renal function
- Monitor peak and trough levels to evaluate drug effectiveness and prevent toxicity; the drug must be given at proper administration times so that accurate blood levels are drawn

TETRACYCLINES

Key facts about tetracyclines

- Bacteriostatic (may be bactericidal with certain organisms)
- Bind reversibly to 30S and 50S ribosomal units, inhibiting bacterial protein synthesis
- Metabolized in the kidneys or not metabolized at all
- Excreted in urine or feces

Mechanism of action

- Tetracyclines are bacteriostatic but may be bactericidal with certain organisms
- They bind reversibly to 30S and 50S ribosomal units, inhibiting bacterial protein synthesis

Pharmacokinetics

- Absorption
  - Absorbed systemically after oral administration
  - Food increases absorption, except for doxycycline and minocycline
  - Calcium and certain other minerals may affect absorption
- Distribution: Widely distributed into body tissues and fluids; all tetracyclines cross the placental barrier
- Metabolism: Metabolized in the kidneys or not metabolized at all; minocycline is metabolized partially by the liver
- Excretion: Excreted in the urine; minocycline is excreted in the feces

Drug examples

- Demeclocycline hydrochloride (Declomycin), doxycycline hyclate (Vibramycin), minocycline hydrochloride (Minocin), oxytetracycline hydrochloride (Terramycin), tetracycline hydrochloride (Sumycin)

When to use tetracyclines

- Gram-positive and gram-negative infections
- Lyme disease
- Gonorrhea
- Syphilis
- *Mycoplasma*, *Chlamydia*, and *Rickettsia* infection
- Acne
- Syndrome of inappropriate antidiuretic hormone

Indications

- Tetracyclines are active against some gram-positive and gram-negative organisms; however, many such organisms are resistant to tetracyclines
- These drugs are commonly used to treat Lyme disease, gonorrhea, and syphilis in penicillin-allergic patients, and infections by unusual organisms *(Mycoplasma, Chlamydia, Rickettsia)*
- They are occasionally prescribed for acne
- Demeclocycline also has been used as a diuretic in treating the syndrome of inappropriate antidiuretic hormone

When NOT to use tetracyclines

- Pregnancy
- Breast-feeding
- Hypersensitivity to tetracyclines
- Children younger than age 8

Contraindications and precautions

- These drugs are contraindicated in pregnant and breast-feeding women and in patients with a hypersensitivity to tetracyclines
- Don't use in children younger than age 8 unless no alternatives exist; may cause permanent tooth discoloration
- Use cautiously in elderly patients

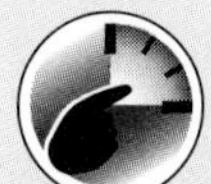

TIME-OUT FOR TEACHING

Teaching about tetracyclines

Include these topics in your teaching plan for the patient receiving a tetracycline.

- Medication regimen, including the drug's name, dosage, frequency, duration, and possible adverse effects
- Signs and symptoms to discuss with the physician
- Avoidance of milk products and drugs containing calcium, magnesium, aluminum, or iron
- Administration on an empty stomach
- Avoidance of direct sunlight and measures to take for sun exposure
- Importance of completing therapy
- Use of alternative contraception during therapy and for 1 week afterward
- Follow-up care, including physician visits

Adverse reactions

- The most common adverse reactions are GI related and include anorexia, GI upset, flatulence, nausea, vomiting, bulky and loose stools, and epigastric burning
- May also cause hypersensitivity reactions, pancreatitis, hepatotoxicity, photosensitivity reaction, rash, pain at I.M. injection site, phlebitis at I.V. infusion site, and mild increase in BUN levels

Interactions

- Antacids, calcium supplements, iron supplements, magnesium-containing laxatives, and milk and dairy products reduce absorption of tetracyclines
- Tetracyclines may increase the effects of oral anticoagulants
- Tetracyclines decrease the effectiveness of hormonal contraceptives
- Tetracyclines decrease the effectiveness of penicillins

Nursing responsibilities

- Obtain urine specimen for culture and sensitivity before starting drug therapy; however, first dose may be given with results pending
- **Because of the risk of thrombophlebitis and hepatotoxicity, only doxycycline and minocycline are given I.V.; if giving drug I.V., monitor I.V. sites often for phlebitis**
- **Instruct the patient not to take antacids, calcium supplements, iron supplements, magnesium-containing laxatives, or milk or dairy products within 2 to 3 hours of taking a tetracycline (for additional teaching tips, see** *Teaching about tetracyclines***)**
- **Teach the patient to use sunscreen and protective clothing to prevent photosensitivity reactions**
- Instruct the patient to discard outdated or decomposed tetracycline because it may be toxic
- **Inform the patient that tetracyclines may cause staining of soft contact lenses**

Topics for patient discussion

- Medication regimen
- Signs and symptoms to discuss with physician
- Avoidance of milk products and drugs containing calcium, magnesium, aluminum, or iron
- Administration on an empty stomach
- Measures to take for sun exposure
- Importance of completing therapy
- Use of alternative contraception during therapy and for 1 week afterward
- Follow-up care
- Importance of discarding outdated or decomposed drug

Adverse reactions to watch for

- GI-related effects, such as anorexia, GI upset, flatulence, nausea, vomiting, bulky and loose stools, epigastric burning; hypersensitivity reactions; pancreatitis; hepatotoxicity; photosensitivity reaction; rash; pain at I.M. injection site; phlebitis at I.V. infusion site; mild increase in BUN levels

Key nursing actions

- Obtain urine specimen for culture and sensitivity before starting drug therapy.
- If giving drug I.V., monitor I.V. sites for phlebitis.

- Instruct the woman taking hormonal contraceptives to use an alternative contraceptive method (barrier method) during the entire course of tetracycline therapy

FLUOROQUINOLONES

Mechanism of action
- Fluoroquinolones are broad-spectrum, systemic antibacterial drugs active against a wide range of organisms
- They produce a bactericidal effect by inhibiting intracellular enzymes essential for the duplication, transcription, and repair of bacterial DNA

Pharmacokinetics
- Absorption: Most are well absorbed rapidly from the GI tract after oral administration; food slows drug absorption
- Distribution: Widely distributed in the body tissues and fluids
- Metabolism: Some undergo partial hepatic metabolism; others aren't metabolized at all
- Excretion: Most are excreted primarily unchanged in the urine

Drug examples
- Ciprofloxacin (Cipro), gatifloxacin (Tequin), gemifloxacin (Factive), levofloxacin (Levaquin), lomefloxacin hydrochloride (Maxaquin), moxifloxacin hydrochloride (Avelox), norfloxacin (Noroxin), ofloxacin (Floxin), sparfloxacin (Zagam)

Indications
- Fluoroquinolones are active against many aerobic gram-positive and gram-negative organisms
- They are commonly used for bone and joint infections, skin and soft-tissue infections, intra-abdominal infections, urinary tract infections, pyelonephritis, pneumonia, acute sinusitis, and chronic bronchitis
- They are also used to treat gonorrhea, endocervical and urethral chlamydial infections, and pelvic inflammatory disease
- They may be used for the prevention of bacterial urinary tract infections

Contraindications and precautions
- Contraindicated in children
- Use very cautiously in patients with cardiovascular disorders, central nervous system disorders, seizures, renal insufficiency, cerebral ischemia, or severe hepatic dysfunction

Adverse reactions
- Nausea, crystalluria, phototoxicity, diarrhea, rash

Interactions
- These drugs may increase serum levels of methylxanthines, causing methylxanthine toxicity
- Antacids may reduce the effectiveness of fluoroquinolones when given within 2 to 8 hours of fluoroquinolone administration

Key facts about fluoroquinolones
- Broad-spectrum, systemic antibacterials
- Active against wide range of organisms
- Produce a bactericidal effect by inhibiting intracellular enzymes
- Most unmetabolized
- Excreted primarily unchanged in urine

When to use fluoroquinolones
- Aerobic gram-positive and gram-negative infections
- Bone and joint infections
- Skin and soft-tissue infections
- Intra-abdominal infections
- Urinary tract infections
- Pyelonephritis
- Pneumonia
- Acute sinusitis
- Chronic bronchitis
- Gonorrhea
- Endocervical and urethral chlamydial infections
- Pelvic inflammatory disease

When NOT to use fluoroquinolones
- Children
- Cardiovascular disorders
- Central nervous system disorders
- Seizures
- Renal insufficiency
- Cerebral ischemia
- Severe hepatic dysfunction

Adverse reactions to watch for
- Nausea, crystalluria, phototoxicity, diarrhea, rash

- Probenecid may decrease renal excretion and increase serum levels of fluoroquinolones

Nursing responsibilities

- Obtain urine for culture and sensitivity testing before starting drug therapy; first dose may be given pending results
- Separate administration times of drug and antacids, calcium, and iron by at least 2 hours
- Tell the patient to take the drug with 8 ounces of water
- Teach the patient to use sunblock and wear protective clothing to prevent photosensitivity reactions
- Monitor the patient's renal function
- Explain to the patient the importance of completing the full course of therapy as prescribed, even if feeling better

Key nursing actions

- Obtain urine for culture and sensitivity testing before starting drug therapy.
- Administer with 8 ounces of water at least 2 hours before or after antacid, calcium, and iron administration.
- Monitor the patient's renal function.
- Explain to the patient the importance of completing the full course of therapy as prescribed.

MISCELLANEOUS ANTI-INFECTIVES

Mechanism of action

- May be bactericidal or bacteriostatic
- Block protein synthesis or may block the synthesis of the cell wall, causing cell lysis and cell death

Pharmacokinetics

- Absorption: Varies with the drug; may be rapidly or poorly absorbed from the GI tract after oral administration
- Distribution: Rapidly distributed throughout the body to all tissues and body fluids: readily penetrates cells
- Metabolism: Varies with drug; may be poorly metabolized or not metabolized at all
- Excretion: Varies with drug
  - Azithromycin is excreted mostly in the feces after excretion in the bile, with less than 10% excreted in the urine
  - Aztreonam is excreted primarily in the urine, with less than 3% excreted in the feces

Key facts about other anti-infectives

- Bactericidal or bacteriostatic
- Block protein synthesis or synthesis of cell wall
- Poorly metabolized or not metabolized at all
- Excreted in urine or feces (varies with drug)

Drug examples

- azithromycin (Zithromax), aztreonam (Azactam), chloramphenicol (Chloromycetin), clarithromycin (Biaxin, Biaxin XL), clindamycin (Cleocin), erythromycin (E-Mycin, Erythrocin), imipenem-cilastatin (Primaxin), metronidazole (Flagyl), pentamidine (NebuPent, Pentam), vancomycin (Vancocin)

Indications

- Aztreonam is used to treat infections caused by gram-negative aerobic bacteria
- Chloramphenicol is used to treat severe infections and ampicillin-resistant *Haemophilus influenzae* infections
- Clindamycin is used to treat infections caused by most aerobic gram-positive organisms

When to use other anti-infectives

- Gram-negative and gram-positive aerobic and anaerobic infections
- Severe infections
- Ampicillin-resistant *Haemophilus influenzae* infections
- Pneumococci
- Group A streptococci
- *Pneumocystis carinii* pneumonia
- Penicillin-resistant staphylococcal infections

- Erythromycin is used to treat infections caused by most gram-positive and gram-negative organisms, pneumococci, and group A streptococci
- Imipenem-cilastatin is used to treat infections caused by gram-positive, gram-negative, and anaerobic organisms
- Metronidazole is used to treat infection caused by anaerobic organisms, including *Bacteroides* and *Trichomonas vaginalis*
- Pentamidine is used to prevent and treat *Pneumocystis carinii* pneumonia in patients who test positive for HIV or who have AIDS
- Vancomycin is used to treat penicillin-resistant staphylococcal infections

Contraindications and precautions

- Azithromycin, clarithromycin, and erythromycin are contraindicated in patients hypersensitive to macrolide antibiotics and in those receiving pimozide; use these drugs cautiously in patients with renal or hepatic dysfunction
- Aztreonam is contraindicated in those with an allergy to the drug; use cautiously in elderly patients and in those with renal or hepatic dysfunction
- Chloramphenicol is contraindicated in those with an allergy to the drug; use cautiously in patients with impaired renal or hepatic function, acute intermittent porphyria, or G6PD deficiency and in those taking drugs that cause bone marrow suppression or blood disorders
- Metronidazole is contraindicated in those with an allergy to the drug and in pregnant patients in their first trimester; use cautiously in patients with a history of blood dyscrasia or CNS disorder, in those with hepatic disease or alcoholism, and in those taking hepatotoxic drugs

When NOT to use other anti-infectives

- Hypersensitivity to macrolide antibiotics
- Pimozide use
- Allergy to anti-infectives
- Pregnancy (first trimester)

Adverse reactions

- Chloramphenicol may cause bone marrow depression
- Clindamycin may cause pseudomembranous colitis
- Erythromycin may cause GI upset and hepatotoxicity
- Vancomycin may cause ototoxicity and nephrotoxicity
- Aztreonam and imipenem-cilastatin may cause seizures, nausea, vomiting, diarrhea, and thrombophlebitis at the infusion site
- Pentamidine may cause nephrotoxicity, bronchospasm, cough (with nebulized administration), and thrombophlebitis at the infusion site
- Metronidazole may cause neuromuscular reactions, nausea, headache, dry mouth, and metallic taste

Adverse reactions to watch for

- Bone marrow depression, pseudomembranous colitis, GI upset, hepatotoxicity, ototoxicity, nephrotoxicity, seizures, nausea, vomiting, diarrhea, thrombophlebitis at infusion site, bronchospasm, cough, neuromuscular reactions, headache, dry mouth, metallic taste

Interactions

- Use of metronidazole with alcohol may cause a disulfiram-like reaction, manifested by nausea, vomiting, tachycardia, flushing, and sweating; use with warfarin may prolong bleeding
- Use of vancomycin with other ototoxic and nephrotoxic drugs may cause additive ototoxicity and nephrotoxicity

Nursing responsibilities

- Institute seizure precautions for the patient receiving aztreonam or imipenem-cilastatin

Key nursing actions

- Institute seizure precautions, if necessary.
- Monitor the patient's renal status.
- Maintain adequate hydration to minimize the risk of nephrotoxicity.
- Monitor the I.V. infusion site for thrombophlebitis.
- Assess the patient for cough or shortness of breath after pentamidine inhalation therapy.

- Monitor the patient's renal status (including urine output and serum BUN and creatinine levels) before, during, and after pentamidine therapy; maintain adequate hydration to minimize the risk of nephrotoxicity
- Monitor the I.V. infusion site for thrombophlebitis
- **Caution the patient to avoid alcohol when taking metronidazole to prevent a disulfiram-like reaction**
- Assess the patient for cough or shortness of breath after pentamidine inhalation therapy

URINARY TRACT ANTISEPTICS

Mechanism of action

- These drugs are bacteriostatic; they inhibit the growth of many species of bacteria in the urine
- They form high concentrations in the urine and provide a local antibacterial effect within the urinary tract

Pharmacokinetics

- Absorption: Well absorbed from the GI tract after oral administration
- Distribution: Distributed widely into tissues and body fluids
- Metabolism: Metabolized in the liver
- Excretion: Excreted in the urine

Drug examples

- Sulfonamides: co-trimoxazole (Bactrim, Bactrim DS, Septra), sulfadiazine, sulfisoxazole
- Miscellaneous: fluoroquinolones, methenamine (Hiprex), nalidixic acid (NegGram), nitrofurantoin (Furadantin, Macrodantin)

Indications

- Sulfonamides are used to treat infections caused by susceptible organisms in the urinary tract; their use may be limited in systemic infections because safe doses of the drugs don't reach effective levels in the plasma
- Methenamine is used to prevent recurrent urinary tract infections

Contraindications and precautions

- Sulfonamides are contraindicated in pregnant and breast-feeding women, in children younger than age 2, and in patients hypersensitive to sulfa drugs or those who have severe renal or hepatic disease, porphyria, or a history of Stevens-Johnson syndrome
- Use sulfonamides cautiously in patients with mild to moderate renal or hepatic disease, severe allergies, asthma, blood dyscrasias, G6PD deficiency, or urinary obstruction

Adverse reactions

- Sulfonamides may cause fever, nausea, vomiting, rash, crystalluria, photosensitivity reaction, blood dyscrasias (such as agranulocytosis and aplastic anemia), rash, Stevens-Johnson syndrome, erythema multiforme, and toxic epidermal necrolysis

Key facts about urinary tract antiseptics

- Bacteriostatic
- Form high concentrations in urine and provide a local antibacterial effect within urinary tract
- Metabolized in the liver
- Excreted in urine

When to use urinary tract antiseptics

- Urinary tract infections

When NOT to use urinary tract antiseptics

- Pregnancy
- Breast-feeding
- Children younger than age 2
- Hypersensitivity to sulfa drugs
- Severe renal or hepatic disease
- Porphyria
- History of Stevens-Johnson syndrome

Adverse reactions to watch for

- Fever, nausea, vomiting, rash, crystalluria, photosensitivity reaction, blood dyscrasias, rash, Stevens-Johnson syndrome, erythema multiforme, toxic epidermal necrolysis

- Nitrofurantoin may cause GI upset, hypersensitivity, peripheral neuropathy, and photosensitivity
- Nalidixic acid and nitrofurantoin also may cause blood dyscrasias

Interactions

- Sulfonamides may increase the effects of oral hypoglycemics
- Sulfonamides may decrease the effectiveness of hormonal contraceptives
- Sulfanomides may increase the risk of bleeding in patients taking oral anticoagulants
- Use of antacids with nitrofurantoin may decrease the extent and rate of nitrofurantoin absorption
- Use of probenecid or sulfinpyrazone with nitrofurantoin may inhibit renal excretion of nitrofurantoin, reduce its efficacy, and increase its toxic potential

Nursing responsibilities

- Assess the patient for signs and symptoms of urinary tract infection, such as urinary frequency and urgency, burning on urination, and flank pain
- Before initiating therapy, obtain specimens for culture and sensitivity tests; the first dose may be given while results are pending
- Instruct the patient to take nitrofurantoin with food or milk to minimize GI irritation
- **Make sure the patient maintains a fluid intake of 2,000 to 3,000 ml/day to reduce crystalluria**
- Teach the patient proper hygiene measures to reduce the chance of reinfection
- Instruct the patient to use sunscreen and protective clothing to prevent photosensitivity reactions
- Monitor the patient's urinary elimination patterns for changes in quantity or frequency and for dysuria
- Inform the patient that nitrofurantoin may turn urine rusty yellow
- **Teach the patient about the importance of complying with the full course of therapy, even if feeling better**
- **Emphasize that sharing antibacterial drugs may be dangerous**
- **Caution the patient that inadequate dosage or premature discontinuation of therapy may exacerbate an infection and lead to resistant organisms**
- Instruct the woman taking hormonal contraceptives to use an alternative contraceptive method (barrier method) during the entire course of sulfonamide therapy

Key nursing actions

- Assess for signs and symptoms of urinary tract infection.
- Before therapy, obtain specimens for culture and sensitivity tests.
- Make sure the patient maintains a fluid intake of 2,000 to 3,000 ml/day to reduce crystalluria.
- Teach about proper hygiene measures to reduce the chance of reinfection.
- Monitor the patient's urinary elimination patterns.
- Teach the patient about the importance of complying with the full course of therapy, even if feeling better.
- Instruct a woman taking hormonal contraceptives to use an alternative contraceptive method (barrier method) during the entire course of therapy.

ANTIFUNGALS

Mechanism of action

- Kill or inhibit fungal growth by inhibiting protein synthesis within the fungal cells or by altering the permeability of the cell membrane

Key facts about antifungals

- Kill or inhibit fungal growth
- Metabolism and excretion vary by drug

Pharmacokinetics

- Absorption: Varies widely, but drugs are usually well absorbed; food may increase or decrease absorption, depending on the drug
- Distribution: Widely distributed in the body tissues and fluid
- Metabolism: Varies widely
- Excretion: Varies widely

Drug examples

- amphotericin B (Fungizone, Amphocin, Abelcet, Amphotec, AmBisome), caspofungin acetate (Cancidas), clotrimazole (Gyne-Lotrimin, Mycelex), econazole (Spectazole), fluconazole (Diflucan), flucytosine (5-FC [Ancobon]), itraconazole (Sporanox), ketoconazole (Nizoral), miconazole (Micatin, Monistat), nystatin (Mycostatin), terbinafine hydrochloride (Lamisil), voriconazole (Vfend)

Indications

- Amphotericin B, caspofungin acetate, fluconazole, flucytosine, and voriconazole are used to treat serious systemic fungal infections
- Clotrimazole, fluconazole, itraconazole, miconazole, and nystatin are used to treat oral and vaginal *Candida* infections
- Econazole is used to treat ringworm, athlete's foot, and jock itch
- Ketoconazole and itraconazole are used to treat pulmonary, subcutaneous, and systemic fungal infections
- Terbinafine hydrochloride and itraconazole are used to treat toenail or fingernail fungus

Contraindications and precautions

- Contraindicated in patients with hypersensitivity to the drugs or their components
- Also contraindicated in pregnant or breast-feeding women

Adverse reactions

- Antifungals may cause hypersensitivity reactions and nausea and vomiting
- Amphotericin B may also cause headache, hypotension, hypokalemia, fever, chills, dyscrasias, phlebitis, and nephrotoxicity
- Amphotericin B and flucytosine may also cause blood dyscrasias
- Caspofungin acetate may also cause fever, tachycardia, tachypnea, and muscle ache
- Miconazole and econazole may also cause pruritus and skin irritation
- Terbinafine hydrochloride may also cause rash, pruritus, diarrhea, dyspepsia, and headache
- Voriconazole may also cause abnormal vision, fever, rash, and photosensitivity reactions

Interactions

- Use of antifungals with other nephrotoxic drugs may cause additive nephrotoxicity
- Use of amphotericin B with diuretics may cause additive hypokalemia

When to use antifungals

- Serious systemic fungal infections
- Oral and vaginal *Candida* infections
- Ringworm
- Athlete's foot
- Jock itch
- Pulmonary, subcutaneous, and systemic fungal infections
- Toenail or fingernail fungus

When NOT to use antifungals

- Hypersensitivity to antifungal drugs or their components
- Pregnancy
- Breast-feeding

Adverse reactions to watch for

- Hypersensitivity reactions, nausea, vomiting, headache, hypotension, hypokalemia, fever, chills, dyscrasias, phlebitis, nephrotoxicity, tachycardia, tachypnea, muscle ache, pruritus, skin irritation, rash, diarrhea, dyspepsia, abnormal vision, photosensitivity reactions

Topics for patient discussion

- Medication regimen and administration
- Signs and symptoms to discuss with the physician
- Avoidance of occlusive dressings
- Importance of compliance with therapy
- Importance of washing personal articles and kitchen utensils in hot, soapy water to prevent the spread of parasites
- Follow-up care

Key nursing actions

- Before initiating therapy, obtain specimens for culture and sensitivity tests.
- Administer amphotericin B by infusion pump, as ordered, to ensure an accurate rate.
- Monitor the patient closely for reactions, such as fever, chills, nausea, vomiting, headache, and phlebitis.
- Assess infected areas for improvement.
- Monitor the patient's renal and electrolyte status.

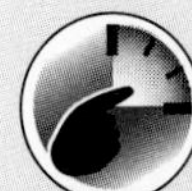

TIME-OUT FOR TEACHING

Teaching about antifungals

Include these topics in your teaching plan for the patient receiving an antifungal.

- Medication regimen, including the drug's name, dosage, frequency, duration, and possible adverse effects
- Signs and symptoms to discuss with the physician, including those related to infection or adverse effects
- Proper procedure for administration
- Avoidance of occlusive dressings
- Importance of compliance with therapy
- Follow-up care, including physician visits

- Use of flucytosine with other bone marrow depressants may cause additive bone marrow depression
- Fluconazole, itraconazole, ketoconazole, and voriconazole may increase the effects of oral anticoagulants by increasing prothrombin time
- Use of itraconazole with antidiabetics may increase the risk of hypoglycemia
- Use of ketoconazole with alcohol may increase hepatotoxicity
- Use of itraconazole or voriconazole with pimozide or quinidine may cause prolongation of the QT interval

Nursing responsibilities

- Before initiating therapy, obtain specimens for culture and sensitivity tests; the first dose may be given pending test results
- Know that amphotericin B is administered only to hospitalized patients or those under close medical supervision
- Administer amphotericin B by infusion pump, as ordered, to ensure an accurate rate (many clinicians order a test dose before full infusion to determine patient tolerance)
- **For 1 to 2 hours after each I.V. amphotericin B dose, monitor the patient closely for reactions to the drug, such as fever, chills, nausea, vomiting, headache, and phlebitis**
- **Assess infected areas during therapy for improvement in the patient's condition**
- Monitor the patient's renal and electrolyte status
- Instruct the patient not to use an occlusive dressing with topical preparations unless otherwise ordered
- If the patient is receiving vaginal cream, ointment, tablets, or suppositories, provide appropriate teaching
  - Teach the patient how to apply the preparation
  - Advise her to use sanitary napkins to help prevent clothing stains
  - Instruct her to continue treatment during menstruation
  - Teach her to avoid sexual contact or to have her partner wear a condom to prevent reinfection until her infection disappears

- Explain that if one member of a family has a parasitic infection, the entire family must be evaluated
- Teach patients and families to wash all personal articles and kitchen utensils in hot, soapy water to prevent spread of parasites
- Instruct the patient receiving voriconazole to use sunscreen and protective clothing to prevent photosensitivity reactions
- Inform the patient that therapy could take weeks or months
- Teach the patient about the importance of complying with the therapeutic regimen (for additional teaching tips, see *Teaching about antifungals*)

ANTHELMINTICS

Mechanism of action

- Anthelmintics achieve their effect by paralyzing the worm, suppressing egg and larva production, causing the head of the parasite to detach from the intestinal wall, or interfering with cellular function
- Ivermectin paralyzes and kills the worm
- Praziquantel and pyrantel paralyze the worm and allow for its expulsion in the stool
- Albendazole and mebendazole interfere with utilization of glucose and cellular processes of the worm
- Thiabendazole interferes with the worm's enzyme systems and suppresses egg and larva production in pork roundworm (trichinella)

Pharmacokinetics

- Absorption: Varies with each drug
- Distribution: Widely distributed
- Metabolism: Varies with each drug
- Excretion: May be excreted in the urine or feces, depending on the drug

Drug examples

- albendazole (Albenza), ivermectin (Stromectol), mebendazole (Vermox), praziquantel (Biltricide), pyrantel (Antiminth), thiabendazole (Mintezol)

Indications

- Anthelmintics treat helminthic or parasitic worm infections
- Mebendazole is used for whipworm, pinworm, roundworm, and hookworm
- Albendazole is used for tapeworms
- Ivermectin is used for onchocerciasis (river blindness) and strongyloidiasis of the intestines
- Pyrantel is used for roundworm and pinworms
- Praziquantel is used for schistosomiasis, flukes, and tapeworm
- Thiabendazole is used for threadworm, rat lungworm, and invasive trichinosis

Contraindications and precautions

- Pyrantel is contraindicated in patients with hepatic disease and in pregnant women

Key facts about anthelmintics

- Paralyze or kill the worm or interfere with its processes
- Metabolism varies by drug
- Excreted in urine or feces

When to use anthelmintics

- Helminthic or parasitic worm infections, such as whipworm, pinworm, roundworm, hookworm, tapeworm, flukes, threadworm, and rat lungworm
- Onchocerciasis
- Strongyloidiasis of the intestines
- Schistosomiasis
- Invasive trichinosis

When NOT to use anthelmintics

- Hepatic disease
- Pregnancy
- Breast-feeding
- Children younger than age 4

Adverse reactions to watch for

- Abdominal pain, anorexia, nausea, vomiting, diarrhea, dizziness, drowsiness, headache, elevated liver enzyme levels

Key nursing actions

- Explain that all family members should be evaluated.
- Teach the patient and family to wash all personal articles and food preparation articles and utensils in hot, soapy water to prevent spread of the parasite.
- Teach the patient and family members to wash hands well, use disposable towels to dry hands, and keep hands away from the mouth.
- Advise the patient to complete the full course of therapy, even if symptoms subside.

Key facts about antivirals

- Inhibit viral replication or prevent viral penetration of host cell
- Metabolism varies by drug
- Excretion varies by drug

- Use praziquantel cautiously in pregnant or breast-feeding women and in children younger than age 4
- Use mebendazole cautiously in children younger than age 2

Adverse reactions

- May cause abdominal pain, anorexia, nausea, vomiting, diarrhea, dizziness, drowsiness, headache, elevated liver enzyme levels

Interactions

- Interactions vary, depending on the drug used

Nursing responsibilities

- Be aware that a purgative to facilitate bowel movements may follow administration of these drugs
- Explain why all family members should be evaluated if one member has a parasitic infection
- Teach the patient and family to wash all personal articles, including sheets and clothes, and food preparation articles and utensils, including cutting boards and knives, in hot, soapy water to prevent spread of the parasite
- Teach the patient and family members to wash hands well, use disposable towels to dry hands, and keep hands away from the mouth
- Advise the patient that dizziness and drowsiness may occur; caution against performing hazardous activities until the drug's effects are known
- Advise the patient to complete the full course of therapy and not to discontinue the drug when symptoms subside
- Advise the patient not to use the drug to treat symptoms of other infections
- Tell the patient that a reevaluation will be performed at the recommended interval and that a second course of treatment may be required

ANTIVIRALS

Mechanism of action

- Antivirals inhibit viral replication or prevent viral penetration into the host cell
- Most antivirals inhibit reverse transcriptase (an enzyme essential for retroviral DNA synthesis), thereby inhibiting viral replication
- Acyclovir, cidofovir, famciclovir, ganciclovir, valacyclovir, and valganciclovir hydrochloride inhibit viral DNA replication
- Amantadine and rimantadine prevent penetration of the virus into host cells
- Vidarabine and trifluridine interfere with DNA synthesis, blocking viral reproduction
- Saquinavir, ritonavir, indinavir sulfate, nelfinavir mesylate, and amprenavir are protease inhibitors that prevent the division of viral polyproteins, which are essential to HIV maturation
- Zanamivir and oseltamivir inhibit neuroaminidase on the surface of the influenza virus, which alters virus particle aggregation and release

Pharmacokinetics

- Vary by drug

Drug examples

- Abacavir sulfate (Ziagen), acyclovir (Zovirax), amantadine (Symmetrel), amprenavir (Agenerase), cidofovir (Vistide), delavirdine mesylate (Rescriptor), didanosine (ddI [Videx]), efavirenz (Sustiva), famciclovir (Famvir), fomivirsen sodium (Vitravene), foscarnet (Foscavir), ganciclovir (DHPG [Cytovene]), indinavir sulfate (Crixivan), lamivudine (3TC, Epivir), nelfinavir mesylate (Viracept), oseltamivir phosphate (Tamiflu), rimantadine (Flumadine), ritonavir (Norvir), saquinavir (Invirase, Fortovase), stavudine (d4T, Zerit), tenofovir disoproxil fumarate (Viread), trifluridine (Viroptic), valacyclovir hydrochloride (Valtrex), valganciclovir hydrochloride (Valcyte), vidarabine (Vira-A), zalcitabine (Hivid, ddC), zanamivir (Relenza), zidovudine (AZT [Retrovir])
- Combination drugs: lopinavir/ritonavir (Kaletra), lamivudine/zidovudine (Combivir), and abacavir sulfate/lamivudine/zidovudine (Trizivir)

Indications

- Acyclovir and valacyclovir are used to treat genital herpes simplex, localized cutaneous herpes zoster infections (shingles), and chickenpox (varicella)
- Acyclovir and vidarabine are used to treat herpes simplex encephalitis and serious herpesvirus infections
- Amantadine and rimantadine are used to prevent influenza A viral infection
- Fomivirsen sodium, ganciclovir, trifluridine, and vidarabine are used to treat ophthalmic herpes simplex
- Cidofovir, ganciclovir, foscarnet, and valganciclovir are used to treat cytomegalovirus retinitis
- Zidovudine, saquinavir, ritonavir, indinavir sulfate, nelfinavir mesylate, amprenavir, and didanosine are used for their virustatic action in HIV infection
- Zalcitabine is used with zidovudine, tenofovir disoproxil fumarate, lamivudine, stavudine, and abacavir sulfate to treat advanced HIV infection
- Zanamivir and oseltamivir phosphate are used to treat influenza A and B viral infections
- Oseltamivir phosphate also is used to prevent influenza A and B viral infections

When to use antivirals

- Genital herpes simplex
- Localized cutaneous herpes zoster infections (shingles)
- Chickenpox (varicella)
- Herpes simplex encephalitis
- Influenza A and B viral infection prevention or treatment
- Ophthalmic herpes simplex
- Cytomegalovirus retinitis
- HIV infection

Contraindications and precautions

- Contraindicated in patients with known or suspected hypersensitivity to these drugs or their components
- Use cautiously in patients with underlying neurologic disease, renal disease, or dehydration, and in those receiving nephrotoxic drugs

When NOT to use antivirals

- Hypersensitivity to antivirals or their components

Adverse reactions to watch for

- Dizziness; ataxia; headache; diarrhea; nausea; vomiting; renal failure; phlebitis at I.V. infusion site; hypotension; anemia; bone marrow depression; granulocytopenia; thrombocytopenia; rash; fever; abnormal liver function test results; vision changes; eye pain; uveitis; vitreitis; pancreatitis; increased intraocular pressure; burning, stinging, tearing, or edema of the eyelid; anorexia; weight loss; weakness; tremor; hallucinations; malaise; confusion; renal toxicity; neuropathy; paresthesia

Key nursing actions

- Administer I.V. infusions by infusion pump, as prescribed.
- Assess lesions daily for changes.
- Monitor the patient's neurologic status.
- Teach the patient how to apply the prescribed topical or ophthalmic drug, as appropriate.
- Caution the patient with infectious skin lesions not to use over-the-counter preparations because they may delay healing.
- Promote abstinence or condom use while lesions are present.

Adverse reactions

- Acyclovir may cause dizziness, ataxia, headache, diarrhea, nausea, vomiting, renal failure, and phlebitis at I.V. infusion site
- Amantadine may cause dizziness, ataxia, headache, and hypotension
- Vidarabine may cause diarrhea, nausea, vomiting, and phlebitis at I.V. infusion site
- Zidovudine may cause anemia and bone marrow depression
- Ganciclovir and valganciclovir may cause granulocytopenia, thrombocytopenia, anemia, rash, fever, diarrhea, headache, and abnormal liver function test results
- Fomivirsen sodium may cause vision changes, eye pain, uveitis, vitreitis, vomiting, bone marrow suppression, pancreatitis, and increased intraocular pressure
- Trifluridine may cause burning, stinging, tearing, edema of the eyelid, and increased intraocular pressure
- Vidarabine may cause nausea, vomiting, diarrhea, anorexia, weight loss, weakness, tremor, ataxia, hallucinations, malaise, and confusion
- Cidofovir and foscarnet may cause fever, nausea, anemia, diarrhea, renal toxicity, headache, and seizures
- Didanosine may cause headache, diarrhea, peripheral neuropathy, and rash
- Zalcitabine may cause neuropathy and pancreatitis
- Saquinavir, ritonavir, nelfinavir, amprenavir, tenofovir, lamivudine, stavudine, abacavir sulfate, nevirapine, delavirdine, and efavirenz may cause nausea, bone marrow suppression, rash, fever, paresthesia, peripheral neuropathy, dizziness, and diarrhea

Interactions

- Use of acyclovir, foscarnet, ganciclovir, or cidofovir with similar-acting drugs may cause additive nephrotoxicity
- Use of amantadine with similar-acting drugs may cause additive anticholinergic effects
- Probenecid increases serum levels of acyclovir, ganciclovir, valganciclovir, valacyclovir, and zidovudine, possibly causing toxicity
- Allopurinol may increase the risk of adverse effects from vidarabine
- Alcohol may increase levels of these drugs, resulting in increased risk of toxicity

Nursing responsibilities

- Administer I.V. infusions around the clock by infusion pump, as prescribed, to ensure accuracy
- **When administering acyclovir, make sure the patient maintains an adequate fluid intake to prevent crystalluria**
- Assess lesions daily for changes in color or amount of drainage
- Monitor the patient's neurologic status, including level of consciousness, for central nervous system adverse effects
- Teach the patient how to apply the prescribed topical or ophthalmic drug, as appropriate

- Instruct the patient to use gloves when applying topical preparations to prevent the spread of infection and to use strict hand-washing technique
- Caution the patient with infectious skin lesions not to use over-the-counter preparations because they may delay healing
- Advise the patient with genital herpes that acyclovir isn't a cure and won't prevent the spread of infection to others
- Promote abstinence or condom use while lesions are present (open lesions are contagious)

ANTITUBERCULOTICS

Mechanism of action

- Kill or inhibit growth of *Mycobacterium* organisms that cause TB

Pharmacokinetics

- Vary by drug

Drug examples

- Aminosalicylate sodium (para-amino salicylate, PAS, Paser), capreomycin (Capastat), cycloserine (Seromycin), ethambutol (Myambutol), ethionamide (Trecator-SC), isoniazid (INH [Nydrazid]), pyrazinamide, rifampin (Rifadin, Rimactane), rifapentine (Priftin), streptomycin sulfate
- Combination drugs: rifampin/isoniazid/pyrazinamide (Rifater) and rifampin/isoniazid (Rifamate)

Indications

- Isoniazid and rifampin are used as first-line drugs to treat TB
- Cycloserine, pyrazinamide, streptomycin, aminosalicylate sodium, capreomycin, ethionamide, rifapentine, and ethambutol are given with first-line drugs to treat TB when the patient is resistant or allergic to less toxic drugs

Contraindications and precautions

- Contraindicated in patients hypersensitive to these drugs and in those with severe liver disease

Adverse reactions

- These drugs cause nausea, vomiting, and hepatitis
- Cycloserine may cause neurotoxicity and deficiencies of vitamin B_{12} and folic acid
- Ethambutol may cause optic neuritis
- Isoniazid may cause peripheral neuropathy
- Rifampin and rifapentine may cause abdominal cramps, diarrhea, headache, hyperuricemia, and ataxia and may turn body fluids red-orange
- Pyrazinamide may cause hepatotoxicity
- Streptomycin may cause ototoxicity

Interactions

- Antacids delay absorption of isoniazid

Key facts about antituberculotics

- Kill or inhibit growth of *Mycobacterium* organisms that cause TB
- Metabolism varies by drug
- Excretion varies by drug

When to use antituberculotics

- TB

When NOT to use antituberculotics

- Hypersensitivity to antituberculotics
- Severe liver disease

Adverse reactions to watch for

- Nausea, vomiting, hepatitis, neurotoxicity, vitamin B_{12} and folic acid deficiencies, optic neuritis, peripheral neuropathy, abdominal cramps, diarrhea, headache, hyperuricemia, ataxia, body fluid color changes, hepatotoxicity, ototoxicity

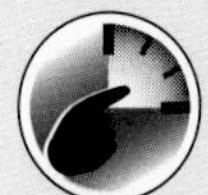

TIME-OUT FOR TEACHING

Teaching about antituberculotics

Include these topics in your teaching plan for the patient receiving an antituberculotic.

- Medication regimen, including the drug's name, dosage, frequency, duration, and possible adverse effects
- Signs and symptoms to discuss with the physician
- Possible changes in color of body secretions
- Infection-control measures
- Need for long-term compliance
- Safety measures
- Follow-up care, including laboratory tests and physician visits

Topics for patient discussion

- Medication regimen
- Signs and symptoms to discuss with the physician
- Body secretion color changes
- Infection-control and safety measures
- Need for long-term compliance
- Importance of avoiding alcohol
- Follow-up care

- Use of isoniazid with other antituberculotics may cause additive neurotoxicity
- Isoniazid inhibits the metabolism of phenytoin and certain other drugs, increasing the risk of toxicity
- Rifampin and rifapentine decrease the effectiveness of estrogens, opioid analgesics, oral anticoagulants, hormonal contraceptives, and oral hypoglycemics by increasing hepatic drug-metabolizing enzyme activity
- Concurrent use with alcohol increases the risk of hepatotoxicity

Key nursing actions

- Assess breath sounds.
- Evaluate sputum for character and amount.
- Before initiating therapy, obtain specimens for culture and sensitivity tests.
- Instruct women to use an effective barrier method of contraception, as appropriate.
- Emphasize the need to comply with therapy, even after the patient feels better.

Nursing responsibilities

- Assess the patient's breath sounds, and evaluate sputum for character and amount
- Before initiating therapy, obtain specimens for culture and sensitivity tests; first dose may be given pending results
- Instruct the patient to avoid alcohol during antitubercular therapy to prevent hepatotoxicity
- **Know that isoniazid is commonly given with pyridoxine (vitamin B_6) to reduce peripheral neuropathy**
- Frequently assess the patient taking ethambutol for visual changes; visual impairment may be permanent unless identified early
- **Teach the patient taking rifampin that this drug may color feces, saliva, sputum, sweat, tears, and urine red-orange to red-brown and may permanently discolor soft contact lenses**
- Instruct women taking rifampin to use an effective barrier method of contraception
- Emphasize the need to comply with therapy, even after the patient feels better; emphasize that 1 to 2 years of therapy may be necessary (for specific teaching tips, see *Teaching about antituberculotics*)

NCLEX CHECKS

It's never too soon to begin your NCLEX preparation. Now that you've reviewed this chapter, carefully read each of the following questions and choose the best answer. Then compare your responses to the correct answers.

1. You're caring for a patient diagnosed with systemic lupus erythematosus. The patient is prescribed prednisone, 20 mg four times daily. When giving discharge instructions, you should teach the patient to avoid eating:

☐ **A.** cold cuts and hot dogs.
☐ **B.** canned peaches and beans.
☐ **C.** white bread and cooked rice.
☐ **D.** fresh fruits and raw vegetables.

2. A patient has been prescribed oral tetracycline (Sumycin) for a skin infection. You should instruct the patient to:

☐ **A.** eat fresh fruit to prevent constipation.
☐ **B.** stay in direct sunlight as much as possible.
☐ **C.** reduce fluid intake to prevent renal failure.
☐ **D.** avoid taking the drug with milk or antacids.

3. Your patient is allergic to penicillin. He also may have a cross-allergy to which class of antibiotics?

☐ **A.** Aminoglycosides
☐ **B.** Cephalosporins
☐ **C.** Macrolides
☐ **D.** Sulfas

4. A physician orders co-trimoxazole (Bactrim) for 10 days for a patient with a urinary tract infection (UTI). The patient also has diabetes and is taking an oral sulfonylurea. Which of the following instructions should you give the patient about this drug?

☐ **A.** Limit fluid intake to 32 oz (1 L) daily.
☐ **B.** Take the co-trimoxazole with an antacid.
☐ **C.** Continue to take the oral antidiabetic as usual.
☐ **D.** Drink at least 64 ounces (eight 8-oz glasses; 240-ml) of fluid daily.

5. A 48-year-old patient is receiving amphotericin B (Fungizone) I.V. for a severe systemic fungal infection. Which adverse reaction is most common?

☐ **A.** Anuria
☐ **B.** Coagulation defects
☐ **C.** Peripheral neuropathies
☐ **D.** Normochromic or normocytic anemia

6. A patient was diagnosed recently with pulmonary tuberculosis. The patient was prescribed a drug regimen of isoniazid (INH), 300 mg P.O. daily; rifampin (Rifadin), 600 mg P.O. daily; pyridoxine (vitamin B_6), 10 mg P.O. daily; ethambutol (Myambutol), 400 mg P.O. daily; and pyrazinamide, 1.5 g P.O. daily.

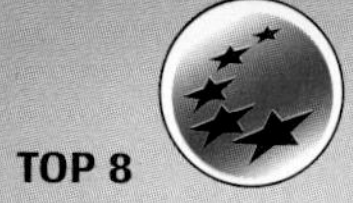

TOP 8

Items to study before your next test on drugs and the immune system

1. Mechanism of action of corticosteroids, immunosuppressants, antibacterials, antifungals, anthelmintics, antivirals, and antituberculotics
2. General characteristics of penicillins, cephalosporins, aminoglycosides, tetracyclines, fluoroquinolones, and urinary tract antiseptics
3. Indications for corticosteroids, immunosuppressants, antibacterials, antifungals, anthelmintics, antivirals, and antituberculotics
4. Common adverse effects of corticosteroids, immunosuppressants, the various classes of antibacterials, antifungals, anthelmintics, antivirals, and antituberculotics
5. Nursing responsibilities when administering corticosteroids, immunosuppressants, antibacterials, antifungals, anthelmintics, antivirals, and antituberculotics
6. Teaching for patients receiving corticosteroids, immunosuppressants, antibacterials, antifungals, antivirals, or antituberculotics
7. Precautions for preventing infection in immunosuppressed patients
8. Teaching for patients infected with helminths and their families

Which of the following statements describes the rationale for giving these drugs at the same time to treat active tuberculosis?

☐ **A.** The drugs are bacteriostatic in usual doses.
☐ **B.** Rifampin increases the activity of isoniazid.
☐ **C.** They're second-line agents and only effective together.
☐ **D.** Combination therapy can prevent or delay bacterial resistance.

7. A human immunodeficiency virus (HIV)–positive patient is beginning an antiretroviral regimen. To reduce the risk of developing HIV infection that is resistant to the drug, he would need to take which of the following drugs without missing doses?

☐ **A.** didanosine (Videx)
☐ **B.** nevirapine (Viramune)
☐ **C.** ritonavir (Norvir).
☐ **D.** zidovudine (AZT)

8. After undergoing small-bowel resection, a patient is prescribed metronidazole (Flagyl) 500 mg I.V. The mixed I.V. solution contains 100 ml. The nurse is to run the drug over 30 minutes. The drip factor of the available I.V. tubing is 15 gtt/ml. What is the drip rate?

____

ANSWERS AND RATIONALES

1. CORRECT ANSWER: D
Because of the immunosuppressive effects of prednisone, the patient is more susceptible to infection. Foods such as fresh fruits and raw vegetables tend to have higher levels of bacteria than cooked foods, thereby increasing the patient's risk of infection. Cold cuts and hot dogs have high levels of sodium, which will increase the fluid retention often associated with prednisone, but this isn't as serious as the potential for life-threatening infections. The other foods listed aren't contraindicated with prednisone therapy.

2. CORRECT ANSWER: D
Milk and antacids reduce the absorption of tetracyclines. Therefore, tetracyclines should be given 1 hour before or 2 hours after ingesting a dairy product or an antacid. Diarrhea, not constipation, is an adverse reaction to tetracyclines. Sunlight should be avoided because tetracycline can cause photosensitivity. Fluid intake should be increased, not reduced, to prevent renal failure.

3. CORRECT ANSWER: B
Cephalosporins and penicillins are chemically related. Cephalosporins have a cross-allergy rate of about 10%. The other classes of antibiotics listed are not chemically related to penicillins.

4. CORRECT ANSWER: D
Sulfonamides such as co-trimoxazole may cause crystalluria. Increasing fluid intake to 64 ounces daily will increase urine output (which should be 1,500 ml daily), possibly preventing crystalluria. Limiting fluid intake is just the opposite of what you want to recommend to your patient. Co-trimoxazole interacts with sulfonylureas to produce increased hypoglycemic effects, so the dose of the oral antidiabetic may have to be adjusted and the patient's glucose level carefully monitored. Co-trimoxazole doesn't need to be taken with an antacid.

5. CORRECT ANSWER: D
Most patients receiving I.V. amphotericin B develop normochromic or normocytic anemia that will significantly decrease hemoglobin level and hematocrit. Although up to 80% of patients receiving amphotericin B may develop some degree of nephrotoxicity, anuria isn't a common complication. Amphotericin B isn't known to cause coagulation defects or peripheral neuropathies.

6. CORRECT ANSWER: D
Mycobacterium tuberculosis can rapidly develop bacterial resistance to isoniazid and rifampin, so they are given with other antituberculotics. Rifampin doesn't increase the activity of isoniazid. All of the drugs listed are bactericidal, except for ethambutol, which is the only one that is bacteriostatic in usual doses. Not all of the drugs listed are second-line agents.

7. CORRECT ANSWER: C
Ritonavir, a protease inhibitor, requires maximum compliance and must be taken consistently. HIV can easily become resistant in the presence of low concentrations of drug, and people who don't take all doses are at risk for developing a resistant organism. Although resistance can develop with the other drugs listed, those drugs aren't as concentration-dependent as are protease inhibitors.

8. CORRECT ANSWER: 50
Use the following equation:

100 ml/30 minutes × 15 gtt/1 ml = 49.9 gtt/minute (50 gtt/minute)

13 Drugs and cancer

LEARNING OBJECTIVES

After studying this chapter, you should be able to:

- Explain the rationale for using antineoplastics to treat cancer.
- List major adverse effects of antineoplastics.
- Identify nursing responsibilities when administering antineoplastics.
- Describe precautions the nurse must take for self-protection when administering antineoplastics.
- Discuss appropriate teaching for the patient who is receiving an antineoplastic.

CHAPTER OVERVIEW

Cancer is a disorder of cell differentiation and replication. It isn't a single disorder, and it may affect any organ or body system. Cancer is one of the leading causes of death in the United States and can affect people of all ages.

Antineoplastics destroy cancer cells and normal tissue, especially rapidly dividing cells. This factor, along with the adverse effects and toxicity of antineoplastics, may limit their dosage or use. Therefore, combination therapy is usually used to kill as many cancerous cells as possible while avoiding toxic effects. The drugs in this chapter are classified by their mechanism of action and source: alkylating drugs, antitumor antibiotics, antimetabolites, hormonal drugs, vinca alkaloids, and natural products. Nursing responsibilities include preventing and treating adverse effects, monitoring laboratory studies, maintaining vascular access and infusion devices, and providing emotional support during the disease process and for changes in body image and sexuality.

ANATOMY AND PHYSIOLOGY

- **Proliferation**
  - Refers to the process of cell renewal and replacement; normally, a balance exists between cell production and cell loss
  - In cancer, the proliferation process becomes unbalanced because normal control mechanisms are unable to halt the process
- **Differentiation**
  - Refers to the process by which cells diversify, acquire specific structural and functional characteristics, and mature;
  - In cancer, cells are poorly differentiated; the more undifferentiated the tumor cell, the more malignant the tumor
  - Cells and tumors may be benign or malignant
- **Other distinguishing characteristics of cancer cells**
  - Uncontrolled proliferation
  - Altered biochemical properties, such as hormone secretion
  - Chromosomal instability: Cell mutations are caused by alterations in DNA; genetic instability causes new mutations with unique characteristics that are increasingly resistant to therapy
  - Capacity to metastasize: Metastasis is the spread of cancer cells from a primary site to distant secondary sites; a correlation exists between the degree of cell malignancy and its metastatic capacity
- **Two types of antineoplastics**
  - Cell-cycle specific: Act on cells undergoing division in the cell cycle
    - Include antimetabolites and vinca plant alkaloids
    - Effective against rapidly growing tumors
  - Cell-cycle nonspecific: Act on cells during any phase of the cell cycle, whether undergoing division or in a resting state
    - Include antitumor antibiotics, alkylating agents, hormones, and steroids
    - Most effective against slow-growing tumors
- **Goal of cancer treatment**
  - To kill cancer cells without destroying normal healthy cells by interfering with cancer-cell replication
- **Combination therapy**
  - Combines different classes of antineoplastics to maximize the therapeutic response; this combining of categories leads to synergistic and additive qualities as well as various toxicities

A&P highlights

- Proliferation: process of cell renewal and replacement
  - In cancer, the proliferation process becomes unbalanced because normal control mechanisms can't halt the process
- Differentiation: process by which cells diversify, acquire specific structural and functional characteristics, and mature
  - In cancer, cells are poorly differentiated
- Cells and tumors may be benign or malignant
- Cells have altered biochemical properties, chromosomal instability, and the capacity to metastasize
- Two types of antineoplastics: cell-cycle specific (act on cells undergoing division in the cell cycle) and cell-cycle nonspecific (act on cells during any phase of the cell cycle)
- Goal of cancer treatment is to kill cancer cells without destroying normal healthy cells by interfering with cancer-cell replication

- Combination therapy is used because single-agent therapy is usually unsuccessful in attaining long-term remission and increases the risk of drug resistance
- Antineoplastics may be combined with other treatments, such as surgery and radiation

Key facts about alkylating drugs

- Affect the synthesis of DNA
- Cell-cycle nonspecific but effective against rapidly growing tumors
- Metabolized in liver
- Excreted in urine

When to use alkylating drugs

- Leukemia
- Brain tumors
- Multiple myeloma
- Hodgkin's disease
- Non-Hodgkin's lymphoma
- Malignant melanoma
- Ovarian cancer
- Lung cancer
- Head and neck tumors
- Breast cancer
- Testicular tumors
- Prostatic cancer
- Osteosarcoma
- Neuroblastoma

When NOT to use alkylating drugs

- Pregnancy
- Renal or liver failure
- Suppressed WBCs, RBCs, and platelets
- Chronic myelogenous leukemia that has shown prior resistance to the drug
- Chronic lymphocytic or acute leukemia, or blastic crisis of chronic myelogenous leukemia
- Infectious disease

ALKYLATING DRUGS

Mechanism of action

- Affect the synthesis of deoxyribonucleic acid (DNA) by causing cross-linking of DNA to inhibit cell reproduction
- These drugs are cell-cycle nonspecific, but are effective against rapidly growing tumors

Pharmacokinetics

- Absorption: Most are rapidly absorbed after oral administration
- Distribution: Distributed throughout the body
- Metabolism: Metabolized in the liver
- Excretion: Excreted in the urine

Drug examples

- Busulfan (Myleran, Busulfex), carboplatin (Paraplatin), carmustine (BiCNU, Gliadel), chlorambucil (Leukeran), cisplatin (cis-platinum [Platinol]), cyclophosphamide (Cytoxan, Neosar), dacarbazine (DTIC [DTIC-Dome]), estramustine phosphate sodium (Emcyt), ifosfamide (Ifex), lomustine (CeeNu), mechlorethamine (nitrogen mustard [Mustargen]), melphalan (Alkeran), procarbazine (Matulane), streptozocin (Zanosar), thiotepa (Thioplex)

Indications

- Indications for each drug differ widely
- Alkylating drugs may be used for many types of cancers, including but not limited to, leukemia, brain tumors, multiple myeloma, Hodgkin's disease, non-Hodgkin's lymphoma, malignant melanoma, ovarian cancer, lung cancer, head and neck tumors, breast cancer, testicular tumors, prostatic cancer, osteosarcoma, and neuroblastoma

Contraindications and precautions

- These drugs are contraindicated in pregnant women and in patients with suppressed white or red blood cells and platelets or renal or liver failure
- Busulfan is contraindicated in patients with chronic myelogenous leukemia that has shown prior resistance to the drug
- Busulfan isn't useful in chronic lymphocytic or acute leukemia or in the blastic crisis of chronic myelogenous leukemia
- Mechlorethamine also is contraindicated in patients with an infectious disease

Adverse reactions

- Primary adverse reactions include nausea and vomiting (which may be severe or protracted), stomatitis, gonadal suppression, bone marrow depression, and pain during I.V. administration
- Busulfan also may cause hyperuricemia and pulmonary fibrosis
- Chlorambucil also may cause gonadal suppression and hyperuricemia
- Cisplatin also may cause ototoxicity, tinnitus, hypocalcemia, hypokalemia, hypomagnesemia, and nephrotoxicity
- Cyclophosphamide also may cause alopecia, gonadal suppression, hemorrhagic cystitis, and hematuria
- Mechlorethamine also may cause gonadal suppression and hyperuricemia
- Melphalan may cause hepatotoxicity, skin reactions, pulmonary fibrosis, bronchospasms, and pneumonitis

Interactions

- Use with other ototoxic and nephrotoxic drugs may cause additive ototoxicity and nephrotoxicity
- Phenobarbital may increase the effect of cyclophosphamide, thereby increasing the risk of toxicity
- Use with anticoagulants, aspirin, and nonsteroidal anti-inflammatories may increase the risk of bleeding

Nursing responsibilities

- Prepare I.V. antineoplastic solutions in a biologic cabinet to ensure safety: always wear gloves, a gown, and a mask when handling antineoplastic I.V. drugs
- Discard drug and any I.V. equipment used in specified containers according to institutional policies
- Reduce pain with I.V. administration, as ordered, by altering the infusion rate, further diluting the drug, or warming the injection site to distend the vein and increase blood flow
- **When administering cisplatin, frequently assess the patient for dizziness, tinnitus, hearing loss, incoordination, and numbness or tingling of extremities; these adverse effects may be irreversible**
- Know that these drugs are given in short, high-dose, intermittent courses to maximize antineoplastic effects while allowing normal cells to recover
- Know that extravasation may cause tissue necrosis; if this occurs, intervene as specified by appropriate institutional protocol
- Monitor the patient's complete blood count (CBC), white blood count (WBC) differential, and platelet count; institute isolation precautions if the patient's WBC count is low
- Assess the patient for nausea and vomiting; give an antiemetic, if needed
- With I.V. administration, monitor the patient for signs and symptoms of phlebitis because many antineoplastics irritate the veins
- Monitor the patient for signs of hemorrhagic cystitis (such as hematuria or dysuria) during cyclophosphamide or ifosfamide therapy

Adverse reactions to watch for

- Nausea and vomiting, stomatitis, gonadal suppression, bone marrow depression, pain during I.V. administration, hyperuricemia, pulmonary fibrosis, ototoxicity, tinnitus, hypocalcemia, hypokalemia, hypomagnesemia, nephrotoxicity, alopecia, hemorrhagic cystitis, hematuria, hepatotoxicity, skin reactions, bronchospasms, and pneumonitis

Key nursing actions

- Reduce pain with I.V. administration by altering the infusion rate, further diluting the drug, or warming the injection site to distend the vein and increase blood flow.
- When administering cisplatin, frequently assess for dizziness, tinnitus, hearing loss, incoordination, and numbness or tingling of extremities.
- Monitor for signs of hemorrhagic cystitis.
- Tell the patient to notify the physician immediately if fever, sore throat, unusual bleeding, or signs and symptoms of infection occur.

- Take bleeding precautions if thrombocytopenia occurs; avoid I.M. injections and venipunctures as much as possible
- Promote fluid intake of at least 2,000 ml daily to maintain adequate renal function
- Teach the patient to notify the physician immediately if fever, sore throat, unusual bleeding, or signs and symptoms of infection occur
- Instruct the patient to avoid crowds and persons with infections to minimize the risk of infection
- Advise the patient to consult the physician before receiving any vaccinations
- Instruct the patient to use a soft toothbrush and an electric razor to decrease the risk of bleeding
- Instruct the patient to avoid alcohol to decrease the risk of toxicity and to avoid aspirin-containing products to decrease the risk of bleeding
- Warn the patient that the drug may cause hair loss, but that hair usually returns
- Know that many antineoplastics have teratogenic effects; teach the patient about the need for contraception during therapy; also discuss the effects of antineoplastics on fertility
- Instruct the patient to inspect the inside of the mouth for redness or ulcers and to rinse his mouth after meals if stomatitis occurs

Key facts about antitumor antibiotics

- Interfere with DNA and ribonucleic acid synthesis
- Cell-cycle nonspecific
- Metabolized by liver
- Excreted in urine as unchanged metabolites

ANTITUMOR ANTIBIOTICS

Mechanism of action

- Interfere with DNA and ribonucleic acid synthesis
- These drugs are cell-cycle nonspecific

Pharmacokinetics

- Absorption: Administered I.V.
- Distribution: Widely distributed
- Metabolism: Metabolized by the liver
- Excretion: Excreted in the urine as unchanged metabolites

Drug examples

- Bleomycin sulfate (Blenoxane), dactinomycin (actinomycin-D [Cosmegen]), daunorubicin citrate [liposomal] (DaunoXome), daunorubicin hydrochloride, doxorubicin (Adriamycin), doxorubicin [liposomal] (Doxil), epirubicin hydrochloride (Ellence), idarubicin (Idamycin), mitomycin (Mutamycin), mitoxantrone (Novantrone), plicamycin (Mithracin), valrubicin (Valstar)

When to use antitumor antibiotics

- Squamous cell carcinoma of the head and neck
- Lymphomas
- Hodgkin's disease
- Embryonal cell carcinoma
- Bone carcinoma
- Kaposi's sarcoma
- Melanoma
- Malignant pleural effusions

Indications

- These drugs are indicated for squamous cell carcinoma of the head and neck, lymphomas, Hodgkin's disease, embryonal cell carcinoma, bone carcinoma, Kaposi's sarcoma, and melanoma
- Bleomycin may also be used for the treatment of malignant pleural effusions and for the prevention of recurrent pleural effusions

Contraindications and precautions

- These drugs are contraindicated during pregnancy
- Dactinomycin is contraindicated in patients with chickenpox or herpes zoster
- Doxorubicin is contraindicated in patients with marked myelosuppression induced by previous antitumor drugs or radiotherapy or who have had a lifetime cumulative dose of 550 mg/m^2 of doxorubicin or daunorubicin
- Use cautiously in patients with liver or renal disease

Adverse reactions

- These drugs may cause alopecia, stomatitis, nausea, vomiting, anorexia, gonadal suppression, hyperuricemia, and phlebitis at the I.V. site
- Daunorubicin, doxorubicin, epirubicin, and idarubicin also may cause heart failure, myocardial toxicity, cardiomyopathy, electrocardiographic changes, and arrhythmias
- Valrubicin also may cause urinary tract infections, bladder pain, incontinence, and cystitis

Interactions

- These drugs may decrease digoxin levels
- Cardiotoxicity may increase if these drugs are given with irradiation or cyclophosphamide
- The use of probenecid with these drugs may increase the risk of hyperuricemia
- Concurrent use with vinca alkaloids may cause serious bronchospasms

Nursing responsibilities

- **When administering daunorubicin or idarubicin, assess the patient for signs and symptoms of heart failure (dyspnea, crackles, peripheral edema, and weight gain)**
- **When administering doxorubicin, epirubicin, or idarubicin, assess the patient for signs and symptoms of myocardial toxicity (dyspnea, arrhythmias, hypotension, and weight gain)**
- Monitor vital signs frequently during administration

ANTIMETABOLITES

Mechanism of action

- Replace normal proteins required for DNA synthesis, thereby interfering with DNA and RNA synthesis
- These drugs are cell-cycle specific

Pharmacokinetics

- Absorption: Absorption varies widely with each drug
- Distribution: Distribution varies widely with each drug
- Metabolism: Metabolized by the liver
- Excretion: Excreted in the urine

When NOT to use antitumor antibiotics

- Pregnancy
- Chickenpox
- Herpes zoster
- Myelosuppression induced by previous antitumor drugs or radiotherapy or a lifetime cumulative dose of 550 mg/m^2 of doxorubicin or daunorubicin

Adverse reactions to watch for

- Alopecia, stomatitis, nausea, vomiting, anorexia, gonadal suppression, hyperuricemia, phlebitis at the I.V. site, heart failure, myocardial toxicity, cardiomyopathy, electrocardiographic changes, arrhythmias, urinary tract infections, bladder pain, incontinence, and cystitis

Key nursing actions

- When administering daunorubicin or idarubicin, assess for signs and symptoms of heart failure.
- When administering doxorubicin, epirubicin, or idarubicin, assess for signs and symptoms of myocardial toxicity.

Key facts about antimetabolites

- Replace normal proteins required for DNA synthesis; interfere with DNA and RNA synthesis
- Cell-cycle specific
- Metabolized by liver
- Excreted in urine

When to use antimetabolites

- Acute myelogenous leukemia
- Acute lymphocytic leukemia
- Acute nonlymphocytic leukemia
- Chronic myelogenous leukemia
- Non-Hodgkin's lymphoma
- GI carcinomas
- Breast and cervical carcinomas
- Painful crises

When NOT to use antimetabolites

- Pregnancy
- Bone marrow suppression
- Resistance to mercaptopurine or thioguanine

Adverse reactions to watch for

- Hepatotoxicity, GI disturbances, myelosuppression, fatigue, paresthesia, abdominal pain, constipation, intestinal obstruction, hyperbilirubinemia, hand-and-foot syndrome, dermatitis, fever, alopecia, stomatitis, hyperuricemia, thrombophlebitis, renal failure, urinary tract infections, myalgia, pneumonia, edema, diarrhea, phototoxicity reactions, bone marrow suppression, cerebellar dysfunction, pulmonary toxicity, seizures, and photosensitivity

Drug examples

- Capecitabine (Xeloda), cytarabine (ARA-C, cytosine arabinoside [Cytosar-U]), floxuridine (FUDR), fludarabine (Fludara), fluorouracil (5-FU [Adrucil]), hydroxyurea (Hydrea), mercaptopurine (6-MP [Purinethol]), methotrexate (Folex), pentostatin (Nipent), thioguanine (6-thioguanine, 6-TG)

Indications

- These drugs are indicated for acute myelogenous, acute lymphocytic, acute nonlymphocytic, and chronic myelogenous leukemia; non-Hodgkin's lymphoma; GI carcinomas; and breast and cervical carcinomas
- Hydroxyurea is also used to treat painful crises and reduce the need for blood transfusions in patients with sickle cell anemia

Contraindications and precautions

- Contraindicated in pregnant women and in patients with bone marrow suppression caused by previous chemotherapy or renal or liver toxicity
- Because cross-resistance to some drugs in this category occurs, a patient with known resistance to mercaptopurine or thioguanine shouldn't receive further therapy with antimetabolites

Adverse reactions

- These drugs may cause hepatotoxicity, GI disturbances, and myelosuppression
- Capecitabine also may cause fatigue, paresthesia, abdominal pain, constipation, intestinal obstruction, hyperbilirubinemia, hand-and-foot syndrome, dermatitis, and fever
- Cytarabine may cause alopecia, stomatitis, hyperuricemia, thrombophlebitis, and hepatotoxicity
- Fludarabine may cause thromboembolic events, GI bleeding, renal failure, urinary tract infections, hepatotoxicity, myalgia, pneumonia, edema, fatigue, and alopecia
- Fluorouracil may cause alopecia, stomatitis, diarrhea, phototoxicity reactions, bone marrow suppression, and cerebellar dysfunction
- Mercaptopurine may cause hyperuricemia and hepatotoxicity
- Methotrexate may cause alopecia, stomatitis, hyperuricemia, hepatotoxicity, pulmonary toxicity, seizures, and photosensitivity

Interactions

- Concurrent use of mercaptopurine or methotrexate with other hepatotoxic drugs causes additive hepatotoxicity
- Allopurinol decreases the metabolism of mercaptopurine, increasing the risk of toxicity
- Chloramphenicol, oral hypoglycemics, phenytoin, probenecid, salicylates, and tetracyclines increase the risk of methotrexate toxicity

Nursing responsibilities

- **When administering fluorouracil, assess the patient for signs and symptoms of cerebellar dysfunction (dizziness, weakness, and atax-**

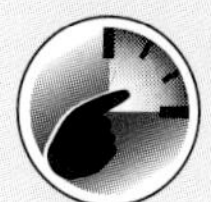

TIME-OUT FOR TEACHING

Teaching about antimetabolites

Include these topics in your teaching plan for the patient receiving an antimetabolite.

- Medication regimen, including the drug's name, dosage, frequency, duration, and possible adverse effects
- Signs and symptoms to discuss with the physician
- Infection-control measures
- Measures to combat common adverse reactions
- Fluid requirements
- Bleeding precautions
- Energy conservation measures
- Follow-up care, including laboratory tests and physician visits
- Community resources for support, guidance, and education

ia) and stomatitis and diarrhea (which may necessitate drug discontinuation); also monitor the patient for bone marrow suppression

- When administering methotrexate in large doses, make sure the patient receives leucovorin (folinic acid or citrovorum factor ["leucovorin rescue"]) to prevent fatal toxicity
- When administering fluorouracil or methotrexate, instruct the patient to use sunscreen and wear protective clothing to prevent photosensitivity reactions (for additional teaching tips, see *Teaching about antimetabolites*)

HORMONAL DRUGS AND DRUGS ALTERING HORMONE RESPONSE

Mechanism of action

- Suppress the immune system and block synthesis of RNA and new proteins
- Alter cell metabolism by changing the hormonal environment of normal hormones in hormone-sensitive tumors

Pharmacokinetics

- Absorption: Absorption is usually rapid
- Distribution: Distributed widely
- Metabolism: Metabolized in the liver
- Excretion: Excreted in the urine, feces, or bile; some may be reabsorbed by the intestines

Drug examples

- Aminoglutethimide (Cytadren), anastrozole (Arimidex), bicalutamide (Casodex), estramustine phosphate sodium (Emcyt), exemestane (Aromasin), flutamide (Eulexin), fulvestrant (Faslodex), goserelin acetate (Zoladex), letrozole (Femara), leuprolide (Lupron), megestrol acetate (Megace), mitotane (Lysodren), nilutamide (Nilandron), prednisone

Topics for patient discussion

- Therapy regimen
- Signs and symptoms
- Infection control measures
- Bleeding precautions

Key nursing actions

- When administering fluorouracil, assess for signs and symptoms of cerebellar dysfunction and stomatitis and diarrhea.
- Monitor the patient for bone marrow suppression.
- When administering methotrexate in large doses, make sure the patient receives leucovorin to prevent fatal toxicity.

Key facts about hormonal drugs and drugs altering hormone response

- Suppress the immune system
- Block synthesis of RNA and new proteins
- Alter cell metabolism
- Metabolized in liver
- Excreted in urine, feces, or bile; some may be reabsorbed by intestines

When to use hormonal drugs and drugs altering hormone response

- Advanced breast cancer (postmenopausal and high-risk)
- Advanced prostate cancer
- Endometriosis and endometrial cancer
- Central precocious puberty
- Anemia related to uterine fibroids
- Anorexia, cachexia, or unexplained weight loss

When NOT to use hormonal drugs and drugs altering hormone response

- Estrogen-dependent neoplasia or thrombophlebitis
- Prostate cancer
- Male breast cancer
- Premenopause
- Genital cancer
- Abnormal vaginal bleeding

Adverse reactions to watch for

- Headache, asthenia, nausea, pain, hot flashes, constipation, diarrhea, nocturia, hematuria, impotence, gynecomastia, dyspnea, asthenia, infection, edema, hypercalcemia, impotence and gynecomastia in males, depression, insomnia, anxiety, fatigue, breast tenderness, thromboembolic events, skin irritations, dizziness, vomiting, cough, heart failure, arrhythmias, cataracts, dry eyes, hepatotoxicity, sweating, and vaginal bleeding or discharge

(Deltasone), tamoxifen citrate (Nolvadex), testolactone (Teslac), testosterone (Delatestryl), toremifene (Fareston), triptorelin pamoate (Trelstar Depot, Trelstar LA)

Indications

- These drugs are used to treat advanced breast cancer in postmenopausal women and advanced prostate cancer
- These drugs are used as palliative treatment in advanced cancers
- Leuprolide acetate is also used to treat endometriosis, central precocious puberty, and anemia related to uterine fibroids
- Megestrol acetate is also used to treat endometrial cancer and anorexia, cachexia, or unexplained weight loss in patients with AIDS
- Tamoxifen is also used as the primary breast cancer prevention in high-risk patients

Contraindications and precautions

- Estrogens are contraindicated in patients with estrogen-dependent neoplasia or thrombophlebitis
- Androgens are contraindicated in patients with prostate cancer or male breast cancer and in premenopausal women
- Progesterones are contraindicated in patients with genital cancer or abnormal vaginal bleeding

Adverse reactions

- Anastrozole may cause headache, asthenia, nausea, pain, and hot flashes
- Bicalutamide, flutamide, and nilutamide may cause constipation, nausea, diarrhea, nocturia, hematuria, impotence, gynecomastia, peripheral edema, dyspnea, back pain, generalized pain, asthenia, pelvic pain, infection, and hot flashes
- Tamoxifen and testosterone may cause edema and hypercalcemia
- Testosterone may cause impotence and gynecomastia in males
- Exemestane may cause depression, insomnia, anxiety, fatigue, pain, nausea, dyspnea, and hot flashes
- Estramustine may cause breast tenderness, painful gynecomastia, edema, thromboembolic events, and skin irritations
- Fulvestrant may cause headache, dizziness, nausea, vomiting, bone pain, asthenia, injection site pain, and cough
- Tamoxifen and letrozole may increase the risk of thromboembolic events
- Toremifene citrate may cause heart failure, arrhythmias, cataracts, dry eyes, thromboembolic events, hepatotoxicity, hypercalcemia, hot flashes, sweating, nausea, and vaginal bleeding or discharge

Interactions

- Testosterone may alter the effects of insulin, oral anticoagulants, and oral hypoglycemics
- Calcium-containing drugs may impair estramustine absorption
- Tamoxifen decreases the effectiveness of estrogens
- Toremifene, testolactone, tamoxifen, and flutamide may increase warfarin's activity and increase the risk of bleeding

Nursing responsibilities

- When administering tamoxifen, warn the patient that it may cause severe bone pain, which is a sign that the drug is effective
- Reassure the patient that such pain will resolve over time and may be controlled with analgesics

VINCA ALKALOIDS AND NATURAL PRODUCTS

Mechanism of action

- Inhibit DNA or RNA synthesis and prevent mitosis, causing cell death
- They are cell-cycle specific

Pharmacokinetics

- Absorption: Most are administered I.V.
- Distribution: Widely distributed
- Metabolism: Metabolized in the liver
- Excretion: Excreted in the urine

Drug examples

- Asparaginase (Elspar), docetaxel (Taxotere), etoposide (VePesid), paclitaxel (Taxol), pegaspargase (Oncaspar), teniposide (Vumon), vinblastine (Velban), vincristine (Oncovin), vindesine (Eldisine), vinorelbine (Navelbine)

Indications

- Testicular cancer, non-Hodgkin's lymphoma, breast cancer, lung cancer, head and neck cancer, and neuroblastomas

Contraindications and precautions

- These drugs are contraindicated in pregnant women and in patients with myelosuppression from previous chemotherapy or radiation
- Also contraindicated in patients with a baseline neutrophil count below 1,500/mm^3, AIDS, or severe bacterial infections
- Pegaspargase is contraindicated in patients with pancreatitis and in those who have suffered a hemorrhagic event with previous L-asparaginase therapy
- Use cautiously in patients with liver impairment

Adverse reactions

- May cause peripheral neuropathy, alopecia, stomatitis, anorexia, constipation, hyperuricemia, phlebitis at the I.V. infusion site, bradycardia, acute bronchospasms, and myelosuppression

Interactions

- Concurrent use of prednisone may enhance hyperglycemia, neurotoxicity, and myelosuppression
- May decrease phenytoin levels when used with phenytoin

Key nursing actions

- When administering tamoxifen, warn that it may cause severe bone pain.
- Reassure patient that such pain will resolve over time and may be controlled with analgesics.

Key facts about vinca alkaloids and natural products

- Inhibit DNA or RNA synthesis
- Prevent mitosis
- Cell-cycle specific
- Metabolized in liver
- Excreted in urine

When to use vinca alkaloids and natural products

- Testicular cancer
- Non-Hodgkin's lymphoma
- Breast cancer
- Lung cancer
- Head and neck cancer
- Neuroblastomas

When NOT to use vinca alkaloids and natural products

- Pregnancy
- Myelosuppression from previous chemotherapy or radiation
- Baseline neutrophil count below 1,500/mm^3
- AIDS or severe bacterial infection
- Pancreatitis
- History of hemorrhagic event

Adverse reactions to watch for

- Peripheral neuropathy, alopecia, stomatitis, anorexia, constipation, hyperuricemia, phlebitis at the I.V. infusion site, bradycardia, acute bronchospasms, and myelosuppression

Key nursing actions

- Premedicate patients receiving paclitaxel with diphenhydramine, dexamethasone, and an H_2 antagonist.
- Always wear gloves when preparing drug.

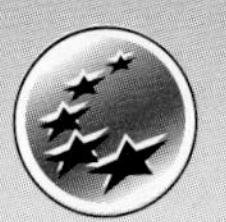

TOP 5

Items to study before your next test on drugs and cancer

1. The rationale for using antineoplastics to treat cancer
2. Major adverse effects of antineoplastics
3. Nursing responsibilities when administering antineoplastics
4. Precautions the nurse must take for self-protection when administering antineoplastics
5. Appropriate teaching for the patient who is receiving an antineoplastic

- **Nursing responsibilities**
  - Premedicate patients receiving paclitaxel with diphenhydramine, dexamethasone, and an H_2 antagonist to prevent hypersensitivity reactions
  - Always wear gloves when preparing drug

NCLEX CHECKS

It's never too soon to begin your NCLEX preparation. Now that you've reviewed this chapter, carefully read each of the following questions and choose the best answer. Then compare your responses to the correct answers.

1. A patient newly diagnosed with lung cancer is beginning chemotherapy. Which of the following instructions is appropriate to give this patient?

☐ A. Increase daily fluid intake to 2 to 3 L.
☐ B. Stay in direct sunlight as much as possible.
☐ C. Avoiding brushing your teeth to prevent gum bleeding.
☐ D. Avoid eating for 6 hours after chemotherapy to prevent nausea.

2. A patient taking antineoplastics develops leukopenia. Which nursing intervention has the highest priority?

☐ A. Assign the patient to a private room.
☐ B. Use an electric shaver to help prevent cuts.
☐ C. Wear a gown and gloves when giving a bed bath.
☐ D. Dispose of the patient's urine in a biohazard container.

3. A patient asks about a drug to prevent breast cancer. Which agent is indicated for the primary prevention of breast cancer in women at high risk for developing breast cancer?

☐ A. Cyclophosphamide (Cytoxan)
☐ B. Ethinyl estradiol (Desogen)
☐ C. Methotrexate (Folex)
☐ D. Tamoxifen (Nolvadex)

4. A 47-year-old patient receives the alkyl sulfonate busulfan (Myleran) for chronic myelogenous leukemia. You assess the patient regularly for adverse drug reactions. You should watch for which adverse respiratory reaction caused by long-term therapy?

☐ A. Asthma attacks
☐ B. Pulmonary fibrosis
☐ C. Pulmonary hypertension
☐ D. Chronic obstructive pulmonary disease (COPD)

5. A patient is taking fluorouracil (Adrucil) for breast cancer. Stomatitis is a common adverse reaction to fluorouracil. You should also assess for which of the following adverse reactions?

☐ A. Heart failure
☐ B. Pulmonary infiltrates
☐ C. Severe renal dysfunction
☐ D. Bone marrow suppression

6. A patient who is receiving chemotherapy for breast cancer develops myelosuppression. Which of the following instructions should the nurse include in the patient's discharge teaching plan?

Select all that apply:

☐ A. Avoid people who have recently received attenuated vaccines.
☐ B. Avoid activities that may cause bleeding.
☐ C. Wash hands frequently.
☐ D. Increase intake of fresh fruits and vegetables.
☐ E. Avoid crowded places such as shopping malls.
☐ F. Treat a sore throat with over-the-counter products.

ANSWERS AND RATIONALES

1. Correct answer: A

Because many antineoplastics are nephrotoxic, increased fluid intake is recommended to decrease the risk of renal toxicity and prevent renal failure. Most chemotherapeutic agents cause photosensitivity, so avoiding exposure to sunlight is recommended. Good oral care and using a soft toothbrush are important. Avoiding food intake for 6 hours after treatment may increase nausea.

2. Correct answer: A

Leukopenia (a low white blood cell count) is a common adverse reaction to many antineoplastics. Patients with leukopenia are more susceptible to infections, so a private room is necessary to reduce the risk of a nosocomial infection. Antineoplastics don't suppress the platelet count, so bleeding precautions aren't warranted. Wearing a gown and gloves isn't necessary; however, practicing good hand-washing technique, using gloves when the risk of contact with any bodily fluids is probable, or wearing a face mask if you have a cough or obvious respiratory tract infection would be adequate. The patient's urine should be handled in the same manner as other body secretions.

3. Correct answer: D

Tamoxifen is indicated for primary breast cancer prevention in high risk patients. How it works isn't fully clear, but it's an estrogen antagonist and may prevent tumor growth resulting from endogenous estrogen. Many breast cancers are estrogen-receptor positive; therefore, giving ethinyl estradiol would stimulate tumor growth. Cyclophosphamide and methotrexate are indicated for chemotherapy, not prevention.

4. Correct answer: B

Pulmonary fibrosis is an adverse reaction to long-term busulfan therapy; pulmonary tissue becomes fibrotic and interferes with normal oxygenation. Busulfan isn't known to cause COPD, pulmonary hypertension, or asthma attacks.

5. CORRECT ANSWER: D

Bone marrow suppression, as evidenced by neutropenia and thrombocytopenia, is an adverse reaction to fluorouracil. Fluorouracil isn't known to cause pulmonary infiltrates, severe renal dysfunction, or heart failure.

6. CORRECT ANSWER: A, B, C, E

Chemotherapy can cause myelosuppression, which is reduced numbers of red blood cells, white blood cells, and platelets. A patient receiving chemotherapy needs to avoid people who have been vaccinated recently because an exaggerated reaction may occur. Because platelet counts are reduced, the patient also needs to avoid activities that could cause trauma and bleeding. The patient should wash her hands frequently because hand washing is the best way to prevent the spread of infection. A patient receiving chemotherapy should avoid crowded places, as well as people with colds during the flu season, because she has a reduced ability to fight infection. Fresh fruits and vegetables should be avoided because they can harbor bacteria that can't be removed easily by washing. Signs and symptoms of infection, such as a sore throat, fever, and a cough, should be reported immediately to the physician.

14 Drugs and the gastrointestinal system

LEARNING OBJECTIVES

After studying this chapter, you should be able to:

- Describe the mechanisms of action of the various types of antiulceratives, antiemetics, emetics, antidiarrheals, and laxatives.
- List the major adverse effects of antiulceratives, antiemetics, emetics, antidiarrheals, and laxatives.
- Identify nursing responsibilities when administering antiulceratives, antiemetics, emetics, antidiarrheals, and laxatives.
- Discuss appropriate teaching for the patient who is receiving antiulceratives, antiemetics, emetics, antidiarrheals, and laxatives.

CHAPTER OVERVIEW

Antiulceratives neutralize or block the release of hydrochloric acid and provide a barrier to the gastric mucosa. Amphojel, used to neutralize hydrochloric acid, may also be used in renal failure to bind phosphate. Nursing responsibilities associated with antiulceratives include monitoring the patient for frank and occult bleeding, constipation, diarrhea, and abdominal or epigastric pain.

Antiemetics are used to prevent or control nausea and vomiting secondary to pathologic conditions, drugs, toxins, radiation, or motion sickness. These drugs may be administered orally, intramuscularly, rectally, or transdermally. Nursing responsibilities include monitoring the patient for fluid and electrolyte imbalances and providing patient safety because many drugs cause dizziness and excessive sedation.

Emetics are used to produce emesis after drug overdose or ingestion of noncaustic poison. These drugs must never be administered to patients with altered levels of consciousness or to those who ingested corrosive substances or petroleum products. Nursing responsibilities include assessing the patient's level of consciousness before administration, giving the drug with water, and observing for toxicity if vomiting doesn't occur. The nurse should also provide mouth care and hygiene after vomiting episodes.

Antidiarrheals are used to control or treat acute or nonspecific diarrhea. Nursing responsibilities include monitoring the patient for abdominal pain and fluid and electrolyte imbalances and assessing stool for frequency, quantity, quality, and occult blood. Patient teaching focuses on dietary modification, including increased fiber intake.

Laxatives are used to treat constipation or to cleanse the bowel before surgery or diagnostic studies. Bulk-forming laxatives may help incorporate water into stool and are occasionally used to treat diarrhea. Lactulose may also be used to decrease ammonia levels in hepatic encephalopathy. Nursing responsibilities include assessing the frequency and consistency of stool and monitoring the patient for fluid and electrolyte imbalances and abdominal pain.

A&P highlights

- The GI system consists of the oral cavity, pharynx, esophagus, stomach, and small and large intestines.
- Accessory organs include gastrin glands, the liver, the gallbladder, and the pancreas.
- Digestion begins in the oral cavity.
- Food and liquid are propelled through the GI tract via peristalsis and segmenting contractions.
- A normally functioning esophageal sphincter keeps swallowed foods and gastric juices in the stomach.
- GI hormones regulate gastric secretions and motility.
- Gastric acid secretion is prompted by the sight, smell, or anticipation of food.
- Once food is in the stomach, gastrin stimulates secretion of gastric acids from the parietal cells.
- Gastric acid also activates pepsinogen to form pepsin, which digests proteins.
- The major nutrients in the body are carbohydrates, proteins, and lipids; they are digested in the GI tract by enzymes and are then absorbed by the small intestines.
- Digested carbohydrates are converted to glucose, which supplies energy.
- Proteins are absorbed as amino acids, which are converted to protein or glucose or catabolized for energy.
- Lipids are stored in adipose tissue for later use as energy.

ANATOMY AND PHYSIOLOGY

Anatomy

- The GI system, a continuous tube that's open at both ends, consists of the oral cavity, pharynx, esophagus, stomach, and small and large intestines; it's surrounded by the peritoneum
  - The small intestines consist of the duodenum, jejunum, and the ileum
  - The large intestines consist of the cecum, vermiform appendix, ascending colon, transverse colon, descending colon, sigmoid colon, rectum, and anus
- Accessory organs to the GI system include gastrin glands, the liver, the gallbladder, and the pancreas

Physiology

- Digestion begins in the oral cavity
- Food and liquid are propelled through the esophagus, into the stomach, and through the small and large intestines via peristalsis — the rhythmic contraction of smooth muscle — and segmenting contractions (alternating contractions and relaxations of adjacent segments of the intestines)
  - A normally functioning esophageal sphincter keeps swallowed foods and gastric juices in the stomach
  - Failure of the esophageal sphincter to close or remain closed causes gastroesophageal reflux disease (GERD)
  - Abnormal peristalsis of the small intestines can lead to constipation, diarrhea, or both, as in irritable bowel syndrome (IBS)
  - Normal peristalsis propels fecal material into the rectum and causes the defecation reflex

- GI hormones, such as gastrin, gastric inhibitory peptides, secretin, and cholecystokinin (CCK), regulate gastric secretions and motility
  - Gastric acid secretion is prompted by the sight, smell, or anticipation of food
  - Once food is in the stomach, gastrin, the GI hormone that's released in response to food in the stomach and the duodenum, stimulates secretion of gastric acids from the parietal cells
  - Gastric acid also activates the gastric enzyme precursor pepsinogen to form pepsin, which digests proteins by breaking peptide bonds
- The major nutrients in the body are carbohydrates, proteins, and lipids; they are digested in the GI tract by enzymes that hydrolyze them into smaller units that are absorbed from the small intestines
- All digested carbohydrates are converted to glucose
- To supply energy, glucose is catabolized in three phases: glycolysis, the citric acid cycle, and the electron transport system
- All ingested proteins are absorbed as amino acids
- Amino acids must be converted to protein or glucose or catabolized for energy, which occurs by deamination and transamination
- Lipids are stored in adipose (fat) tissue; when the body needs energy, lipid molecules are hydrolyzed

Function

- The GI system obtains and processes almost all of the nutrients the body intakes and needs; it supplies the body with all of the energy and building materials required by the body for daily activities, growth, and repair
  - The stomach serves as a temporary storage area for food, which remains there until it's partially digested
  - The small intestines' main function is to complete digestion of the food; most of the nutrients, water, and electrolytes in foods are digested and absorbed in the small intestines
  - The large intestines' main function is to absorb water and minerals and eliminate digestive waste products; intestinal bacteria in the large intestines also release intestinal gases and synthesize vitamin K and some B vitamins, which are absorbed in the colon
  - The peritoneum lines the walls of the abdominal cavity; the folds of the peritoneum (mesenteries) hold the intestines and other GI organs in place
- The accessory organs produce or store secretions used in digestion
  - The liver has digestive, metabolic, and regulatory functions
    - Its chief digestive function is to produce bile, which acts as a fat emulsifier in the small intestines
    - The liver produces blood proteins, such as albumin and globulin, lipoproteins, and proteins involved with blood coagulation
    - It stores a small reserve of fat, glycogen, iron, and vitamins A, B_{12}, D, E, and K
    - It detoxifies or excretes many wastes and toxins; it also excretes cholesterol

Functions of GI structures

- The stomach is a temporary storage and digestion area for food.
- The small intestines complete the digestion of food; they are also the site of nutrient, water, and electrolyte absorption.
- The large intestines absorb water and minerals and eliminate digestive waste products; intestinal bacteria in the large intestines release intestinal gases and synthesize vitamin K and some B vitamins.
- The peritoneum lines the walls of the abdominal cavity; the folds of the peritoneum hold the intestines and other GI organs in place.

Functions of accessory GI organs

- The liver produces bile, blood proteins, lipoproteins, and proteins involved with blood coagulation. It also stores fat, glycogen, iron, and vitamins A, B_{12}, D, E, and K; detoxifies and excretes wastes and toxins; and excretes cholesterol.
- The gallbladder stores and concentrates bile.
- The exocrine pancreas secretes digestive enzymes.
- The endocrine pancreas secretes hormones.

- The gallbladder stores and concentrates the bile secreted by the liver
- The exocrine pancreas contains cells that secrete digestive enzymes into the duodenum via the pancreatic duct; pancreatic fluid contains amylase to digest starch; trypsin, chymotrypsin, and carboxypeptidase to digest proteins; lipase to digest certain lipids; cholesterol esterase to digest cholesterol esters; and ribonuclease and deoxyribonuclease to digest nucleic acids
- The endocrine pancreas secretes hormones (glucagon, insulin, and somatostatin) directly into the bloodstream

- Glucagon, epinephrine, growth hormone, cortisol, and thyroxine increase the blood glucose level; insulin is the only hormone that lowers it

ANTIULCERATIVES

ANTACIDS

Key facts about antacids

- They neutralize gastric acid, thereby increasing the pH of the stomach and duodenal bulb.
- Metabolism action unknown
- Excreted in feces and breast milk

When to use antacids

- Indigestion
- Reflux esophagitis
- Peptic ulcers
- Renal failure

When NOT to use antacids

- Abdominal pain of unknown origin

Adverse reactions to watch for

- Constipation, hypophosphatemia, diarrhea, hypermagnesemia

Mechanism of action

- Drugs used to treat gastric hyperacidity and ulcers achieve their effects by neutralizing gastric acid, inhibiting gastric acid secretions, or providing direct mucosal protection
- Antacids neutralize gastric acid, thereby increasing the pH of the stomach and duodenal bulb

Pharmacokinetics

- Absorption: Minimally absorbed
- Distribution: Distributed throughout the GI tract
- Metabolism: Unknown
- Excretion: Excreted in the feces; some may be excreted in breast milk

Drug examples

- Aluminum hydroxide (ALternaGEL, Amphojel), magaldrate (aluminum-magnesium complex [Riopan]), magnesium hydroxide (Milk of Magnesia); aluminum hydroxide and magnesium hydroxide combinations (Gelusil, Maalox, Mylanta)

Indications

- All antacids are used for indigestion, reflux esophagitis, and peptic ulcers
- Amphojel may be used to bind dietary phosphate in renal failure

Contraindications and precautions

- Antacids are contraindicated in abdominal pain of unknown origin
- Antacids containing magnesium must be used with caution in renal failure

Adverse reactions

- Constipation, hypophosphatemia (with aluminum hydroxide); diarrhea, hypermagnesemia (with magnesium hydroxide)

Interactions

- Antacids decrease absorption of sucralfate, anticholinergics, histamine$_2$-receptor antagonists, fluoroquinolones, iron, isoniazid, phenothiazines, and tetracyclines

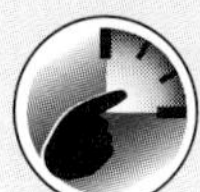

TIME-OUT FOR TEACHING

Teaching about antacids

Include these topics in your teaching plan for the patient receiving an antacid.
- Medication regimen, including the drug's name, dose, frequency, duration, and possible adverse effects
- Signs and symptoms to discuss with the physician
- How and when to take the medication
- Possible dietary interactions
- Measures to promote bowel elimination
- Avoidance of over-the-counter self-medication
- Follow-up care

- Antacids cause premature dissolution of enteric-coated tablets

Nursing responsibilities

- Know that antacids containing both aluminum and magnesium hydroxide balance the constipating effects of aluminum with the laxative effects of magnesium
- Instruct the patient to shake the suspension well, or, if taking chewable tablets, to chew them thoroughly and then drink half a glass of water to promote passage to the stomach
- Give antacids at least 1 hour apart from enteric-coated tablets
- Teach the patient who has heart failure or hypertension or who must restrict sodium intake to check antacid labels for sodium content and to use only low-sodium preparations
- Instruct the patient not to take antacids for more than 2 weeks or for recurring problems without consulting a physician (for additional teaching tips, see *Teaching about antacids*)
- Assess the patient for epigastric or abdominal pain, frank bleeding, and occult bleeding
- Teach the patient to avoid gastric irritants, such as alcohol, smoking, aspirin-containing products, caffeine, nonsteroidal anti-inflammatory drugs (NSAIDs), and foods that cause GI irritation, because these may counteract the effects of the drug and worsen the ulcer

HISTAMINE$_2$-RECEPTOR ANTAGONISTS

Mechanism of action

- Inhibit gastric acid secretion by inhibiting the action of histamine at histamine$_2$-receptors in gastric parietal cells

Pharmacokinetics

- Absorption: Cimetidine, nizatidine, and ranitidine are absorbed rapidly and completely; famotidine is 60% to 75% absorbed after oral administration; food and antacids may impair drug absorption

Topics for patient discussion

- Medication regimen
- Signs and symptoms to discuss with the physician
- Possible dietary interactions
- Measures to promote bowel elimination
- Avoidance of over-the-counter self-medication
- Avoidance of gastric irritants, such as alcohol, smoking, aspirin-containing products, caffeine, nonsteroidal anti-inflammatory drugs, and foods that cause GI irritation
- Follow-up care

Key nursing actions

- Instruct the patient to shake the suspension well, or, if taking chewable tablets, to chew them thoroughly and then drink half a glass of water to promote passage to the stomach.
- Give antacids at least 1 hour apart from enteric-coated tablets.
- Assess the patient for epigastric or abdominal pain, frank bleeding, and occult bleeding.

Key facts about histamine$_2$-receptor antagonists

- Inhibit gastric acid secretion by inhibiting the action of histamine at histamine$_2$-receptors in gastric parietal cells
- Metabolized by the liver
- Primarily excreted in the liver

- Distribution: Cimetidine crosses the placental barrier and appears in breast milk; these drugs are distributed widely throughout the body
- Metabolism: Metabolized by the liver
- Excretion: Primarily excreted in the liver

Drug examples

- Cimetidine (Tagamet, Tagamet HB), famotidine (Pepcid, Pepcid AC), nizatidine (Axid), ranitidine (Zantac)

Indications

- These drugs are used for active duodenal ulcers and gastric hypersecretory states (Zollinger-Ellison syndrome) and as prophylaxis for stress ulcer (unlabeled use)
- Over-the-counter preparations are used for heartburn, acid indigestion, and sour stomach

Contraindications and precautions

- These drugs are contraindicated in breast-feeding women and in those with known hypersensitivity
- Use these drugs with caution in pregnant women and in those with impaired renal or hepatic function
- These drugs may cause dizziness and confusion; use them cautiously in elderly patients because of an increased risk of CNS effects

Adverse reactions

- Headache, dizziness, confusion

Interactions

- Cimetidine inhibits hepatic drug-metabolizing enzymes and may cause increased serum levels and consequent toxicity of chlordiazepoxide, diazepam, lidocaine, metoprolol, oral anticoagulants, phenytoin, propranolol, quinidine, and theophylline
- Antacids may inhibit absorption of histamine$_2$-receptor antagonists
- Cigarette smoking increases gastric acid secretion and may decrease the effectiveness of histamine$_2$-receptor antagonists

Nursing responsibilities

- Teach the patient that smoking worsens ulcer disorders and counteracts the effects of histamine$_2$-receptor antagonists
- Don't give an antacid within 1 hour of administering histamine$_2$-receptor antagonists; this may decrease the latter's absorption
- Caution the patient about possible dizziness, and recommend avoidance of hazardous activities that require alertness
- Assess the patient for epigastric or abdominal pain, frank bleeding, and occult bleeding
- Teach the patient to avoid gastric irritants, such as smoking, alcohol, aspirin-containing products, caffeine, NSAIDs, and foods that cause GI irritation, because these may counteract the effect of the drug and worsen the ulcer

When to use histamine$_2$-receptor antagonists

- Active duodenal ulcers
- Gastric hypersecretory states
- Prophylaxis for stress ulcer
- Heartburn
- Acid indigestion
- Sour stomach

When NOT to use histamine$_2$-receptor antagonists

- Pregnancy
- Breast-feeding
- Hypersensitivity to histamine$_2$-receptor antagonists

Adverse reactions to watch for

- Headache, dizziness, confusion

Key nursing actions

- Don't give an antacid within 1 hour of administering histamine$_2$-receptor antagonists.
- Assess the patient for epigastric or abdominal pain, frank bleeding, and occult bleeding.
- Teach the patient to avoid gastric irritants, such as smoking, alcohol, aspirin-containing products, caffeine, NSAIDs, and foods that cause GI irritation.

PROTON PUMP INHIBITORS

Mechanism of action

- Block gastric acid secretions by inhibiting the acid pump in the gastric parietal cells

Pharmacokinetics

- Varies with each drug
- Absorption: Omeprazole and lansoprazole are rapidly absorbed in the small intestines
- Distribution: Highly protein-bound
- Metabolism: Extensively metabolized in the liver
- Excretion: Eliminated by the kidneys

Drug examples

- Esomeprazole (Nexium), lansoprazole (Prevacid), omeprazole (Prilosec, Prilosec OTC), pantoprazole (Protonix), rabeprazole (Aciphex)

Indications

- Proton pump inhibitors are used to treat erosive esophagitis and GERD
- Lansoprazole, omeprazole, and rabeprazole are used to treat duodenal ulcer
- Lansoprazole and omeprazole are used to treat gastric ulcer
- All drugs except esomeprazole are used to treat hypersecretory conditions
- All drugs except pantoprazole are used to eradicate *H. pylori*
- Lansoprazole is used to prevent and treat NSAID-related gastric ulcers

Contraindications and precautions

- These drugs are contraindicated in patients with known hypersensitivity
- Use these drugs cautiously in pregnant and breast-feeding women

Adverse reactions

- Omeprazole may cause headache, diarrhea, abdominal pain, nausea and vomiting, dizziness, rash, and constipation
- Lansoprazole may cause abdominal pain, diarrhea, and nausea
- Esomeprazole may cause headache, dry mouth, diarrhea, abdominal pain, nausea, vomiting, flatulence, and constipation
- Pantoprazole may cause headache, insomnia, chest pain, nausea, vomiting, constipation, abdominal pain, rhinitis, dizziness, and anxiety
- Rabeprazole may cause headache

Interactions

- May interfere with the metabolism of diazepam, phenytoin, and warfarin, increasing their half-lives and plasma levels
- May interfere with the absorption of drugs (such as ketoconazole, ampicillin, and iron) that depend on gastric pH for absorption

Nursing responsibilities

- Monitor the patient for diarrhea and abdominal pain
- Teach the patient to swallow capsules whole and not to chew or crush them

Key facts about proton pump inhibitors

- Block gastric acid secretions by inhibiting the acid pump in the gastric parietal cells
- Extensively metabolized in the liver
- Eliminated by the kidneys

When to use proton pump inhibitors

- Erosive esophagitis
- GERD
- Duodenal ulcer
- Gastric ulcer
- Hypersecretory conditions
- *H. pylori*
- NSAID-related gastric ulcers

When NOT to use proton pump inhibitors

- Hypersensitivity to proton pump inhibitors
- Pregnancy
- Breast-feeding

Adverse reactions to watch for

- Headache, diarrhea, abdominal pain, nausea, vomiting, dizziness, rash, constipation, dry mouth, flatulence, insomnia, chest pain, rhinitis, anxiety

Key nursing actions

- Monitor the patient for diarrhea and abdominal pain.
- Teach the patient to swallow capsules whole.
- Teach the patient to avoid gastric irritants, such as smoking, alcohol, aspirin-containing products, caffeine, NSAIDs, and foods that cause GI irritation.

- Teach the patient to avoid gastric irritants, such as smoking, alcohol, aspirin-containing products, caffeine, NSAIDs, and foods that cause GI irritation, because these may counteract the effect of the drug and worsen the ulcer

LOCAL-ACTING DRUGS

Key facts about local-acting drugs

- Protect the gastric mucosa by coating the ulcer crater
- Metabolism is unknown
- Excreted in feces

When to use local-acting drugs

- Gastric, duodenal, and stress ulcers

When NOT to use local-acting drugs

- Hypersensitivity
- Pregnancy
- Breast-feeding
- Chronic renal failure

Adverse reactions to watch for

- Constipation

Key nursing actions

- Assess the patient for epigastric or abdominal pain, frank bleeding, occult bleeding, and constipation.
- Teach the patient to avoid gastric irritants, such as smoking, alcohol, aspirin-containing products, caffeine, NSAIDs, and foods that cause GI irritation.

Mechanism of action

- Protect the gastric mucosa by coating the ulcer crater

Pharmacokinetics

- Absorption: Only 3% to 5% of the drug is absorbed after oral administration
- Distribution: Acts locally at the ulcer site
- Metabolism: Unknown
- Excretion: Excreted in the feces

Drug examples

- Sucralfate (Carafate)

Indications

- Sucralfate is used for short-term treatment and prevention of gastric, duodenal, and stress ulcers

Contraindications and precautions

- Sucralfate is contraindicated in patients with known hypersensitivity
- Use sucralfate with caution in pregnant or breast-feeding women and in those with chronic renal failure

Adverse reactions

- Constipation

Interactions

- Sucralfate binds with other drugs in the GI tract and may decrease absorption of cimetidine, phenytoin, tetracyclines, and warfarin
- Antacids increase gastric pH and may decrease the effectiveness of sucralfate
- Sucralfate decreases absorption of lansoprazole; separate doses of these drugs by giving lansoprazole 30 minutes before sucralfate

Nursing responsibilities

- Give sucralfate at least 2 hours apart from cimetidine, phenytoin, tetracyclines, or warfarin
- Don't administer an antacid with sucralfate; separate administration times by at least 30 minutes
- For maximum effectiveness, administer sucralfate at least 1 hour before meals and at bedtime
- Assess the patient for epigastric or abdominal pain, frank bleeding, occult bleeding, and constipation
- Teach the patient to avoid gastric irritants, such as smoking, alcohol, aspirin-containing products, caffeine, NSAIDs, and foods that cause GI irri-

tation, because these may counteract the effects of the drug and worsen the ulcer
- Know that sucralfate is poorly water-soluble; if it is to be administered through a nasogastric tube, it requires special preparation by a pharmacist

CHOLINERGIC BLOCKERS

Mechanism of action
- Anticholinergics inhibit GI motility and gastric secretions

Pharmacokinetics
- Absorption: Poorly absorbed from the GI tract (about 10% to 25%)
- Distribution: Rapidly distributed; doesn't cross the blood brain barrier
- Metabolism: Unknown
- Excretion: Unknown

Drug examples
- Glycopyrrolate (Robinul), mepenzolate bromide (Cantil), methscopolamine bromide (Pamine), propantheline (Pro-Banthine)

Indications
- Adjunctive therapy for peptic ulcer disease

Contraindications and precautions
- Contraindicated in angle-closure glaucoma, uncontrolled tachycardia, urinary or GI tract obstruction, hypersensitivity, severe ulcerative colitis, myasthenia gravis, tachycardia caused by cardiac insufficiency or thyrotoxicosis, acute or severe hemorrhage, or unstable cardiovascular status
- Also contraindicated in children and breast-feeding women

Adverse reactions
- Tachycardia, dry mouth, constipation, urine retention, urinary hesitancy

Interactions
- Use with similar-acting drugs causes additive anticholinergic effects
- Antacids may decrease the absorption of anticholinergic antiulceratives

Nursing responsibilities
- Assess the patient for epigastric or abdominal pain, frank bleeding, and occult bleeding
- Teach the patient to avoid gastric irritants, such as smoking, alcohol, aspirin-containing products, caffeine, NSAIDs, and foods that cause GI irritation, because these may counteract the effects of the drug and worsen the ulcer

MISCELLANEOUS ANTIULCERATIVES

Mechanism of action
- Bismuth subsalicylate reduces GI motility and gastric secretions
- Misoprostol replaces gastric prostaglandins and enhances natural local protective mechanisms

Key facts about cholinergic blockers
- Inhibit GI motility and gastric secretions
- Metabolism and excretion are unknown

When to use cholinergic blockers
- Peptic ulcer disease

When NOT to use cholinergic blockers
- Angle-closure glaucoma
- Uncontrolled tachycardia
- Urinary or GI tract obstruction
- Hypersensitivity
- Severe ulcerative colitis
- Myasthenia gravis
- Tachycardia caused by cardiac insufficiency or thyrotoxicosis
- Acute or severe hemorrhage
- Unstable cardiovascular status
- Children
- Breast-feeding

Adverse reactions to watch for
- Tachycardia, dry mouth, constipation, urine retention, urinary hesitancy

Key nursing actions
- Assess the patient for epigastric or abdominal pain, frank bleeding, occult bleeding, and constipation.
- Teach the patient to avoid gastric irritants, such as smoking, alcohol, aspirin-containing products, caffeine, NSAIDs, and foods that cause GI irritation.

Key facts about antiulceratives

- Reduce GI motility and gastric secretions, replace gastric prostaglandins, and enhance natural local protective mechanisms
- Metabolism and excretion unknown

When to use antiulceratives

- *Helicobacter-pylori* ulcers
- Gastric ulcer prevention related to NSAID use
- Duodenal ulcers

When NOT to use antiulceratives

- Hypersensitivity
- Pregnancy
- Breast-feeding
- Chronic renal failure
- Liver impairment
- Allergy to prostaglandins

Adverse reactions to watch for

- Darkened tongue or stools, diarrhea, abdominal pain, flatulence, dyspepsia, infertility, nausea, vomiting, vaginal spotting, uterine cramping, miscarriage

Key nursing actions

- Watch for diarrhea.
- Know that women of childbearing age should be assessed for pregnancy before receiving misoprostol
- Assess the patient for epigastric or abdominal pain, frank bleeding, and occult bleeding.
- Teach the patient to avoid gastric irritants, such as smoking, alcohol, aspirin-containing products, caffeine, NSAIDs, and foods that cause GI irritation.

Pharmacokinetics

- Absorption: Misoprostol is extensively and rapidly absorbed
- Distribution: Unknown
- Metabolism: Unknown
- Excretion: Unknown

Drug examples

- Bismuth subsalicylate (Pepto-Bismol), misoprostol (Cytotec)

Indications

- Bismuth subsalicylate may be used with antibiotics to eradicate *Helicobacter pylori,* which has been implicated as a cause of ulcers
- Misoprostol is used to prevent gastric ulcers resulting from use of NSAIDs or to treat duodenal ulcers not responding to other medication regimens

Contraindications and precautions

- These drugs are contraindicated in patients with known hypersensitivity
- Use these drugs cautiously in pregnant or breast-feeding women and in those with chronic renal failure or liver impairment
- Misoprostol is contraindicated in patients who are allergic to prostaglandins and in pregnant or breast-feeding women

Adverse reactions

- Bismuth subsalicylate may darken tongue or stools
- Misoprostol may cause diarrhea (most common adverse reaction); it may also cause abdominal pain, flatulence, dyspepsia, infertility, nausea and vomiting, vaginal spotting, uterine cramping, and miscarriage

Interactions

- Bismuth subsalicylate increases the action of warfarin and oral hypoglycemic agonists
- Bismuth subsalicylate and misoprostol decrease absorption of tetracyclines

Nursing responsibilities

- Administer misoprostol with food or after meals and at bedtime to decrease the risk of diarrhea
- Observe the patient for diarrhea
- Know that women of childbearing age should be assessed for pregnancy before receiving misoprostol
  - Begin therapy on the second or third day of the menstrual period following a negative pregnancy test
  - Encourage the woman to use contraception throughout therapy
- Assess the patient for epigastric or abdominal pain, frank bleeding, and occult bleeding
- Teach the patient to avoid gastric irritants, such as smoking, alcohol, aspirin-containing products, caffeine, NSAIDs, and foods that cause GI irritation, because these may counteract the effects of the drug or worsen the ulcer

ANTIEMETICS AND EMETICS

ANTIEMETICS

Mechanism of action

- Mechanisms vary
- Aprepitant, dronabinol, granisetron, ondansetron, palonosetron, phenothiazines, and trimethobenzamide act on the CNS to prevent nausea and vomiting
- Dimenhydrinate, meclizine, and scopolamine reduce motion sickness by inhibiting impulses from the inner ear to the vestibular pathway
- Metoclopramide increases the rate of gastric emptying and enhances gastroesophageal sphincter tone

Pharmacokinetics

- Absorption: Usually well absorbed from the GI tract
- Distribution: Unknown
- Metabolism: Extensively metabolized by the liver
- Excretion: Excreted in the urine and the feces

Drug examples

- Aprepitant (Emend), dimenhydrinate (Dramamine), dronabinol (THC [Marinol]), granisetron (Kytril), meclizine (Antivert, Bonine), metoclopramide (Reglan), ondansetron (Zofran), palonosetron (Aloxi), phenothiazines (chlorpromazine [Thorazine], perphenazine [Trilafon], prochlorperazine [Compazine], promethazine [Phenergan], thiethylperazine [Torecan]), trimethobenzamide (Tigan)

Indications

- Aprepitant, palonosetron, ondansetron, granisetron, and dronabinol are used in the management of nausea and vomiting associated with chemotherapy
- Dimenhydrinate is used in motion sickness
- Metoclopramide promotes gastric emptying in patients receiving tube feedings and in patients with diabetic gastroparesis

Contraindications and precautions

- Metoclopramide is contraindicated in suspected GI obstruction; use cautiously and at a reduced dose in patients with renal impairment
- Phenothiazines are contraindicated in angle-closure glaucoma, bone marrow depression, and severe liver or heart disease
- Dimenhydrinate is contraindicated in patients hypersensitive to the drug or its components; the I.V. product contains benzyl alcohol, which has been associated with fatal "gasping syndrome" in neonates

Adverse reactions

- Phenothiazines may cause hypotension, constipation, blurred vision, dryness of the eyes and mouth, extrapyramidal reactions, and photosensitivity reactions

Key facts about antiemetics

- Mechanisms vary; some act on CNS to prevent nausea and vomiting, some reduce motion sickness, some increase the rate of gastric emptying and enhance gastroesophageal sphincter tone
- Extensively metabolized by the liver
- Excreted in urine and feces

When to use antiemetics

- Nausea and vomiting associated with chemotherapy
- Motion sickness
- Tube feedings
- Diabetic gastroparesis

When NOT to use antiemetics

- Suspected GI obstruction
- Angle-closure glaucoma
- Bone marrow depression
- Severe liver or heart disease
- Hypersensitivity

Adverse reactions to watch for

- Hypotension, constipation, blurred vision, dryness of the eyes and mouth, extrapyramidal reactions, photosensitivity reactions, hypotension, pain at I.M. injection site, rectal irritation, drowsiness

Topics for patient discussion

- Medication regimen, including proper timing of and technique for administration
- Signs and symptoms to discuss with the physician
- Safety measures
- Measures to alleviate anticholinergic effects and bowel elimination
- Importance of changing position slowly and wearing sunscreen and protective clothing as appropriate
- Ways to reduce dry mouth
- Follow-up care

Key nursing actions

- Assess the patient for nausea and vomiting and fluid and electrolyte imbalances.
- Instruct the patient not to consume alcohol when taking an antiemetic.
- Teach the patient to take oral antiemetics 1 hour before exposure to conditions causing motion sickness.

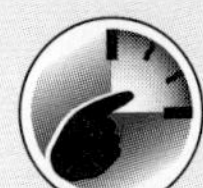

TIME-OUT FOR TEACHING

Teaching about antiemetics

Include these topics in your teaching plan for the patient receiving an antiemetic.

- Medication regimen, including the drug's name, dosage, frequency, duration, and possible adverse effects
- Signs and symptoms to discuss with the physician
- Proper timing of and technique for administration
- Safety measures
- Measures to alleviate anticholinergic effects and bowel elimination
- Follow-up care, including physician visits

- Trimethobenzamide may cause hypotension, pain at the I.M. injection site, and rectal irritation (with suppositories)
- Antiemetics may cause drowsiness

Interactions

- Use with antihistamines, other central nervous system (CNS) depressants, including opioids, and sedative-hypnotic drugs causes additive CNS depression
- Use of phenothiazines with other hypotensive drugs causes additive hypotension
- Use of phenothiazines or meclizine with anticholinergic drugs causes additive anticholinergic effects
- Metoclopramide affects GI motility, possibly altering GI absorption of other drugs, such as salicylates, diazepam, levodopa, lithium, tetracycline, and digoxin

Nursing responsibilities

- Decrease initial dose of metoclopramide by 50% of usual recommended dose if creatinine clearance is less than 40 ml/minute
- When administering phenothiazines, instruct the patient to change position slowly to minimize orthostatic hypotension and to wear sunscreen and protective clothing to prevent photosensitivity reactions (for additional teaching tips, see *Teaching about antiemetics*)
- Assess the patient for nausea and vomiting and fluid and electrolyte imbalances
- Caution the patient to avoid activities requiring alertness until the response to the drug is known
- Inform the patient that frequent mouth rinses, good oral hygiene, and sugarless gum or candy may reduce dry mouth
- Instruct the patient not to consume alcohol when taking an antiemetic to prevent additive CNS depression
- Teach the patient to take oral antiemetics 1 hour before exposure to conditions causing motion sickness

EMETICS

Mechanism of action
- Stimulate the chemoreceptor trigger zone and gastric mucosa to induce vomiting

Pharmacokinetics
- Unknown

Drug examples
- Ipecac syrup

Indications
- To induce emesis to treat poisoning
- In early management of drug overdose in conscious patients after recent ingestion of a noncaustic substance

Contraindications and precautions
- Emetics are contraindicated in semicomatose or unconscious patients
- These drugs are also contraindicated in patients who are inebriated or have a history of seizures and in those who have ingested caustic substances or petroleum products

Adverse reactions
- Arrhythmias, cardiotoxicity, diarrhea, drowsiness

Interactions
- Emetics cause a reduced emetic effect when used with activated charcoal

Nursing responsibilities
- Assess the patient's level of consciousness before administering the drug; if the patient is unconscious, perform gastric lavage instead
- Obtain a history to find out if caustic substances were ingested and to determine possible antidotes
- Follow administration of ipecac syrup with one or two glasses of tepid water or other clear liquid; milk may counteract the effect of the drug and delay or prevent vomiting
- Know that lavage is necessary if a second dose doesn't produce vomiting; ipecac may be cardiotoxic if absorbed
- Instruct parents with children over age 1 to keep a small amount of ipecac syrup on hand for emergencies; however, warn them *not* to administer ipecac syrup to a child who has ingested a caustic substance
- **Don't confuse ipecac syrup with ipecac fluid extract, which is rarely used but is 14 times more potent than ipecac syrup**

Key facts about emetics
- Stimulate the chemoreceptor trigger zone and gastric mucosa to induce vomiting
- Metabolism and excretion unknown

When to use emetics
- Poisoning
- Drug overdose

When NOT to use emetics
- Semicomatose state or unconsciousness
- Inebriation
- History of seizures
- Ingestion of caustic substance or petroleum

Adverse reactions to watch for
- Arrhythmias, cardiotoxicity, diarrhea, drowsiness

Key nursing actions
- Assess the patient's level of consciousness before administering the drug.
- Obtain a history to find out if caustic substances were ingested and to determine possible antidotes.
- Follow administration of ipecac syrup with one or two glasses of tepid water or other clear liquid.

Key facts about antidiarrheals

- Reduce fluid content of stool
- Decrease the volume of gastric and intestinal secretions
- Metabolized by the liver
- Excreted by kidneys or in feces

When to use antidiarrheals

- Acute or chronic nonspecific diarrhea

When NOT to use antidiarrheals

- Abdominal pain of unknown cause

Adverse reactions to watch for

- Constipation, drowsiness, nausea, abdominal pain, pain at injection site, gallstones

ANTIDIARRHEALS AND LAXATIVES

ANTIDIARRHEALS

Mechanism of action

- Camphorated opium tincture, difenoxin, diphenoxylate, and loperamide slow intestinal motility, ultimately reducing water absorption from stool
- Bismuth subsalicylate, kaolin and pectin mixture, and polycarbophil reduce the fluid content of the stool
- Octreotide is used to decrease the volume of gastric and intestinal secretions and diarrhea secondary to vasoactive intestinal tumors such as carcinoid tumor

Pharmacokinetics

- Absorption: Opium preparations are absorbed systemically; others are absorbed readily from the GI tract, except for loperamide
- Distribution: Varies
- Metabolism: Metabolized by the liver
- Excretion: Opium preparations are excreted by the kidneys; others are excreted primarily in the feces

Drug examples

- Bismuth subsalicylate (Pepto-Bismol), camphorated opium tincture (Paregoric), difenoxin (with atropine [Motofen]), diphenoxylate (with atropine [Lomotil]), kaolin and pectin mixture (Kapectolin), loperamide (Imodium), octreotide (Sandostatin), polycarbophil (FiberCon)

Indications

- To control and relieve symptoms of acute or chronic nonspecific diarrhea

Contraindications and precautions

- These drugs are contraindicated in abdominal pain of unknown cause, especially if the patient has a fever

Adverse reactions

- Constipation, drowsiness (with camphorated opium tincture, difenoxin, diphenoxylate, and loperamide), nausea, abdominal pain, pain at the injection site, gallstones (with octreotide)

Interactions

- Use of camphorated opium tincture, difenoxin, diphenoxylate, or loperamide with other CNS depressants causes additive CNS depression
- Use of difenoxin, diphenoxylate, or loperamide with similar-acting drugs causes additive anticholinergic effects
- Concurrent use of kaolin with digoxin may decrease digoxin absorption

Nursing responsibilities

- Assess the patient's skin turgor and monitor fluid and electrolyte balance for evidence of dehydration resulting from diarrhea

- Assess for abdominal pain and distention, nausea and vomiting, and frank or occult bleeding; auscultate for bowel sounds; and evaluate stools for frequency and consistency
- Know that high-dose, long-term use of difenoxin or diphenoxylate may cause dependence (atropine has been added to these preparations to discourage abuse)
- Don't confuse camphorated opium tincture with deodorized tincture of opium, which is 25 times more potent
- When administering camphorated opium tincture, difenoxin, diphenoxylate, or loperamide, caution the patient to avoid activities requiring alertness until the response to the drug is known; also instruct the patient to avoid alcohol and CNS depressants
- Instruct the patient to notify the physician if diarrhea persists or fever occurs

Key nursing actions

- Assess patient's skin turgor and monitor fluid and electrolyte balance for evidence of dehydration.
- Assess for abdominal pain and distention, nausea and vomiting, and frank or occult bleeding.
- Auscultate for bowel sounds.
- Evaluate stools for frequency and consistency.
- Instruct patient to notify physician if diarrhea persists or fever occurs.

LAXATIVES

Mechanism of action

- Bulk-forming laxatives increase the water content of stool, forming a viscous solution that promotes peristalsis and improves the elimination rate
- Lubricant laxatives increase water retention in the stool, prevent water absorption from the stool, and lubricate and soften intestinal contents
- Hyperosmotic laxatives increase water content of the stool and soften the stool; lactulose also inhibits diffusion of ammonia from the colon into the blood, reducing serum ammonia levels in patients with liver dysfunction
- Saline cathartic laxatives draw water into the bowel, increasing the bulk of intestinal contents and stimulating peristalsis
- Stimulant laxatives stimulate peristalsis and inhibit water and electrolyte reabsorption from the intestine
- Stool softeners allow more fluid and fat to penetrate the feces, producing a softer fecal mass

Key facts about laxatives

- Increase water content of stool, prevent water absorption from stool, and lubricate and soften intestinal contents to promote peristalsis and improve elimination
- Allow fluid and fat to penetrate the feces, producing a softer fecal mass
- Metabolized by microflora of the intestines
- Excreted in feces

Pharmacokinetics

- Absorption: Minimally absorbed
- Distribution: Distributed in the intestines
- Metabolism: Metabolized by the microflora of the intestines
- Excretion: Excreted in the feces

Drug examples

- Bulk-forming laxatives include methylcellulose (Citrucel), polycarbophil (FiberCon), psyllium (Fiberall, Konsyl, Metamucil, Perdiem)
- Lubricant laxatives include mineral oil (Kondremul, Fleet Mineral Oil Enema)
- Hyperosmotic laxatives include lactulose (Cephulac, Chronulac)
- Saline cathartic laxatives include magnesium citrate, magnesium hydroxide (Milk of Magnesia), magnesium sulfate, polyethylene glycol-electrolyte solution (GoLYTELY), and sodium phosphates (sodium phosphate and sodium biphosphate [Fleet Phospho-soda])

- Stimulant laxatives include bisacodyl (Biscolax, Dulcolax), cascara sagrada, castor oil (Alphamul), glycerin suppositories, phenolphthalein (Ex-Lax), and senna (Senokot)
- Stool softeners include docusate calcium (Surfak), docusate potassium (Dialose), and docusate sodium (Colace)

Indications

- To treat or prevent constipation and to prepare the bowel for radiologic or endoscopic procedures
- Methylcellulose and psyllium also are used to manage chronic watery diarrhea
- Lactulose also is used as an adjunctive drug in managing hepatic encephalopathy

Contraindications and precautions

- These drugs are contraindicated in patients with persistent or severe abdominal pain of unknown cause, especially when accompanied by fever

Adverse reactions

- May cause nausea, vomiting, abdominal cramping; esophageal obstruction or intestinal obstruction (with bulk-forming laxatives); lipid pneumonia, nutritional deficiencies (with lubricant laxatives); cramps, distention, flatulence, belching (with osmotic laxatives); dehydration, electrolyte imbalance (with saline cathartic laxatives)
- Long-term use and abuse of laxatives may cause permanent loss of colonic motility, laxative dependence, and electrolyte imbalances

Interactions

- Laxatives reduce intestinal transit time and may decrease absorption of orally administered drugs

Nursing responsibilities

- Assess for abdominal pain and distention, nausea and vomiting, and frank or occult bleeding; auscultate for bowel sounds; and evaluate stools for frequency and consistency
- Monitor the patient for fluid and electrolyte imbalances
- Mix bulk-forming laxatives in a full glass of water or juice; give an additional glass of fluid after administering
- When administering laxatives as adjunctive drugs for hepatic encephalopathy, assess the patient's mental status, including level of consciousness and orientation
- Dilute sodium phosphates with water before giving and monitor the patient for electrolyte disturbances
- Teach the patient that most laxatives are for short-term use only and that long-term use may cause electrolyte imbalances and laxative dependence by causing a permanent loss of colonic motility; encourage the patient to use other methods to regulate bowels, such as increasing dietary bulk and fluid intake and engaging in exercise (for additional teaching tips, see *Teaching about laxatives*)

When to use laxatives

- Constipation
- Radiologic and endoscopic procedures
- Chronic watery diarrhea
- Hepatic encephalopathy

When NOT to use laxatives

- Persistent or severe abdominal pain of unknown cause

Adverse reactions to watch for

- Nausea, vomiting, abdominal cramping, esophageal or intestinal obstruction, lipid pneumonia, nutritional deficiencies, cramps, distention, flatulence, belching, dehydration, electrolyte imbalance, loss of colonic motility, dependence

Key nursing actions

- Assess for abdominal pain and distention, nausea and vomiting, and frank or occult bleeding.
- Auscultate for bowel sounds.
- Evaluate stools for frequency and consistency.
- Monitor patient for fluid and electrolyte imbalances.
- Mix bulk-forming laxatives in full glass of water or juice; give additional glass of fluid after administration.

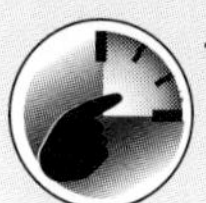

TIME-OUT FOR TEACHING

Teaching about laxatives

Include these topics in your teaching plan for the patient receiving a laxative.
- Medication regimen, including the drug's name, dosage, frequency, duration, and possible adverse effects
- Signs and symptoms to discuss with the physician
- Proper timing of and technique for administration
- Nonpharmacologic bowel elimination measures, including diet and exercise
- Dietary fibers and fluids
- Follow-up care

NCLEX CHECKS

It's never too soon to begin your NCLEX preparation. Now that you've reviewed this chapter, carefully read each of the following questions and choose the best answer. Then compare your responses to the correct answers.

1. A patient is using aluminum hydroxide (Amphojel) as an antacid. You should warn the patient about which adverse reaction?

☐ A. Black stools
☐ B. Constipation
☐ C. Acid rebound
☐ D. Reduced iron absorption

2. As part of the treatment regimen for a patient with a peptic ulcer, the physician orders cimetidine (Tagamet), 300 mg P.O., before meals and at bedtime. Your best response to the order is to:

☐ A. give the drug as ordered.
☐ B. change the drug times to be given with meals.
☐ C. hold the drug and check the dosage with the physician.
☐ D. hold the drug and ask the physician to change it to twice daily.

3. A 48-year-old patient takes large doses of a nonsteroidal anti-inflammatory drug (NSAID) for rheumatoid arthritis. Misoprostol (Cytotec) is prescribed with food to prevent NSAID-induced ulcers. Which common dose-related adverse reaction to misoprostol do you need to discuss with your patient?

☐ A. Diarrhea
☐ B. Dyspepsia
☐ C. Headache
☐ D. Tinnitus

4. A 3-year-old child has just ingested a large but unknown number of iron tablets at home. His mother phones the emergency department concerning the use of syrup of ipecac for her child. You should instruct the mother to:

Topics for patient discussion

- Medication regimen, including proper timing and technique for administration
- Signs and symptoms to discuss with the physician
- Nonpharmacologic bowel elimination measures
- Dietary fibers and fluids
- Follow-up care

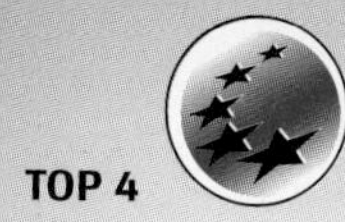

TOP 4

Items to study before your next test on drugs and the gastrointestinal system

1. Mechanisms of action of the various types of antiulceratives, antiemetics, emetics, antidiarrheals, and laxatives
2. Major adverse effects of antiulceratives, antiemetics, emetics, antidiarrheals, and laxatives
3. Nursing responsibilities when administering antiulceratives, antiemetics, emetics, antidiarrheals, and laxatives
4. Teaching for the patient receiving antiulceratives, antiemetics, emetics, antidiarrheals, or laxatives

- ☐ A. give the drug with a glass of milk.
- ☐ B. not give the drug because iron isn't that toxic.
- ☐ C. wait at least 30 minutes before giving the drug.
- ☐ D. have the child drink a large glass of tepid water after taking the drug.

5. A patient complains of severe nausea and vomiting from radiotherapy for metastatic breast cancer. Which antiemetic will be most effective?

- ☐ A. Chlorpromazine (Thorazine)
- ☐ B. Meclizine (Antivert)
- ☐ C. Ondansetron (Zofran)
- ☐ D. Trimethobenzamide (Tigan)

6. You suspect that a patient has been poisoned. An emetic is contraindicated when:

- ☐ A. the patient is a child.
- ☐ B. the patient is elderly.
- ☐ C. a caustic substance has been ingested.
- ☐ D. ingestion occurred less than 1 hour ago.

7. You advise a patient not to take a stimulant laxative for an extended period. Which of the following conditions could result from the long-term use of a stimulant laxative?

- ☐ A. Hepatotoxicity
- ☐ B. Small-intestine blockage
- ☐ C. Permanent loss of colonic motility
- ☐ D. Withdrawal reactions when the laxative is stopped

8. A patient returns from the operating room after receiving extensive abdominal surgery. He has 1,000 ml of lactated Ringer's solution infusing via a central line. The physician orders the I.V. fluid to be infused at 125 ml/hour plus the total output of the previous hour. The drip factor of the tubing is 15 gtt/minute and the output for the previous hour was 75 ml via Foley catheter, 50 ml via nasogastric tube, and 10 ml via Jackson Pratt tube. For how many drops per minute should the nurse set the I.V. flow rate to deliver the correct amount of fluid? ______

ANSWERS AND RATIONALES

1. CORRECT ANSWER: B
Aluminum is considered constipating. It doesn't change stool color. It neutralizes acid without rebound and has little impact on iron absorption unless taken in excessive amounts. Many antacids will include magnesium (which may cause diarrhea) along with aluminum to prevent this adverse reaction.

2. CORRECT ANSWER: A
Cimetidine inhibits gastric acid secretions and works best when the stomach is empty, so giving it before meals and at bedtime is correct. The dosage is also correct. Changing the times is inappropriate and would require a physician's or-

der. Holding the drug and getting the order changed would interfere with the maximum effectiveness of the drug.

3. CORRECT ANSWER: A
Diarrhea is the most common adverse reaction to misoprostol. The patient can minimize the reaction by taking the drug after meals and at bedtime and by avoiding magnesium-containing antacids. The patient should contact his physician if the diarrhea becomes severe. Dyspepsia, headache, and tinnitus aren't common adverse reactions to misoprostol.

4. CORRECT ANSWER: D
Syrup of ipecac will induce vomiting best when taken with 1 to 2 glasses of tepid water or other clear liquids. Milk may counteract the effects of the drug and delay or prevent vomiting. Iron is highly toxic to children (and to adults), and excessive oral iron must be removed quickly to prevent serious harm. Syrup of ipecac needs to be given as soon as possible to prevent absorption of the ingested drug.

5. CORRECT ANSWER: C
Ondansetron is used specifically for nausea and vomiting due to radiotherapy. Trimethobenzamide is indicated for general mild to moderate nausea and vomiting, while chlorpromazine is used for severe nausea and vomiting. Meclizine is used for motion sickness.

6. CORRECT ANSWER: C
The only contraindication for an emetic is use with caustic agents or petroleum distillate because trauma to the esophagus would be heightened. Emetics are used in pediatric and elderly patients without adverse consequences as long as the patients are monitored appropriately. Emetics are appropriate if the substance has been ingested less than 1 hour before administration.

7. CORRECT ANSWER: C
Prolonged use or abuse of stimulant laxatives may lead to permanent loss of colonic motility. Prolonged use can lead to laxative dependence as a result of chronic stimulation of smooth-muscle activity. In general, these drugs aren't hepatotoxic, don't significantly affect the small intestines, and aren't associated with withdrawal reactions.

8. CORRECT ANSWER: 65
First, calculate the volume to be infused (in milliliters):

75 ml + 50 ml + 10 ml = 135 ml total output for the previous hour

135 ml + 125 ml ordered as a constant flow =
260 ml to be infused over the next hour.

Next, use the formula:

Volume to be infused/Total minutes to be infused × Drip factor =
Drops per minute.

In this case, 260 ml divided by 60 minutes x 15 gtt/minute = 65 gtt/minute

15 Drugs and the reproductive system

LEARNING OBJECTIVES

After studying this chapter, you should be able to:

- Describe the mechanisms of action of androgens, estrogens, and progestins.
- Identify indications for male and female hormonal drugs.
- List common adverse effects of male and female hormonal drugs.
- Identify nursing responsibilities when administering male and female hormonal drugs.
- Discuss patient teaching related to male and female hormonal drugs.

CHAPTER OVERVIEW

This chapter reviews the use of androgens, estrogens and progestins, fertility drugs, and obstetric drugs. Androgens are used to provide replacement therapy for hormonal deficiencies in men and to create an environment unfavorable for tissue or tumor growth. Finasteride specifically decreases prostate size and improves urine flow in patients with benign prostatic hyperplasia (BPH).

Estrogens and progestins are used for contraception, treatment of hormone-sensitive tissue or tumors, restoration of hormone balance during menopause, and treatment of osteoporosis.

Lactation suppressants, fertility drugs, oxytocics, and labor suppressants are used during the childbearing cycle.

Nursing responsibilities for all these drugs include assessing for weight gain, observing for thromboembolism (with estrogens), and monitoring fetal and maternal heart rate (with obstetric drugs). Patient teaching includes proper use of these drugs and information on adverse effects.

ANATOMY AND PHYSIOLOGY

Anatomy

- The male reproductive system includes the scrotum, testes, duct system, accessory reproductive glands, and penis
- The female reproductive system includes the ovaries, fallopian tubes, uterus, vagina, external genitalia, and mammary glands

Physiology

- Hormones and puberty
  - During puberty, the hypothalamus begins to release the gonadotropin-releasing hormones: follicle-stimulating hormone (FSH) and luteinizing hormone (LH)
  - These hormones stimulate the gonads to release sex hormones
    - Testosterone is released in men; estrogen and progesterone are released in women
    - These sex hormones induce sexual development and body changes characteristic of sexual maturity
  - Puberty is marked by the production of mature spermatozoa in males and the onset of menarche in females
- Male hormones
  - Male testicular function is regulated by the two gonadotropic hormones: FSH and LH
  - FSH maintains normal spermiogenesis (production of sperm)
  - LH maintains normal spermiogenesis and promotes testosterone secretion, which is responsible for sexual drive, development of secondary sex characteristics, and growth
- Female reproductive hormones
  - LH and FSH promote follicle maturation and ovarian secretion of estrogen and progesterone
  - Estrogen is responsible for secondary sex characteristics
    - It stimulates endometrial growth during the first half of the menstrual cycle
    - It stimulates cervical secretion of mucus that facilitates passage of sperm into the uterus and fallopian tubes
    - It stimulates bone growth
  - Progesterone prepares the endometrium for implantation of the fertilized ovum during the second half of the menstrual cycle; it also causes breast development
  - The gonadotropic hormones (LH and FSH) have a reciprocal relationship with the ovarian hormones (estrogen and progesterone)

A&P highlights

- Male reproductive system: scrotum, testes, duct system, accessory reproductive glands, and penis
- Female reproductive system: ovaries, fallopian tubes, uterus, vagina, external genitalia, and mammary glands
- During puberty, the hypothalamus releases FSH and LH; these hormones stimulate gonads to release sex hormones
- Male testicular function is regulated by FSH and LH
- In females, LH and FSH promote follicle maturation and ovarian secretion of estrogen and progesterone
- Estrogen is responsible for secondary sex characteristics in females

Key facts about the menstrual cycle

- Menstrual cycle beginning is dated from the first day of the menstrual flow
- Ovulation occurs around the middle of the cycle
- Preovulatory stage varies
- Postovulatory phase is usually constant and lasts for about 14 days

Key facts about childbirth

- Labor – the process by which the fetus is expelled from the uterus
- Oxytocin receptors, uterine stretch, and fetal stimulation of oxytocin and estrogen contribute to the onset of labor
- Labor is maintained by cervical dilation

Key facts about lactation

- Milk produced by mammary glands in the breasts
- Regulated by estrogen, progesterone, prolactin, and oxytocin

    - A high estrogen level inhibits FSH output, stabilizing estrogen levels, and stimulates LH release, which in turn increases progesterone output
    - A high progesterone level inhibits LH output
- The menstrual cycle
  - The beginning of the menstrual cycle is dated from the first day of the menstrual flow
  - Ovulation occurs around the middle of the cycle, which is divided into preovulatory (follicular) and postovulatory (luteal) phases
  - The preovulatory (follicular) phase varies among individuals
    - The pituitary gland releases FSH, which stimulates a group of ovarian follicles to grow
    - One follicle will grow faster and reach maturity; the others will atrophy
    - Soon after FSH levels increase, LH levels rise; together, these hormones promote estrogen secretion by the ovarian follicle
    - The LH surge lasts for about 24 hours and causes the mature follicle to rupture, leading to ovulation
  - The postovulatory (luteal) phase is usually constant and lasts for about 14 days
    - This phase is characterized by the conversion of the ruptured follicle into the corpus luteum, which produces estrogen and progesterone
    - The corpus luteum reaches maturity 8 to 9 days after ovulation and begins to degenerate if pregnancy hasn't occurred
    - The decline in corpus luteum activity, which reduces estrogen and progesterone output, results in menstruation
    - Eventually, when estrogen and progesterone levels have fallen, FSH and LH are released again and a new menstrual cycle begins
- Childbirth
  - Labor is the process by which the fetus is expelled from the uterus by uterine contractions
  - Several factors contribute to the onset of labor
    - Oxytocin receptors on uterine muscle fibers
    - Uterine stretch that stimulates oxytocin secretion
    - Fetal stimulation of oxytocin and estrogen with decreased progesterone secretion
  - Once labor begins, it's maintained by cervical dilation, which increases oxytocin secretion
- Lactation
  - Lactation is milk production by the mammary glands in the breasts
  - Lactation is regulated by estrogen and progesterone (which stimulate proliferation of breast tissue), prolactin (which causes milk production when stimulated by estrogen and progesterone), and oxytocin (which helps expel the milk during breast-feeding)

- The high prolactin level in the postpartum woman inhibits FSH and LH release
- If the woman doesn't breast-feed, the prolactin level declines, FSH and LH levels rise, and the cyclic release soon follows
- The amount of prolactin released in response to breast-feeding gradually decreases, and ovulation and the menstrual cycle resume

- Hormones and aging
  - With age, the hormones of the reproductive system slowly decline
  - Decreased testosterone secretion in males leads to a decrease in sex drive and spermatogenesis
  - As females age, the ovarian follicles gradually degenerate and don't produce any more mature egg cells; thus by age 45, few follicles remain
  - The aging ovaries no longer produce sufficient hormones to stimulate cyclic changes in the endometrium, and menstruation ceases; this process is known as menopause

Key facts about hormones and aging

- Reproductive hormones decline with age
- As females age, ovarian follicles gradually degenerate
- Menopause occurs

Function

- The primary role of the reproductive system is to produce offspring
- The reproductive system also has endocrine functions
- The reproductive system forms an integral part of each person's self-concept

ANDROGENS

Key facts about androgens

- Simulate the action of endogenous hormone
- Stimulate production of RBCs
- Metabolism varies
- Excretion varies

Mechanism of action

- Simulate the action of endogenous hormone to replace deficient hormones or treat hormone-sensitive disorders
- Stimulate the production of red blood cells by enhancing the production of the erythropoietic stimulating factor
- Danazol is an antigonadotropin that suppresses the production of LH and FSH, reducing engorgement in the ectopic endometrial tissue and the accompanying pain; it also decreases ovarian activity and estrogen production

Pharmacokinetics

- Absorption
  - Oral testosterone is absorbed by the GI tract
  - I.M. injections of esters in oil are absorbed slowly; they can be given at 2- to 4-week intervals
  - Topical testosterone is absorbed by the skin, and effects continue for 24 hours after application
- Distribution: Varies by drug
- Metabolism: Varies by drug
- Excretion: Varies by drug

When to use androgens

- Hypogonadism
- Delayed puberty
- Postpartum breast engorgement
- Androgen-sensitive inoperable metastatic breast cancer (palliative care)
- Endometriosis
- Fibrocystic breast disease
- Hereditary angioedema
- Advanced disseminated breast carcinoma (palliative care)

When NOT to use androgens

- Cardiac disease
- Hepatic disease
- Renal disease
- Prostate or breast cancer
- Hypersensitivity
- Pregnancy

Adverse reactions to watch for

- Nausea, vomiting, diarrhea, sodium and water retention, edema, weight gain, mood swings, changes in libido, impotence, precocious puberty, priapism, premature epiphyseal closure, breast tenderness, impotence, sterility, hirsutism, reduced breast size, and hoarseness

Drug examples

- Danazol (Danocrine), fluoxymestrone, methyltestosterone (Methitest, Testred, Virilon), testolactone (Teslac), testosterone (Androderm, Androgel 1%, Delatestryl, Depo-Testosterone, Testoderm, Testopel)

Indications

- Testosterone and methyltestosterone are used to treat hypogonadism, delayed puberty, and postpartum breast engorgement; they are also prescribed as palliative treatment for androgen-sensitive inoperable metastatic (skeletal) breast cancer in women 1 to 5 years postmenopause
- Danazol is used to treat endometriosis, as palliative treatment for fibrocystic breast disease, and as prophylaxis for hereditary angioedema
- Fluoxymesterone is used to treat androgen deficiencies and inoperable breast cancer that is androgen-responsive
- Testolactone is used as adjunctive therapy in the palliative treatment of advanced disseminated breast carcinoma in postmenopausal women when hormonal therapy is indicated and in premenopausal women with disseminated breast carcinoma in whom ovarian function has been terminated

Contraindications and precautions

- Contraindicated in patients with serious cardiac, hepatic, or renal diseases
- Contraindicated in patients with hypersensitivity to the drug or its components
- Contraindicated in men with known or suspected cancer of the prostate or breast
- Contraindicated in pregnant women; pregnant women should also avoid skin contact with Androgel
- Testosterone transdermal systems and the gel are contraindicated in women

Adverse reactions

- These drugs may cause nausea, vomiting, diarrhea, sodium and water retention, edema, weight gain, mood swings, changes in libido, and impotence
- In boys, precocious puberty, priapism, and premature epiphyseal closure may occur
- In men, breast tenderness, impotence, and sterility may occur
- In women, hirsutism, reduced breast size, and hoarseness may occur

Interactions

- Concurrent use with glucocorticoids increases the risk of edema
- Androgens will increase cyclosporin levels and the risk of cyclosporine toxicity
- Androgens may decrease serum glucose levels, thereby reducing insulin requirements
- These drugs may increase the effects of anticoagulants

- **Nursing responsibilities**
  - **Know that most androgens, including all anabolic steroids such as testolactone, are Schedule III controlled substances**
  - Use deep I.M. injections for parenteral forms, preferably into a large muscle mass
  - **Testosterone *must* be administered I.M. only**
  - Give fluoxymesterone with food to reduce abdominal discomfort
  - Assess the patient for weight gain and edema
  - Monitor the patient's blood pressure, weight, electrolyte and lipid levels, and liver function test results
  - Instruct women to use a nonhormonal contraceptive (barrier method) during therapy
  - Advise women taking danazol to expect amenorrhea
  - **Warn women that androgen therapy may cause hoarseness, deeper voice, facial hair, acne, and menstrual irregularities; advise them to notify their physician if these effects occur**
  - **Advise male adolescents receiving androgens for delayed puberty to have bone development checked every 6 months**

ANDROGEN HORMONE INHIBITORS

- **Mechanism of action**
  - Finasteride inhibits steroid 5alpha-reductase, which is an enzyme that converts testosterone into 5alpha-dihydrotestosterone (DHT)
  - Thus, finasteride leads to a decrease in the high levels of DHT found in men with an enlarged prostate or balding scalp
- **Pharmacokinetics**
  - Absorption: Well absorbed orally
  - Distribution: Approximately 90% is protein-bound; crosses the blood-brain barrier
  - Metabolism: Undergoes hepatic metabolism
  - Excretion: Excreted in the bile and the feces
- **Drug examples**
  - Finasteride (Propecia, Proscar)
- **Indications**
  - To treat benign prostatic hyperplasia (BPH)
  - To treat androgenic alopecia (male-pattern baldness)
- **Contraindications and precautions**
  - Contraindicated in patients with hypersensitivity to the drug
  - Contraindicated in women and children
  - **Pregnant women shouldn't handle or come in contact with crushed or broken tablets**
- **Adverse reactions**
  - Adverse reactions to finasteride are generally mild and transient and include erectile dysfunction, decreased libido, breast tenderness and en-

Key nursing actions

- Know that most androgens are Schedule III controlled substances.
- Testosterone must be administered I.M. only.
- Warn women that androgen therapy may cause hoarseness, deeper voice, facial hair, acne, and menstrual irregularities.
- Advise male adolescents receiving androgens for delayed puberty to have bone development checked every 6 months.

Key facts about androgen hormone inhibitors

- Finasteride inhibits steroid 5alpha-reductase
- Finasteride leads to a decrease in high levels of DHT found in some men
- Undergoes hepatic metabolism
- Excreted in bile and feces

When to use androgen hormone inhibitors

- Benign prostatic hyperplasia
- Androgenic alopecia

When NOT to use androgen hormone inhibitors

- Hypersensitivity
- Women
- Children
- Pregnancy

Adverse reactions to watch for

- Erectile dysfunction, decreased libido, breast tenderness and enlargement, testicular pain, and hypersensitivity reactions

largement, testicular pain, and hypersensitivity reactions, such as lip swelling and rash
- Finasteride may cause hepatic impairment because the liver extensively metabolizes it

Interactions
- None reported

Nursing responsibilities
- **Warn men that women who are or may become pregnant shouldn't come in contact with crushed or broken tablets because of the risk to the male fetus**
- Warn men that they may have a decreased volume of ejaculate during treatment and that impotence and decreased libido may occur
- Explain that treatment for alopecia is long-term and discontinuing the drug will cause balding to resume
- **Know that men treated for BPH still must be evaluated for prostate cancer before and during therapy because finasteride doesn't protect against prostate cancer; finasteride decreases prostate-specific antigen (PSA) levels, even in the presence of prostate cancer**

Key nursing actions
- Warn that women who are or may become pregnant shouldn't come in contact with crushed or broken tablets because of the risk to the male fetus.
- Know that men treated for BPH still must be evaluated for prostate cancer before and during therapy.

ANABOLIC STEROIDS

Mechanism of action
- Anabolic steroids promote body tissue-building processes and reverse catabolic or tissue-depleting processes, such as anemias, trauma, surgery, arthritis, and osteoporosis
- During exogenous administration of anabolic steroids, testosterone release is inhibited through the inhibition of pituitary LH
- Large doses of anabolic steroids may suppress spermatogenesis through feedback inhibition of pituitary FSH

Pharmacokinetics
- Unknown

Drug examples
- Nandrolone decanoate (Deca-Durabolin), oxandrolone (Oxandrin), oxymetholone (Anadrol-50), stanozolol (Winstrol)

Indications
- Oxymetholone is used to treat anemias
- Oxandrolone is used as adjunctive therapy to promote weight gain after weight loss from catabolic disorders, such as surgery, severe trauma, anemia, arthritis, chronic infections, and osteoporosis
- Stanozolol is used prophylactically to decrease frequency and severity of attacks from hereditary angioedema
- Nandrolone decanoate is used to treat renal insufficiency–induced anemia

Key facts about anabolic steroids
- Promote body tissue-building processes
- Reverse catabolic or tissue-depleting processes
- Large doses may suppress spermatogenesis
- Metabolism and excretion are unknown

When to use anabolic steroids
- Anemia, including renal insufficiency-induced anemia
- Promote weight gain
- Hereditary angioedema

When NOT to use anabolic steroids
- Hypersensitivity
- Prostate carcinoma
- Breast carcinoma
- Hypercalcemia
- Nephrosis
- Pregnancy

Contraindications and precautions

- Contraindicated in patients hypersensitive to anabolic steroids
- Contraindicated in men with prostate or breast carcinoma
- Contraindicated in women with breast carcinoma and hypercalcemia, nephrosis, or the nephrotic phase of nephritis; also contraindicated in pregnant women
- These drugs shouldn't be used to enhance physical appearance or athletic performance
- **Anabolic steroids are classified as Schedule III Controlled Substances because of their potential for abuse, especially among athletes**
- Elderly patients using anabolic steroids may be at an increased risk for the development of prostatic hypertrophy and prostatic carcinoma
- Anabolic steroids may stunt growth when given to young children

Adverse reactions

- **Virilization is the most common adverse effect; acne occurs mostly in women and prepubertal males**
- Because these drugs suppress gonadotropic functions of the pituitary, they may have a direct effect on the testes and cause serious disturbances of growth and development if given to young children
- In postpubertal males, these drugs may cause acne, inhibition of testicular function with oligospermia, gynecomastia, testicular atrophy, chronic priapism, epididymitis, bladder irritability, change in libido, and impotence
- In females, these drugs may cause irreversible hirsutism, acne, hoarseness or deepening of the voice, clitoral enlargement, change in libido, and menstrual irregularities
- Anabolic steroids have been associated with peliosis hepatitis (blood-filled cysts in the liver and spleen) and liver cell tumors, which may cause liver failure or malignant and fatal tumors
- They have been linked with blood lipid changes associated with increased risk of atherosclerosis and increased cholesterol and low-density lipoprotein levels
- Anabolic steroids may also cause insomnia, edema from sodium retention, ankle swelling, nausea, vomiting, and diarrhea

Interactions

- Anabolic steroids increase the effects of anticoagulants
- These drugs may increase the hypoglycemic effects of sulfonylureas

Nursing responsibilities

- **Warn athletes that the use of anabolic steroids to improve physical appearance or athletic performance is contraindicated and that adverse effects may be serious and irreversible**
- **Warn women that virilization may occur while on drug therapy; tell these patients to contact their physician and discontinue the drug if amenorrhea, menstrual irregularities, hoarseness, hirsutism, or acne occurs**

Adverse reactions to watch for

- Virilization, acne, disturbances of growth and development in children, inhibition of testicular function with oligospermia, gynecomastia, testicular atrophy, chronic priapism, epididymitis, bladder irritability, change in libido, impotence, irreversible hirsutism, hoarseness or deepening of the voice, clitoral enlargement, menstrual irregularities, peliosis hepatitis, liver cell tumors, blood lipid changes, insomnia, edema from sodium retention, ankle swelling, nausea, vomiting, and diarrhea

Key nursing actions

- Warn that using anabolic steroids to improve physical appearance or athletic performance is contraindicated; adverse effects may be serious and irreversible.
- Warn that virilization may occur while on drug therapy.

- Monitor glucose levels in patients with diabetes carefully because glucose tolerance may be altered in these patients
- Monitor liver function test results

ESTROGENS, PROGESTINS, AND PROLACTIN SECRETION INHIBITORS

ESTROGENS AND PROGESTINS

Key facts about estrogens and progestins

- Simulate endogenous hormones to restore hormonal balance and treat hormone-sensitive tumors
- Metabolized in liver and skin
- Excretion varies

When to use estrogens and progestins

- Contraception
- Hormonal deficiencies
- Breast cancer
- Endometriosis
- Menopausal hot flashes and atrophic vaginitis
- Calcium restoration
- Menstrual cycle regulation or restoration
- Endometrial or renal cancer
- Premenstrual syndrome

When NOT to use estrogens and progestins

- Embolism
- Thrombophlebitis
- Breast cancer
- History of cerebrovascular accident
- Unexplained abnormal genital bleeding
- Pregnancy
- Obstetric emergencies
- Maternal hypertension
- Toxemia
- Cardiovascular disease prevention

Mechanism of action

- Simulate the endogenous hormones to restore hormonal balance and treat hormone-sensitive tumors

Pharmacokinetics

- Absorption: Well absorbed from the GI tract
- Distribution: Largely protein-bound; distributed into virtually all body tissues
- Metabolism: Metabolized in the liver; the skin metabolizes transdermal systems to a small extent
- Excretion: Some estrogens are excreted in bile, reabsorbed from the intestines, and returned to the liver; water-soluble estrogens are excreted in the urine and tubular reabsorption is minimal

Drug examples

- Conjugated estrogenic substances (Premarin), estradiol (Estrace, Estraderm, Delestrogen, Depo-Estradiol), medroxyprogesterone acetate (Provera), megestrol (Megace), norethindrone/mestranol (Norinyl, Ortho-Novum), progesterone

Indications

- Estrogens are used to provide contraception; to treat hormonal deficiencies, breast cancer, endometriosis, and (during menopause) hot flashes and atrophic vaginitis; and to restore positive calcium balance in postmenopausal osteoporosis
- Progestins are used to provide contraception; to regulate or restore the menstrual cycle; and to treat endometrial or renal cancer, endometriosis, and premenstrual syndrome

Contraindications and precautions

- Estrogens and progestins are contraindicated in patients with embolism, thrombophlebitis, breast cancer, history of cerebrovascular accident, unexplained abnormal genital bleeding, and known or suspected pregnancy
- Oxytocic drugs are contraindicated in obstetric emergencies, maternal hypertension, and toxemia
- Estrogens and progestins should be used with caution in patients with asthma, epilepsy, migraine, or heart or kidney disease
- Estrogens and progestins should not be used to prevent cardiovascular disease

Adverse reactions

- Adverse effects include nausea, vomiting, diarrhea, weight gain, edema, rash, headache, insomnia, hypertension, and thromboembolic disorders, including deep vein thrombosis and pulmonary embolism
- Estrogen use is associated with an increased risk of endometrial and breast cancer, gallbladder disease requiring surgery in postmenopausal women, thromboembolic disease, hepatic adenoma, and massive elevations in triglyceride levels that lead to pancreatitis in patients with a family history of lipoprotein metabolism
- Estrogens may increase the risk of depression

Adverse reactions to watch for

- Nausea, vomiting, diarrhea, weight gain, edema, rash, headache, insomnia, hypertension, thromboembolic disorders, endometrial and breast cancer, gallbladder disease, thromboembolic disease, hepatic adenoma, massive elevations in triglyceride levels that lead to pancreatitis, and depression

Interactions

- Penicillins, sulfonamides, and tetracyclines alter normal GI flora, decreasing the effects of estrogen
- Estrogens decrease the effects of barbiturates, anticonvulsants, antidiabetics, and oral anticoagulants
- Estrogens may increase the effects and risk of toxicity of corticosteroids
- Hydantoins may decrease the effects of estrogens and cause breakthrough bleeding, spotting, and pregnancy

Nursing responsibilities

- Assess the patient for edema; monitor blood pressure, weight, and cholesterol and triglyceride levels
- Teach the patient the appropriate administration technique (for oral, intravaginal, or transdermal use)
- Teach the patient about the importance of complying with therapy (for additional teaching tips, see *Teaching about estrogen replacement therapy*)
- Warn the patient not to smoke while taking these drugs because smoking increases the risk of thromboembolism (especially in women older than age 35)

Key nursing actions

- Assess for edema; monitor blood pressure, weight, and cholesterol and triglyceride levels.
- Warn not to smoke while taking these drugs because smoking increases the risk of thromboembolism.
- Ensure that the patient knows the procedure for missed doses and understands the need to use another form of contraception for that cycle.

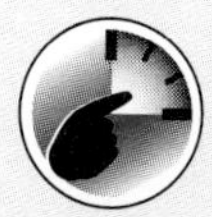

TIME-OUT FOR TEACHING

Teaching about estrogen replacement therapy

Include these topics in your teaching plan for the patient receiving estrogen replacement therapy.

- Medication regimen, including the drug's name, dosage, frequency, duration, and possible adverse effects
- Signs and symptoms to discuss with the physician, including headache, shortness of breath, chest pain, breast lumps, and calf tenderness or swelling
- Proper administration technique
- Cyclic nature of therapy
- Self-breast examination
- Follow-up care, including breast and pelvic examinations, Pap smears, and physician visits

Topics for patient discussion

- Therapy regimen
- Signs and symptoms
- Proper administration technique

- Advise the patient to receive routine breast, pelvic, and blood pressure examinations and Pap smears to detect adverse effects
- **Ensure that the patient taking hormonal contraceptives knows the procedure for missed doses and understands the need to use another form of contraception for that cycle**
- Advise a woman who suspects she is pregnant to notify her physician immediately
- **Urge women to notify their physician immediately if they experience pain in the groin or calves, sharp chest pain or sudden shortness of breath, abnormal bleeding, sudden severe headaches, dizziness, fainting, vision or speech disturbance, weakness in the arms or legs, severe abdominal pain, yellowing of the skin or eyes, or severe depression**

PROLACTIN SECRETION INHIBITORS

Key facts about prolactin secretion inhibitors

- Decrease the serum prolactin level
- Metabolized in liver
- Excreted primarily in feces

Mechanism of action

- Decrease the serum prolactin level in patients with hyperprolactinemia

Pharmacokinetics

- Absorption: Bromocriptine is poorly (about 28%) absorbed in the GI tract; bioavailability of cabergoline is unknown
- Distribution: Unlike cabergoline, bromocriptine is highly (90% to 96%) protein-bound to albumin
- Metabolism: Completely metabolized by the liver
- Excretion: Primarily excreted in the feces with minor excretion in the urine; the major route of excretion is in the bile

When to use prolactin secretion inhibitors

- Idiopathic or pituitary adenoma–induced hyperprolactinemia
- Hyperprolactinemia-associated dysfunctions
- Acromegaly
- Parkinson's disease

Drug examples

- Bromocriptine mesylate (Parlodel); cabergoline (Dostinex)

Indications

- These drugs are used to inhibit prolactin secretion in idiopathic or pituitary adenoma–induced hyperprolactinemia
- Parlodel is used to treat hyperprolactinemia-associated dysfunctions, including amenorrhea with or without galactorrhea, infertility, or hypogonadism
- Parlodel is also used to treat acromegaly and Parkinson's disease
- **Parlodel had been used to treat postpartum lactation, but this indication has been withdrawn by the manufacturer because of the risk of hypertension, stroke, and seizures; Parlodel should no longer be used for that indication**

When NOT to use prolactin secretion inhibitors

- Hypersensitivity
- Uncontrolled hypertension
- Severe ischemic heart disease
- Peripheral vascular disease

Contraindications and precautions

- These drugs are contraindicated in patients with hypersensitivity to ergot alkaloids
- **Cabergoline is contraindicated in patients with uncontrolled hypertension**

- Parlodel is also contraindicated in patients with severe ischemic heart disease or peripheral vascular disease

Adverse reactions

- These drugs may cause orthostatic and symptomatic hypotension
- Bromocriptine mesylate causes many adverse reactions, but they usually range from mild to moderate and include nausea, headache, dizziness, vertigo, fatigue, light-headedness, vomiting, abdominal cramps, nasal congestion, constipation, diarrhea, psychosis, and hypotension
- Long-term treatment with bromocriptine has been associated with pulmonary infiltrates, pleural effusion, and pleural thickening
- Cabergoline has a lower rate of adverse events; some common adverse events are headache, nausea, and vomiting

Adverse reactions to watch for

- Orthostatic and symptomatic hypotension, nausea, headache, dizziness, vertigo, fatigue, light-headedness, vomiting, abdominal cramps, nasal congestion, constipation, diarrhea, psychosis, hypotension, pulmonary infiltrates, pleural effusion, pleural thickening

Interactions

- Erythromycin may increase bromocriptine mesylate levels
- Sympathomimetics exacerbate the adverse effects of bromocriptine
- Phenothiazines decrease the efficacy of bromocriptine and cabergoline
- Cabergoline has additive hypotensive effects when given with antihypertensive medications

Nursing responsibilities

- Know that for patients being treated for amenorrhea and galactorrhea, bromocriptine suppresses galactorrhea and reinitiates normal ovulatory menstrual cycles, usually in 6 to 8 weeks; however, some patients may respond in as little as a few days, whereas others may take up to 8 months
- Pituitary evaluation must be performed before the start of treatment because bromocriptine has been associated with pituitary tumors
- Give bromocriptine with food or with meals
- Know that dizziness and fainting may occur, particularly following the first dose or if the patient stands up too quickly; instruct the patient to take the first dose lying down and to avoid sudden changes in posture, such as rising from a sitting position

Key nursing actions

- Know that for patients being treated for amenorrhea and galactorrhea, bromocriptine suppresses galactorrhea and reinitiates normal ovulatory menstrual cycles; some may respond in a few days, others may take up to 8 months.
- Know that dizziness and fainting may occur.

FERTILITY DRUGS (OVULATION STIMULANTS)

Mechanism of action

- Stimulate ovarian function by increasing levels of pituitary gonadotropins, which stimulates the maturation and endocrine activity of ovarian follicles and the subsequent development and function of the corpus luteum

Pharmacokinetics

- Absorption: Clomiphene is readily absorbed orally; follitropins have absorption-rate limitations and the absorption rate following I.M. and S.C. administration is slower than the excretion rate
- Distribution: Unknown
- Metabolism: Unknown
- Excretion: Excreted in the feces

Key facts about fertility drugs

- Stimulate ovarian function by increasing levels of pituitary gonadotropins
- Metabolism unknown
- Excreted in feces

When to use fertility drugs

- Infertility
- Follicle stimulation
- Spermatogenesis stimulation (with primary or secondary hypogonadotropic hypogonadism)
- Prepubertal cryptorchidism and hypogonadism
- Ovulation

When NOT to use fertility drugs

- Pregnancy
- Precocious puberty
- Prostatic carcinoma or other androgen-dependent neoplasm
- Allergies to HCG
- High gonadotropin levels (women)
- Normal or elevated gonadotropin levels (men)
- High levels of FSH
- Liver disease
- History of liver dysfunction
- Abnormal bleeding
- Organic intracranial lesion
- Ovarian cysts
- Uncontrolled thyroid or adrenal dysfunction

Adverse reactions to watch for

- Ovarian enlargement, cyst formation, hot flushes, dizziness, light-headedness, nausea, vomiting, bloating, abnormal uterine bleeding, pulmonary and vascular complications, adnexal torsion, breast pain, gynecomastia, mastitis, and abnormal liver enzyme levels

Drug examples

- Choriogonadotropin alfa (Ovidrel), clomiphene citrate (Clomid, Milophene, Serophene), follitropin alfa (Gonal-F), follitropin beta (Follistim), human chorionic gonadotropin (HCG [Chorex-5, Choron 10, Gonic, Pregnyl, Profasi]), human menopausal gonadotropin (HMG [Pergonal]), menotropins (Pergonal, Repronex), urofollitropin (Bravelle, Fertinex)

Indications

- To treat infertility secondary to anovulation (through stimulation of endocrine gland)
- For follicle stimulation in patients undergoing in vitro fertilization (IVF) or other assisted reproductive technology
- Pergonal (menotropins) only is used with concomitant human chorionic gonadotropin (HCG) in men for the stimulation of spermatogenesis with primary or secondary hypogonadotropic hypogonadism
- Urofollitropin may also be used to treat infertility in women with polycystic ovary syndrome
- Chorionic gonadotropin is used to treat prepubertal cryptorchidism and hypogonadism in males and to induce ovulation in women

Contraindications and precautions

- HCG is contraindicated in pregnant women and in patients with precocious puberty, prostatic carcinoma or other androgen-dependent neoplasm, or prior allergic reaction to HCG
- Menotropins are contraindicated in pregnant women and in women with high gonadotropin levels indicating primary ovarian failure, overt thyroid dysfunction, any cause of infertility other than anovulation, abnormal bleeding, ovarian cysts or enlargement not due to polycystic ovary syndrome, or organic intracranial lesion such as pituitary tumor
- Menotropins are contraindicated in men with normal gonadotropin levels, or elevated gonadotropin levels indicating primary testicular failure, and infertility disorders other than hypogonadotropic hypogonadism
- Follitropins are contraindicated in patients with high levels of FSH indicating primary ovarian failure, uncontrolled thyroid or adrenal dysfunction, infertility not due to anovulation, abnormal vaginal bleeding, ovarian cysts or enlargement not due to polycystic ovary syndrome, tumors of the breast, ovary, uterus, hypothalamus, or pituitary gland, and during pregnancy
- Clomiphene is contraindicated in patients with liver disease, history of liver dysfunction, abnormal bleeding, organic intracranial lesion, ovarian cysts, uncontrolled thyroid or adrenal dysfunction, and during pregnancy
- Use HCG cautiously in patients with epilepsy, migraine, asthma, or cardiac or renal disease because androgens may cause fluid retention

Adverse reactions

- **Using ovarian stimulants may result in multiple births, ovarian enlargement, and cyst formation**

- Ovarian stimulants may also cause hot flushes, dizziness, light-headedness, nausea, vomiting, bloating, and abnormal uterine bleeding
- Follitropins may also cause pulmonary and vascular complications and adnexal torsion as a complication of ovarian enlargement
- **In men, menotropin may cause breast pain, gynecomastia, mastitis, nausea, and abnormal liver enzyme levels**

Interactions

- None significant

Nursing responsibilities

- Instruct the patient in infertility measures and the importance of complying with therapy
- Offer emotional support
- Encourage compliance with follow-up diagnostic testing to evaluate drug effectiveness
- Warn the patient of the risk of ovarian hyperstimulation syndrome and multiple births with treatment

ABORTIFACIENTS

Mechanism of action

- Compete with progesterone at progesterone receptor sites, resulting in inactivity of progesterone and termination of pregnancy

Pharmacokinetics

- Absorption: Rapidly absorbed following oral administration
- Distribution: 98% protein-bound
- Metabolism: Primarily metabolized in the liver
- Excretion: Primarily excreted in the feces

Drug examples

- Mifepristone (Mifeprex), prostaglandins, carboprost tromethamine (Hemabate), dinoprostone (prostaglandin E_2, [Prostin E2])

Indications

- To terminate pregnancy
- Dinoprostone also is used for uterine content evacuation and for the management of nonmetastatic gestational trophoblastic disease (benign hydatidiform mole)

Contraindications and precautions

- Mifepristone is contraindicated in patients with IUD, ectopic pregnancy, adnexal mass, chronic adrenal failure, concurrent long-term corticosteroid therapy, hemorrhagic disorders, concurrent anticoagulation therapy, allergy to drug or other prostaglandin, or inherited prophyrias
- Prostaglandins are contraindicated in patients with hypersensitivity, acute pelvic inflammatory disease, and active cardiac, pulmonary, hepatic, or renal disease

Adverse reactions

- May cause nausea and vomiting, diarrhea, headache

Key nursing actions

- Instruct in infertility measures and the importance of complying with therapy.
- Warn of the risk of ovarian hyperstimulation syndrome and multiple births.

Key facts about abortifacients

- Compete with progesterone at progesterone receptor sites
- Result is termination of pregnancy
- Primarily metabolized in liver
- Primarily excreted in feces

When to use abortifacients

- Pregnancy termination
- Uterine content evacuation
- Nonmetastatic gestational trophoblastic disease management

When NOT to use abortifacients

- Ectopic pregnancy
- Adnexal mass
- IUD
- Chronic adrenal failure
- Concurrent long-term corticosteroid therapy
- Hemorrhagic disorders
- Concurrent anticoagulation therapy
- Drug allergy
- Inherited prophyrias
- Hypersensitivity
- Acute pelvic inflammatory disease
- Active cardiac, pulmonary, hepatic, or renal disease

Adverse reactions to watch for

- Nausea, vomiting, diarrhea, and headache

Key nursing actions

- Warn patient that surgical intervention may be needed in cases of incomplete abortion or severe bleeding.
- Explain that she may experience bleeding or spotting for 9 to 16 days after treatment.

Key facts about oxytocic drugs

- Enhance uterine mobility by stimulating uterine and smooth-muscle contraction
- Metabolism unknown
- Excreted through kidneys, liver, and mammary glands

When to use oxytocic drugs

- Postpartum hemorrhage
- Labor promotion
- Milk letdown reflex initiation
- Therapeutic abortion
- Uteroplacental respiratory reserve test

When NOT to use oxytocic drugs

- Obstetric emergencies
- Maternal hypertension
- Toxemia
- Significant cephalopelvic proportions
- Unfavorable fetal positions
- Fetal distress
- Drug hypersensitivity

Adverse reactions to watch for

- Nausea, vomiting, bradycardia, hypertension, and anaphylaxis; fetal: bradycardia, hypoxia, intracranial hemorrhage; maternal: tetanic contractions and arrhythmias

Interactions
- Don't use with oxytocics because oxytocic effects may be enhanced

Nursing responsibilities
- Explain to the patient that treatment with abortifacients requires three office visits
- **Warn the patient that surgical intervention may be needed in cases of incomplete abortion or severe bleeding; other measures may need to be taken to ensure complete abortion**
- Explain to the patient that she may experience bleeding or spotting for 9 to 16 days or up to 30 days after treatment; urge the patient to seek medical treatment if she experiences persistent moderate to heavy vaginal bleeding
- Once treatment is completed, teach the patient about the use of a contraceptive method that is appropriate for her

OBSTETRIC DRUGS

OXYTOCIC DRUGS

Mechanism of action
- Enhance uterine motility by directly stimulating uterine and smooth-muscle contraction

Pharmacokinetics
- Absorption: Immediate after I.M. or I.V. administration
- Distribution: Unknown
- Metabolism: Unknown
- Excretion: Eliminated through the kidneys, liver, and mammary glands

Drug examples
- Ergonovine maleate (Ergotrate Maleate), methylergonovine maleate (Methergine), oxytocin (Pitocin), prostaglandin E_2 (PGE_2 [Dinoprostone])

Indications
- To manage postpartum hemorrhage
- Oxytocin also is used to promote labor, initiate the milk letdown reflex, induce therapeutic abortion, and test uteroplacental respiratory reserve (unlabeled use)

Contraindications and precautions
- Contraindicated in obstetric emergencies, maternal hypertension, and toxemia
- Contraindicated in patients with significant cephalopelvic proportions, unfavorable fetal positions, fetal distress, or hypersensitivity to drug

Adverse reactions
- These drugs may cause nausea, vomiting, bradycardia, hypertension, and anaphylaxis

- Fetal adverse effects of oxytocin include bradycardia, hypoxia, and intracranial hemorrhage; maternal adverse effects of oxytocin include tetanic contractions and arrhythmias

Interactions

- Use of dopamine or other vasoconstrictors with ergonovine or methylergonovine may increase peripheral vasoconstriction
- Use of ergonovine or methylergonovine with a vasoconstrictor or regional anesthetic may cause severe hypertension

Nursing responsibilities

- **Oxytocin is given I.V. only when used to induce labor; I.V. oxytocin requires continuous monitoring and observation and a physician must be immediately available**
- Monitor the patient's blood pressure, pulse rate, urine output, uterine contractions, and vaginal bleeding
- Monitor the fetal heart rate
- Know that hypocalcemia may decrease the patient's response to ergonovine maleate; administer I.V. calcium salts, if necessary

LABOR SUPPRESSANTS (UTERINE RELAXANTS)

Mechanism of action

- Relax uterine muscles and decrease uterine contractions
- Exert beta-adrenergic agonist effects on uterine smooth muscles, thereby inhibiting uterine contractions

Pharmacokinetics

- Absorption: Administered I.V.
- Distribution: 100% bioavailable and 32% is protein-bound; drug crosses the placental barrier
- Metabolism: Unknown
- Excretion: Primarily excreted in the urine

Drug examples

- Terbutaline (Brethine)

Indications

- To prevent premature labor from 29 to 36 weeks of gestation

Contraindications and precautions

- Contraindicated in patients with ruptured membranes, abruptio placentae, hypertension, preeclampsia, fetal distress, or pregnancy of less than 20 weeks
- **Patients may develop transient cerebral ischemia, chorioamnionitis, and intrauterine growth retardation; use these drugs only if the benefits outweigh the risks**

Adverse reactions

- Maternal effects include widening pulse pressure, hypotension, tachycardia, and electrolyte imbalances

Key nursing actions

- Oxytocin is given I.V. only when inducing labor.
- I.V. oxytocin requires continuous monitoring and observations.
- Monitor the fetal heart rate.

Key facts about labor suppressants

- Relax uterine muscles
- Decrease uterine contractions
- Metabolism unknown
- Excreted primarily in urine

When to use labor suppressants

- Premature labor prevention

When NOT to use labor suppressants

- Ruptured membranes
- Abruptio placentae
- Hypertension
- Preeclampsia
- Fetal distress
- Pregnancy of less than 20 weeks
- Transient cerebral ischemia
- Chorioamnionitis
- Intrauterine growth retardation

Adverse reactions to watch for

- Maternal: widening pulse pressure, hypotension, tachycardia, electrolyte imbalances; fetal: increased heart rate, hypotension, and hypocalcemia

- Fetal effects include increased heart rate, hypotension, and hypocalcemia

Interactions

- Use of terbutaline with beta-adrenergic blockers interferes with the uterine-inhibiting action of terbutaline
- Use of terbutaline with corticosteroids may cause pulmonary edema

Nursing responsibilities

- **Place the patient in a left lateral recumbent position to promote venous return to the heart and decrease hypotension**
- Monitor the patient and fetus closely for adverse effects
- Know that the patient initially will receive the drug by the I.V. route but will be switched to oral administration when stable

Key nursing actions

- Place in left lateral recumbent position to promote venous return to the heart and decrease hypotension.
- Monitor patient and fetus closely.

GONADOTROPIN-RELEASING HORMONES

Mechanism of action

- These hormones are gonadotropin-releasing hormones (GnRH) agonists that at first stimulate the release of pituitary gonadotropins, LH and FSH, resulting in an increase in steroidogenesis
- Repeated doses inhibit the stimulatory effects on the pituitary gland and lead to a decreased secretion of gonadal steroids after about 4 weeks of therapy

Pharmacokinetics

- Absorption: Nafarelin is rapidly absorbed systemically after intranasal administration
- Distribution: About 80% protein-bound
- Metabolism: Unknown
- Excretion: Excreted in the urine and feces

Key facts about gonadotropin-releasing hormones

- GnRH agonists that at first stimulate release of pituitary gonadotropins, LH and FSH
- Result is steroidogenesis increase
- Repeated doses inhibit stimulatory effect on pituitary gland
- Metabolism unknown
- Excreted in urine and feces

Drug examples

- Gonadorelin (Lutrepulse), goserelin (Zoladex), histrelin acetate (Supprelin), leuprolide (Lupron), nafarelin acetate (Synarel)

Indications

- Leuprolide and nafarelin are used to treat endometriosis
- Nafarelin and histrelin are used to treat central precocious puberty
- Goserelin and leuprolide are used as palliative treatment for advanced prostatic cancer
- Gonadorelin is used to treat primary hypothalamic amenorrhea

When to use gonadotropin-releasing hormones

- Endometriosis
- Central precocious puberty
- Advanced prostatic cancer
- Primary hypothalamic amenorrhea

Contraindications and precautions

- Contraindicated in patients hypersensitive to GnRH-agonist, in those with undiagnosed abnormal vaginal bleeding, and in pregnant and breast-feeding women
- **Repeated uses aren't recommended for patients who have major risk factors for decreased bone mineral content, such as with alcoholism, drug use, or tobacco use, or a strong family history of osteoporosis**

When NOT to use gonadotropin-releasing hormones

- Drug hypersensitivity
- Undiagnosed abnormal vaginal bleeding
- Pregnancy
- Breast-feeding

- **Adverse reactions**
  - Hot flashes, headache, nausea, vomiting, constipation, emotional lability, vaginitis, and decreased libido
- **Interactions**
  - None reported
- **Nursing responsibilities**
  - Administer these drugs by the appropriate route: nafarelin, by nasal spray; leuprolide, by subcutaneous or I.M. injection; gonadorelin, by I.V. injection; goserelin, by subcutaneous injection
  - Monitor hydration status to prevent fluid loss from vomiting
  - **Closely monitor the patient's cardiac status during goserelin therapy because goserelin has been associated with cardiac complications, including heart failure and arrhythmias**

Adverse reactions to watch for

- Hot flashes, headache, nausea, vomiting, constipation, emotional lability, vaginitis, and decreased libido

Key nursing actions

- Monitor hydration status to prevent fluid loss from vomiting.
- Closely monitor cardiac status during goserelin therapy.

NCLEX CHECKS

It's never too soon to begin your NCLEX preparation. Now that you've reviewed this chapter, carefully read each of the following questions and choose the best answer. Then compare your responses to the correct answers.

1. A patient asks, "Why is the doctor prescribing danazol (Danocrine) for my endometriosis?" Your best answer would be that the drug:

☐ **A.** increases the activity of the ovaries.
☐ **B.** increases the production of estrogen.
☐ **C.** causes the body to release a luteinizing hormone (LH) surge.
☐ **D.** decreases the secretion of follicle-stimulating hormone (FSH) and LH.

2. A patient with metastatic breast cancer is prescribed testosterone, an androgenic steroid. Although androgenic and anabolic steroids produce similar effects, which rationale correctly describes how they differ?

☐ **A.** Androgenic steroids produce masculinizing effects; anabolic steroids build muscle mass.
☐ **B.** Androgenic steroids promote a positive nitrogen balance; anabolic steroids stimulate cellular protein synthesis.
☐ **C.** Androgenic steroids promote tissue growth; anabolic steroids stimulate the development of male sex characteristics.
☐ **D.** Androgenic steroids promote the development of female sex characteristics; anabolic steroids suppress their development.

3. You're giving a postmenopausal woman prescribed estrogen therapy. Which of the following adverse reactions should you include in your teaching plan?

☐ **A.** Renal calculi
☐ **B.** Uterine atony
☐ **C.** Deep-vein thrombosis
☐ **D.** Narrowing of the visual fields

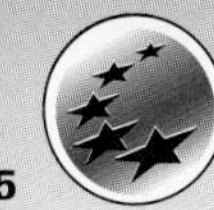

TOP 5

Items to study for your next test on drugs and the reproductive system

1. Mechanisms of action of androgens, estrogens, and progestins
2. Indications for male and female hormonal drugs
3. Common adverse effects of male and female hormonal drugs
4. Nursing responsibilities when administering male and female hormonal drugs
5. Patient teaching related to male and female hormonal drugs

4. A pregnant patient experiences fetal demise during the 30th week of gestation. She asks you why she's being given a prostaglandin E2 suppository at this time. You respond by saying prostaglandin suppositories:

- ☐ A. cause labor to start.
- ☐ B. prevent postpartum infections in cases like this.
- ☐ C. help relieve the pain when the baby is delivered.
- ☐ D. allow the patient to relax and decrease her anxiety.

5. Your patient is taking a hormonal oral contraceptive. You must instruct her about the possibility of decreased effectiveness of hormonal contraceptives if she's also taking:

- ☐ A. an anticoagulant.
- ☐ B. a benzodiazepine.
- ☐ C. a corticosteroid.
- ☐ D. a tetracycline.

6. The nurse is monitoring a patient who is receiving oxytocin (Pitocin) to induce labor. The nurse should be prepared for which of the following maternal adverse reactions?

Select all that apply:

- ☐ A. Hypertension
- ☐ B. Jaundice
- ☐ C. Dehydration
- ☐ D. Fluid overload
- ☐ E. Uterine tetany
- ☐ F. Bradycardia

ANSWERS AND RATIONALES

1. CORRECT ANSWER: D

Danazol is an antigonadotropin that suppresses the production of LH and FSH, reducing engorgement in the ectopic endometrial tissue and the accompanying pain. The drug decreases the activity of the ovaries, decreases estrogen production, and reduces LH.

2. CORRECT ANSWER: A

Androgenic steroids produce masculinizing effects; anabolic steroids build muscle mass. Androgenic steroids don't promote the development of female sex characteristics, a positive nitrogen balance, or tissue growth. Anabolic steroids don't suppress female sex characteristics, stimulate cellular protein synthesis, or stimulate the development of male sex characteristics.

3. CORRECT ANSWER: C

Estrogen therapy increasing clotting tendencies. If the woman has leg pain, redness, or swelling, she needs to call the physician because she may have developed deep-vein thrombosis. Also, you should warn her that smoking increases the risk of blood clots and that she should avoid smoking during drug therapy.

Estrogen therapy doesn't cause narrowing of the visual fields, uterine atony, or renal calculi.

4. CORRECT ANSWER: A
Prostaglandin vaginal suppositories or gel are used to induce labor in cases of second- or third-trimester fetal demise. They stimulate smooth muscle and cause the uterus to contract. They're also sometimes used before induction of normal pregnancies. Prostaglandin has no analgesic, anxiolytic, or antimicrobial effects.

5. CORRECT ANSWER: D
Tetracycline, ampicillin, and penicillin V cause alterations in the normal flora of the GI tract that lead to a decreased efficacy of the contraceptive agent and may cause the woman to become pregnant. The other drugs interact with hormonal contraceptives, but these agents, not the hormonal contraceptives, are affected, resulting in either increased or decreased drug levels.

6. CORRECT ANSWER: A, D, E
Adverse reactions to oxytocin in the mother include hypertension, fluid overload, and uterine tetany. The antidiuretic effect of oxytocin increases renal reabsorption of water, leading to fluid overload — not dehydration. Jaundice and bradycardia are adverse reactions that may occur in the neonate. Tachycardia, not bradycardia, is reported as a maternal adverse reaction.

16

Drugs and the integumentary system

LEARNING OBJECTIVES

After studying this chapter, you should be able to:

- Describe the mechanisms of action of various topical drugs.
- List common adverse effects of topical drugs.
- Identify nursing responsibilities when administering topical drugs.
- Discuss appropriate teaching for the patient receiving a topical drug.

CHAPTER OVERVIEW

This chapter reviews the fundamental mechanism of action and indications for topical drugs. Applied to the skin, topical drugs are used to treat various dermatologic conditions. In the form of lotions and ointments, they include emollients, keratolytics, antibacterial drugs, antifungals, antivirals, antiparasitics, anti-inflammatories, debriding drugs, antipruritics, and acne products.

Nursing responsibilities include thoroughly cleaning the affected area (including removing the remains of previously applied medication), teaching the patient the importance of using topical drugs properly, and providing necessary emotional support to the patient with a skin disorder.

ANATOMY AND PHYSIOLOGY

Anatomy

- The integumentary system consists of the skin and its derivatives, such as hair, nails, the sudoriferous (sweat) glands, sebaceous (oil) glands, and ceruminous glands
- The skin is the largest and most visible organ of the body; every square inch of skin contains blood vessels, nerves, sweat glands, oil glands, sensory receptors, and cells
- The epidermis is the skin's surface layer and the body's outermost protective covering
- The dermis lies just below the epidermis and constitutes the bulk of the skin
- Beneath the dermis is subcutaneous tissue, also called the hypodermis or the superficial fascia; subcutaneous tissue isn't skin but is loose connective tissue that attaches the skin to underlying structures

Physiology

- Chemically, acidic skin secretions inhibit bacteria from multiplying on the body's surface
- Physically, keratinized cells of the epidermis, hair, and nails provide a barrier to invading organisms
- Biologically, the skin contains macrophage-like Langerhans' cells that attack bacteria and viruses
- When exposed to ultraviolet light, the skin converts cholesterol to vitamin D
- Thermoregulation is a homeostatic process whereby the skin maintains the body's temperature at about 98.6° F (37° C)
  - Thermoregulation is a negative feedback mechanism
  - When skin receptors sense a temperature stimulus (heat or cold), they send impulses to the control center of the brain
  - The brain transmits impulses to effector organs (sweat glands and blood vessels)
  - The effector organs respond accordingly to the brain's message
    - When the body is hot, the sweat glands produce perspiration and the blood vessels dilate
    - Evaporation of sweat from the surface dissipates heat; vasodilation brings more warm blood to the skin, where it's cooled
    - When the body is cold, blood vessels constrict to prevent heat loss
- Nutrition and hormones influence hair growth, hair distribution, and sebaceous gland secretions

Function

- The skin has six major functions
  - To protect the body chemically, physically, and biologically
  - To excrete waste products from the body
  - To help regulate body temperature
  - To provide cutaneous sensation
  - To promote vitamin D synthesis

A&P highlights

- The integumentary system consists of the skin and its derivatives, such as hair, nails, and sweat, sebaceous, and ceruminous glands.
- The epidermis is the skin's surface layer and the body's outermost protective covering.
- The dermis lies just below the epidermis and constitutes the bulk of the skin.
- Beneath the dermis is subcutaneous tissue that attaches the skin to underlying structures.
- Chemically, acidic skin secretions inhibit bacteria from multiplying on the body's surface.
- Keratinized cells of the epidermis, hair, and nails provide a barrier to invading organisms.
- Macrophage-like Langerhans' cells attack bacteria and viruses.
- The skin maintains body temperature at about 98.6° F (37° C) via thermoregulation.
- When the body is hot, sweat glands produce perspiration and blood vessels dilate.
- When the body is cold, blood vessels constrict to prevent heat loss.

Functions of skin

- Protects the body
- Excretes waste products
- Helps regulate body temperature
- Provides cutaneous sensations
- Promotes vitamin D synthesis
- Acts as a reservoir for blood

- To act as a reservoir for blood
- The hair protects the body from heat loss and ultraviolet rays, shields the eyes, and helps keep dust out of the upper respiratory tract
- Nails protect the ends of fingers and toes
- Sudoriferous glands help maintain normal body temperatures
- Sebaceous glands secrete sebum that softens and lubricates the hair and skin, impedes water loss from the skin, and acts as a bacteriocide
- Ceruminous glands line the external ear canal; ceruminous and sebaceous gland secretions combine to form cerumen (earwax)

TOPICAL DRUGS

Key facts about topical drugs

- Allow skin to retain water
- Break down protein in keratin, causing a loss of the stratum corneum skin layer
- Bactericidal or bacteriostatic
- Kill or inhibit growth of fungi and viruses
- Kill parasitic arthropods
- Decrease inflammation and itching and cause vasoconstriction
- Digest necrotic collagenous tissue
- Relieve itching
- Clean and dry skin and reduce the size and activity of sebaceous glands
- Metabolism varies by drug
- Excretion varies by drug

Mechanism of action

- Emollients allow the skin to retain water
- Keratolytics break down protein in keratin, causing a loss of the stratum corneum skin layer
- Antibacterial drugs kill (bactericidal) or inhibit the growth (bacteriostatic) of susceptible bacteria
- Antifungals kill or inhibit the growth of susceptible fungi
- Antivirals kill or inhibit the growth of susceptible viruses
- Antiparasitics kill parasitic arthropods
- Anti-inflammatories decrease inflammation and itching and cause vasoconstriction
- Debriding and wound-healing agents digest necrotic collagenous tissue, thereby removing the substances necessary for bacterial growth and allowing better access to the site for antibodies, leukocytes, and anti-infectives
- Antipruritics relieve itching of the skin and mucous membranes
- Acne products clean and dry the skin (cleaner and antiseptic drugs), reduce bacteria that cause infection (antibiotics), and reduce the size and activity of sebaceous glands (isotretinoin)

Pharmacokinetics

- Absorption: Varies with individual drug
  - Some topical drugs are systemically absorbed through the skin
  - Some are minimally absorbed or not absorbed at all
- Distribution: Varies with individual drug.
- Metabolism: Varies with individual drug
- Excretion: Varies with individual drug; may be excreted in the urine and feces

Drug examples

- Emollients: lanolin, mineral oil
- Keratolytics and antipsoriatics: resorcinol, salicylic acid (Oxy Clean, PROPApH Astringent, Clearasil, Salacid, Stri-Dex Pads), coal tar preparations (AquaTar, Estar, Fototar, Oxipor VHC, Polytar, PsoriGel)
- Antibacterial drugs: bacitracin (Baciguent); gentamicin sulfate (Garamycin), mafenide acetate (Sulfamylon), neomycin sulfate (My-

ciguent), silver sulfadiazine (Silvadene); neomycin sulfate, polymyxin B, and bacitracin combination (Neosporin); neomycin sulfate, gramicidin, and polymyxin B combination
- Antifungals: clotrimazole (Lotrimin, Mycelex), griseofulvin (Fulvicin-U/F, Grifulvin, Grisactin), ketoconazole (Nizoral), miconazole nitrate (Monistat-Derm, Micatin), nystatin (Mycostatin)
- Antivirals: acyclovir (Zovirax), penciclovir (Denavir)
- Antiparasitics: crotamiton (Eurax), lindane (G-well), malathion (Ovide), permethrin (Nix, Elimite, Acticin), pyrethrin (RID)
- Anti-inflammatories: betamethasone valerate (Valisone), coal-tar (Fototar, Balnetar), dexamethasone (Decaderm, Decadron), hydrocortisone (Cort-Dome), triamcinolone (Aristocort, Kenalog)
- Debriding and wound-healing drugs: becaplermin (Regranex), Chlorophyll derivatives (Chloresium), dextranomer (Debrisan), trypsin (Granulex)
- Antipruritics: calamine lotion, cyproheptadine (Periactin), diphenhydramine (Benadryl), oatmeal (Aveeno Colloidal)
- Acne products: antibiotics (clindamycin [Cleocin T], erythromycin [Ery-Derm], tetracycline [Topicycline]), cleaners/antiseptic drugs (azelaic acid [Azelex], benzoyl peroxide, isotretinoin [Accutane]), tretinoin [Retin-A])

Indications

- Emollients are used to lubricate and moisturize the skin to treat dryness and itching
- Keratolytics and antipsoriatics are used to treat superficial fungal infections, psoriasis, seborrheic dermatitis, corns, and calluses
- Antibacterial drugs fight bacterial skin infections; mafenide and silver sulfadiazine are used to treat burn wounds
- Antifungals are used to treat fungal skin infections
- Antivirals are used to treat types 1 and 2 herpes simplex virus infections
- Antiparasitics are used to treat scabies (mites), pediculosis (lice), and their eggs
- Anti-inflammatories are used to treat dermatitis and allergic skin reactions
- Debriding drugs are used to treat and clean decubitus ulcers, venous and peripheral vascular ulcers, burns, infected traumatic or surgical wounds, and other skin injuries
- Antipruritics are used to treat pruritus
- Acne products are used to treat acne vulgaris

Contraindications and precautions

- These drugs are contraindicated in patients with hypersensitivity to the drugs or their components
- **Mafenide, silver sulfadiazine, isotretinoin, and tretinoin are contraindicated in pregnant and breast-feeding women**

Adverse reactions

- All topical drugs, especially antiacne agents, may cause skin irritation

When to use topical drugs

- Dryness and itching
- Psoriasis
- Seborrheic dermatitis
- Corns
- Calluses
- Bacterial and fungal skin infections
- Burns
- Types 1 and 2 herpes simplex virus infections
- Scabies
- Pediculosis
- Dermatitis
- Allergic skin reactions
- Decubitus ulcers
- Venous and peripheral vascular ulcers
- Infected traumatic or surgical wounds
- Pruritus
- Acne vulgaris

When NOT to use topical drugs

- Hypersensitivity
- Pregnancy
- Breast-feeding

Adverse reactions to watch for

- Skin irritation; metabolic acidosis; hemolytic anemia; bone marrow suppression; leukopenia; behavioral changes; fluid and electrolyte imbalances; impaired wound healing; suppressed immune response; nosebleeds; burning, redness, or itching of the eyes; scaling, redness, burning, or pain of the lips; photosensitivity reactions

Key nursing actions

- Before applying a topical drug, assess skin and remove remains of previously applied medication.
- Use aseptic technique when applying medications to open lesions.
- As appropriate, provide psychological support.

- **Mafenide may cause metabolic acidosis, hemolytic anemia, and bone marrow suppression**
- **Silver sulfadiazine may cause leukopenia**
- Anti-inflammatories may cause systemic adverse effects with absorption of large quantities (behavioral changes, fluid and electrolyte imbalances, impaired wound healing, suppressed immune response)
- Acne products
  - **These drugs may cause nosebleeds; burning, redness, or itching of the eyes; and scaling, redness, burning, or pain of the lips**
  - **Isotretinoin and tretinoin may cause photosensitivity reactions**

Interactions

- No significant drug interactions have been reported
- Increased use of antiacne products may increase skin irritation

Nursing responsibilities

- Before applying a topical drug to treat a skin disorder, assess the skin lesion and remove the remains of previously applied medication
- Use aseptic technique when applying medication to open lesions
- As appropriate, provide psychological support to the patient with a skin disorder
- Teach the patient how to apply the medication
- Teach the patient that topical drugs are for external use only and to avoid contact with the eyes
- **Warn women not to breast-feed while using mafenide or silver sulfadiazine**
- Assess respiratory status and blood pH level for signs of metabolic acidosis in patients using mafenide
- **Family members of a patient with parasites may also need to be treated with antiparasitics to control spread of infestation**
- Follow these guidelines when applying acne products
  - Clean the affected area before applying the drug
  - **Advise the patient using isotretinoin or tretinoin to apply sunscreen and wear protective clothing to prevent photosensitivity reactions**
  - **Advise women using isotretinoin or tretinoin to use contraception (severe fetal abnormalities may occur in pregnant women using these drugs); all patients should be instructed not to give blood during or for 30 days after therapy (to prevent pregnant women from receiving the blood)**
- Teach the patient using topical tetracycline to be careful to cover the entire affected area (for additional teaching tips, see *Teaching about acne products*)

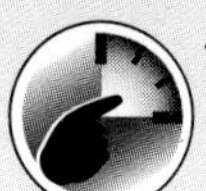

TIME-OUT FOR TEACHING

Teaching about acne products

Include these topics in your teaching plan for the patient receiving an acne product.

- Medication regimen, including the drug's name, dosage, frequency, duration, and possible adverse effects
- Signs and symptoms to discuss with the physician
- Proper administration technique
- Skin care measures
- Normal skin reactions
- Follow-up care, including physician visits

Topics for patient discussion

- Medication regimen, including proper administration
- Signs and symptoms to discuss with the physician
- Skin care measures
- Normal skin reactions
- Follow-up care

NCLEX CHECKS

It's never too soon to begin your NCLEX preparation. Now that you've reviewed this chapter, carefully read each of the following questions and choose the best answer. Then compare your responses to the correct answers.

1. Your patient has third-degree burns of the upper torso. The treatment plan includes applying mafenide (Sulfamylon) 10% cream to the burn twice daily. After three applications of the cream, you note a significant increase in the patient's respiratory rate. Arterial blood gas analysis shows the following values: pH, 7.30; $Paco_2$, 35 mm Hg; Pao_2, 90 mg Hg; and HCO_3^-, 10 mEq/L. Based on these findings, which acid-base disturbance has occurred as a result of Sulfamylon therapy?

☐ **A.** Metabolic acidosis
☐ **B.** Metabolic alkalosis
☐ **C.** Respiratory acidosis
☐ **D.** Respiratory alkalosis

2. A patient has had athlete's foot for 12 weeks that hasn't responded to undecylenic acid (Desenex). Which of the following drugs would you anticipate as the most appropriate at this time?

☐ **A.** Aluminum acetate (Domeboro) soaks
☐ **B.** Hydrocortisone cream (Cortaid)
☐ **C.** Miconazole cream (Micatin)
☐ **D.** Neomycin ointment (Neosporin)

3. While obtaining a history from the parents of a 4-year-old child, you discover the child has been recently treated with permethrin (Nix). Which of the following nursing actions should you do in response to this information?

☐ **A.** Carefully check the hair and scalp.
☐ **B.** Obtain a stool sample for ova and parasites.
☐ **C.** Assess the child for age-appropriate cognitive ability and motor development.
☐ **D.** Put on a mask and sterile gown to keep the child from getting a respiratory infection.

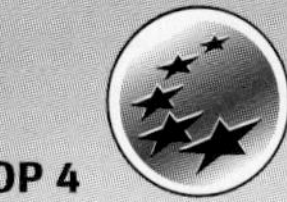

TOP 4

Items to study before your next test on drugs and the integumentary system

1. Mechanisms of action of various topical drugs
2. Common adverse effects of topical drugs
3. Nursing responsibilities when administering topical drugs
4. Teaching for the patient receiving a topical drug

4. Your patient has a viral infection. You expect the physician to prescribe which dermatologic agent?

- ☐ A. Acyclovir (Zovirax)
- ☐ B. Bacitracin (Baciguent)
- ☐ C. Hydrocortisone (Acticort)
- ☐ D. Silver sulfadiazine (Silvadene)

5. When applying a dermatologic agent, what's the first and last thing you should do?

- ☐ A. Wash your hands.
- ☐ B. Check the medication label.
- ☐ C. Keep the medication in a cool place.
- ☐ D. Wash the affected area with soap and water.

6. A patient is admitted to the burn unit with third-degree burns of his left leg. Silver sulfadiazine (Silvadene) 1% cream is applied to the burn twice daily. What abnormal laboratory findings can result from therapy with silver sulfadiazine?

- ☐ A. Decreased blood pH
- ☐ B. Decreased sodium level
- ☐ C. Increased blood glucose level
- ☐ D. Decreased white blood cell (WBC) count

7. A patient returns from the operating room with a partial-thickness skin graft on her left arm. The donor tissue was taken from her left hip. In planning her immediate postoperative care, which of the following interventions should the nurse include?

Select all that apply:

- ☐ A. Change the dressing every 8 hours on the graft site.
- ☐ B. Elevate the left arm and provide complete rest of the grafted area.
- ☐ C. Administer pain medication every 4 hours as ordered for pain in donor site.
- ☐ D. Perform range-of-motion (ROM) exercises to the left arm every 4 hours.
- ☐ E. Monitor the pulse in the left arm every 4 hours.
- ☐ F. Encourage the patient to ambulate as desired the first postoperative day.

ANSWERS AND RATIONALES

1. CORRECT ANSWER: A

Sulfamylon is a carbonic anhydrase inhibitor and retards the production of the enzyme that breaks down carbonic acid. Thus, it increases carbonic acid levels in the body and causes metabolic acidosis. The increased respiratory rate is a compensatory mechanism to try to reduce the $Paco_2$ level. The less-than-normal pH and HCO_3^- (bicarbonate) levels are consistent with metabolic acidosis.

2. Correct answer: C

Miconazole, a broad-spectrum antifungal, should be more effective against the organism causing this problem than undecylenic acid. Hydrocortisone isn't indicated as the sole agent for fungal infections because it doesn't kill the organism and may compromise the immune response. Soaks with aluminum acetate, an astringent, may help with the itching but won't effectively treat the fungus. Neomycin is an antibacterial, and therefore won't be effective against this fungal infection.

3. Correct answer: A

Permethrin is a topical agent that's used to treat head lice and scabies in children and adults. A careful examination of the patient's hair and scalp is indicated. The drug has no effect on intestinal parasites. Assessing the child for mental ability and motor development level is an appropriate action, but it isn't related to the drug's effects. It isn't necessary to use a mask and sterile gown with this patient.

4. Correct answer: A

Acyclovir is an antiviral dermatologic agent. Bacitracin and silver sulfadiazine are both antibacterial agents. Hydrocortisone is an anti-inflammatory.

5. Correct answer: A

While standard precautions require gloves when touching broken or excoriated skin, hand washing is still imperative before and after applying the medication to the skin. The medication label should be checked before the procedure begins. It's important to keep the medication in a cool area, but that isn't an action at these points. Soap and water are often detrimental to the skin being treated, and washing the area after applying the agent would wash away the drug.

6. Correct answer: D

Leukopenia (a decrease in WBC count) commonly occurs with the initiation of silver sulfadiazine therapy. The WBC count usually returns to normal after the first few days of therapy. Acid-base disturbances and changes in blood pH aren't associated with silver sulfadiazine therapy. The drug doesn't interfere with blood glucose or sodium levels.

7. Correct answer: B, C, E

The left arm should be elevated to reduce edema. Complete rest of the arm is needed to allow the graft to adhere. The donor site is usually more painful than the graft site and the patient will require pain medication to obtain relief. Because adequate circulation is needed for graft healing, it's important to monitor for pulse presence. Changing the dressing every 8 hours, performing ROM exercises, and ambulating are inappropriate because postoperative graft sites require immobilization for 3 to 5 days.

Drugs and the sensory system

LEARNING OBJECTIVES

After studying this chapter, you should be able to:

- Describe the mechanisms of action of ophthalmic and otic drugs.
- Explain the rationales for using anti-infectives, anti-inflammatories, anesthetics, lubricants, miotics, beta-adrenergic blockers, mydriatics, and cycloplegics to treat eye disorders.
- List common adverse effects of ophthalmic and otic drugs.
- Compare the correct technique for instilling eardrops in children to the technique used with adults.
- Know the proper administration of the different types of eye medications.
- Identify nursing responsibilities when administering ophthalmic and otic drugs.
- Discuss appropriate teaching for the patient who is receiving an ophthalmic or otic drug.

CHAPTER OVERVIEW

Ophthalmic drugs are applied onto the conjunctival sac. These drugs may be anti-infective, anti-inflammatory, anesthetic, lubricating, miotic, mydriatic, cycloplegic, or diuretic. Generally, mydriatic drugs are contraindicated in glaucoma. Nursing responsibilities focus on proper drug administration, effective patient teaching, and promotion of compliance with therapy.

Otic medications (also called aural medications) help to treat infection and inflammation of the ear, remove excess cerumen, and provide anesthesia. Antihistamines and decongestants may help to clear obstruction of a eustachian tube. Locally instilled otic medications may be administered to treat pain associated with infection or to reduce excess cerumen. For locally instilled otic medications, nursing responsibilities may include warming the drops to room temperature before administration.

ANATOMY AND PHYSIOLOGY

Anatomy

- The sensory system includes vision, hearing, equilibrium, smell, and taste (the special senses) and touch, pressure, temperature, and pain (the general senses); the focus of this chapter is on vision, hearing, and equilibrium
- The eyes are complex, sensory organs for vision
  - The eyes are spherical complex structures composed of three layers of tissues (the cornea and sclera, a middle choroid coat, and an inner retina) and a lens
  - The retina contains receptor cells (rods and cones)
  - The space between the cornea and the lens is divided by the iris into the anterior and posterior chambers
  - These chambers contain aqueous humor, a clear, watery fluid
    - Aqueous humor flows into the Schlemm's canal
    - **If aqueous humor secretion doesn't balance with absorption, intraocular pressure in the anterior chamber may build up, which may lead to vision impairment and loss when the pressure is transmitted to the vitreous humor in the posterior cavity, thereby damaging the retina**
  - The accessory structures of the eye include the eyebrows, eyelids, eyelashes, conjunctivae, lacrimal glands, and eye muscles
    - The eyebrows, eyelids, and eyelashes keep debris from entering the eye
    - The conjunctivae are thin vascular membranes that line the inner surface of the eyelids and sclerae
    - The lacrimal glands discharge fluid secretions to moisten the conjunctivae
    - The eye muscles are paired and work together to perform eye movement
- The ears consist of the external (outer) ear, the middle ear, and the inner ear
  - The external ear consists of the auricle (pinna) and the external auditory canal
  - The middle ear (or the tympanic cavity) is a mucosa-lined structure that contains three small bones called the malleus (hammer), stapes (stirrup), and incus (anvil)
    - The malleus is attached to the tympanic membrane
    - The stapes is attached to the oval window

A&P highlights

- The sensory system includes vision, hearing, equilibrium, smell, taste, touch, pressure, temperature, and pain.
- The eyes are complex, sensory organs for vision composed of three layers of tissues and a lens.
- The accessory structures of the eye include the eyebrows, eyelids, eyelashes, conjunctivae, lacrimal glands, and eye muscles.
- The eyebrows, eyelids, and eyelashes keep debris from entering the eye.
- The conjunctivae line the inner surface of the eyelids and sclerae.
- The lacrimal glands discharge fluid secretions to moisten the conjunctivae.
- Eye muscles allow eye movement.
- The external ear consists of the auricle and the external auditory canal.
- The middle ear is a mucosa-lined structure that contains three small bones: the malleus, stapes, and incus.
- The inner ear consists of the vestibule, semicircular canals, and cochlea.
- When stimulated, the eye receptors collect light waves and transmit them as nerve impulses along the visual pathways to the brain, which translates them into images.
- The eye with normal refractive powers can form clear images of an object 20 feet away.
- When stimulated, the ear receptors gather sound waves and transmit them as nerve impulses to the brain; the brain interprets these impulses as hearing.

- The incus is located between the malleus and the stapes and articulates with these two structures when vibrations from the eardrum to the fluid of the inner ear transmit; the vibration excites receptor nerve endings in the inner ear
- The inner ear, also known as the osseus canal, consists of the vestibule, semicircular canals, and cochlea

Physiology

- When stimulated, the eye receptors collect light waves and transmit them as nerve impulses along the visual pathways to the brain, which translates them into images
  - An image forms on the retina when light stimulates the rods and cones
  - The eye with normal refractive powers can form clear images of an object 20 feet away
  - The eyes must make many changes, such as accommodation, papillary constriction, and eye convergence, to adapt and form clear images of objects that are closer than 20 feet (near vision)
  - Binocular vision contributes to depth perception, that is, the ability to judge relative distances of objects
- When stimulated, the ear receptors gather sound waves and transmit them as nerve impulses to the brain; the brain interprets these impulses as hearing
- The sense of equilibrium is controlled by the semicircular canals of the inner ear

Function

- The eye is for vision
  - The rods are photoreceptors that provide vision when it's dark
  - The cones provide colored vision when it is light
- The ear is for hearing and maintaining balance
  - The external ear collects sound
  - The middle ear conducts sound
  - The inner ear contains structures that transmit sound waves and maintain equilibrium

Functions of eye structures

- Rods are photoreceptors that provide vision when it's dark.
- Cones provide colored vision when it is light.

Functions of ear structures

- External ear collects sound.
- Middle ear conducts sound.
- Inner ear contains structures that transmit sound waves and maintain equilibrium.

OPHTHALMIC DRUGS

Mechanism of action

- Anti-infectives kill or inhibit growth of susceptible bacteria, fungi, and viruses
- Anti-inflammatories control inflammation, thereby reducing vision loss and scarring
- Anesthetics produce corneal anesthesia
- Lubricants replace tears or add moisture to the eye
- Topical ophthalmic drugs used to treat glaucoma achieve their effects by opening the anterior chamber angle and increasing the outflow or decreasing the production of aqueous humor

- Systemic ophthalmic drugs used to treat glaucoma decrease aqueous humor production or reduce intraocular pressure by increasing intravascular osmotic pressure, creating an osmotic gradient that draws fluid from the eye
- Miotics reduce intraocular pressure by constricting the pupil, contracting ciliary muscles, opening the anterior chamber angle, and increasing outflow of aqueous humor
  - Miotic cholinergic agonists reduce intraocular pressure by mimicking the action of acetylcholine
  - Miotic acetylcholinesterase inhibitors reduce intraocular pressure by inhibiting the action of cholinesterase
- Beta-adrenergic blockers reduce intraocular pressure by decreasing sympathetic impulses to the eye and decreasing aqueous humor production without affecting accommodation or pupil size
- Mydriatics and cycloplegics dilate and paralyze the pupil
  - Cholinergic blockers (anticholinergics) inhibit the parasympathetic nervous system, producing mydriasis (pupil dilation) and cycloplegia
  - Adrenergic agonists mimic the actions of the sympathetic nervous system, causing mydriasis
- Antiallergic drugs prevent the release of histamine, thereby diminishing the allergic response
- Diuretics reduce aqueous humor production and decrease intraocular pressure
  - Carbonic anhydrase inhibitors decrease intraocular pressure by decreasing aqueous humor production
  - Osmotic agents decrease intraocular pressure by reducing the volume of vitreous humor

Pharmacokinetics

- Absorption: Some drugs are systemically absorbed
- Distribution: Varies with each drug; may penetrate the cornea, conjunctiva, and aqueous humor
- Metabolism: Varies with each drug
- Excretion: Varies with each drug; some anti-infectives are excreted through the nasolacrimal duct while the excretion of other drugs is unknown

Drug examples

- Anti-infectives
  - Antibacterial drugs: bacitracin (AK-Tracin), chloramphenicol (Chloromycetin), ciprofloxacin (Ciloxan), erythromycin (Ilotycin Ophthalmic), gatifloxacin (Zymar), gentamicin (Garamycin, Gentak), levofloxacin (Quixin), moxifloxacin (Vigamox), neomycin sulfate (AK-Spore), ofloxacin (Ocuflox), polymyxin B sulfate, sulfacetamide (Bleph-10, Sulamyd), sulfisoxazole (Gantrisin Ophthalmic), and tobramycin (Tobrex)
  - Antifungals: amphotericin B (Fungizone) and natamycin (Natacyn)

Key facts about ophthalmic drugs

- Kill or inhibit growth of susceptible bacteria, fungi, and viruses
- Control inflammation, thereby reducing vision loss and scarring
- Produce corneal anesthesia
- Replace tears or add moisture to the eye
- Reduce intraocular pressure
- Dilate and paralyze the pupil
- Diminish allergic response
- Reduce aqueous humor production
- Metabolism varies by drug
- Excretion varies by drug

- Antivirals: fomivirsen (Vitravene), trifluridine (Viroptic), and vidarabine (Vira-A)

- Anti-inflammatories: dexamethasone sodium phosphate (Decadron Phosphate Ophthalmic), diclofenac (Voltaren Ophthalmic), fluorometholone (FML), flurbiprofen sodium (Ocufen Liquifilm), ketorolac (Acular), Loteprednol (Lotemax), medrysone (HMS), prednisolone acetate (Pred-Forte), suprofen (Profenal), combination products, corticosteroids with antibiotics (such as dexamethasone and neomycin [Maxitrol])
- Anesthetics: proparacaine (Ophthaine), tetracaine (Pontocaine)
- Lubricants: hydroxypropyl cellulose (Lacrisert), petroleum-based ointment, polyvinyl alcohol for hard contact lenses (artificial tears [Liquifilm Tears, Tears Naturale])
- Miotics
  - Cholinergic agonists (direct-acting): acetylcholine, carbachol (Carboptic), and pilocarpine hydrochloride (Isopto Carpine)
  - Acetylcholinesterase inhibitors: physostigmine, demecarium bromide (Humorsol)
- Beta-adrenergic blockers: betaxolol (Betoptic), carteolol (Ocupress), levobetaxolol (Betaxon), levobunolol (Betagan), metipranolol (OptiPranolol), timolol maleate (Timoptic)
- Mydriatics and cycloplegics
  - Cholinergic blockers: atropine sulfate (Isopto Atropine), cyclopentolate (Cyclogyl), homatropine (Isopto Homatropine), scopolamine (Isopto Hyoscine) and tropicamide (Mydriacyl)
  - Adrenergic agonists: dipivefrin (Propine), epinephrine borate (Epinal), epinephrine hydrochloride (Epifrin), hydroxyamphetamine (Paredrine), and phenylephrine hydrochloride (Neo-Synephrine)
- Mast cell stabilizers: cromolyn sodium (Crolom), lodoxamide tromethamine (Alomide), nedocromil (Alocril), pemirolast potassium (Alamast); H1-receptor agonist antiallergy drug example: azelastine hydrochloride (Optivar), emedastine difumarate (Emadine); ketotifen fumarate (Zaditor); levocabastine hydrochloride (Livostin); olopatadine (Patanol)
- Diuretics
  - Carbonic anhydrase inhibitors: acetazolamide (Diamox), brinzolamide (Azopt), dichlorphenamide (Daranide), dorzolamide (Trusopt), methazolamide
  - Osmotic agents: glycerin (Osmoglyn), isosorbide (Ismotic)

Indications

- Anti-infectives are used to treat various infections
  - Antibacterial drugs are used to treat susceptible ocular bacterial infections
  - Antifungals are used to treat susceptible ocular fungal infections
  - Antivirals are used to treat susceptible ocular viral infections
- Anti-inflammatories are used to treat nonpyogenic inflammatory ocular conditions

When to use ophthalmic drugs

- Susceptible ocular bacterial, fungal, or viral infections
- Nonpyogenic inflammatory ocular conditions
- Anesthesia
- Dilation and lubrication for eye examination or surgery
- Glaucoma
- Inflammatory eye conditions
- Adhesion prevention
- Allergic ocular disorders
- Allergic conjunctivitis and itching

- Anesthetics are used for anesthesia during eye examinations and eye surgery
- Lubricants are used to treat keratitis, to moisten contact lenses or artificial eyes, as a tear replacement, or to protect the eye during surgery or diagnostic procedures
- Miotics are used to treat chronic open-angle glaucoma and acute and chronic angle-closure glaucoma
- Beta-adrenergic blockers are used to treat glaucoma
  - Betaxolol, levobunolol, and timolol are used to treat chronic open-angle glaucoma
  - Timolol is also used to treat aphakic glaucoma
- Mydriatics and cycloplegics are used to treat inflammatory eye conditions, to prevent adhesions, to dilate the pupils during eye examinations, and to prepare the patient for surgery
- Mast cell stabilizers are used to treat allergic ocular disorders and symptomatic itching caused by allergic conjunctivitis
- Diuretics are used to treat glaucoma and to prepare the patient for surgery

Contraindications and precautions

- Anti-inflammatory ophthalmic drugs are contraindicated in acute eye infections
- Miotics are contraindicated in secondary glaucoma, acute iritis, and inflammatory diseases
- Mydriatics are contraindicated in angle-closure glaucoma

Adverse reactions

- Anti-infectives may cause superinfection and local irritation
- Anti-inflammatories may cause cataracts, increased intraocular pressure, impaired healing, and masking of signs and symptoms of infection
- Anesthetics may cause temporary stinging or burning of the eye and temporary loss of the corneal reflex
- Lubricants may cause discomfort, burning, or pain on instillation
- Miotics can cause ocular and systemic adverse effects
  - Ocular adverse effects include myopia, decreased vision in poor light, eye ache, and local irritation
  - Systemic adverse effects include headache, flushing, diaphoresis, GI upset, and diarrhea
- Beta-adrenergic blockers may cause ocular irritation and visual disturbances
- Mydriatics and cycloplegics can cause ocular and systemic adverse effects
  - Ocular adverse effects include increased intraocular pressure, eye ache, hypersensitivity, and photophobia
  - Systemic adverse effects include tachycardia, hypertension, headache, and dry mouth
- Mast cell stabilizers may cause headache, dizziness, and lacrimation
- Diuretics may cause GI upset
  - Carbonic anhydrase inhibitors may also cause diarrhea, paresthesia, lethargy, and weakness

When NOT to use ophthalmic drugs

- Acute eye infections
- Secondary glaucoma
- Acute iritis
- Inflammatory diseases
- Angle-closure glaucoma

Adverse reactions to watch for

- Superinfection, local irritation, cataracts, increased intraocular pressure, impaired healing, masking of signs and symptoms of infection, temporary stinging or burning, temporary loss of corneal reflex, discomfort, pain on instillation, myopia, decreased vision in poor light, eye ache, local irritation, headache, flushing, diaphoresis, GI upset, diarrhea, hypersensitivity, photophobia, tachycardia, hypertension, dry mouth, dizziness, lacrimation, paresthesia, lethargy, weakness, dehydration, hyperglycemia, glycosuria

Topics for patient discussion

- Medication regimen, including proper administration
- Signs and symptoms to discuss with the physician
- Proper handling of eye dropper
- Hand washing
- Importance of carrying identification describing disorder and drug therapy, if appropriate
- Importance of wearing eye patch or dark glasses after medication administration, if appropriate
- Follow-up care

Key nursing actions

- Assess patient for signs and symptoms of eye disorders and adverse effects.
- If patient is using more than one topical ophthalmic medication, wait at least 5 minutes before instilling second eye medication, as prescribed.
- Keep eye medications sterile; avoid skin or eye contact with applicator.
- Don't give ophthalmic anesthetics to patient for home use.
- After mydriatic or cycloplegic eyedrop administration, minimize systemic absorption by applying pressure to the lacrimal sac for 3 to 5 minutes.

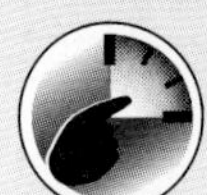

TIME-OUT FOR TEACHING

Teaching about ophthalmic drugs

Include these topics in your teaching plan for the patient receiving an ophthalmic.

- Medication regimen, including the drug's name, dosage, frequency, duration, and possible adverse effects
- Signs and symptoms to discuss with the physician
- Proper timing of and technique for administration
- Proper handling of eye dropper
- Hand washing
- Follow-up care

  – Osmotic diuretics may also cause dehydration, hyperglycemia, and glycosuria (glycerin)

Interactions

- None significant

Nursing responsibilities

- Assess the patient for signs and symptoms of eye disorders and adverse effects
- **If the patient is using more than one topical ophthalmic medication, wait at least 5 minutes before instilling a second eye medication, as prescribed**
- Keep all eye medications sterile; avoid skin or eye contact with the applicator
- Teach the patient how to instill eye medications properly (for additional teaching tips, see *Teaching about ophthalmic drugs*)
- Instruct the patient with glaucoma to carry identification describing the disorder and drug therapy
- Know that ophthalmic anesthetics are used only for eye examinations and surgery and shouldn't be given to the patient for home use
- **Inform the patient receiving an eye anesthetic that an eye patch may be necessary after administration to protect the eye from injury until the corneal reflex returns (about 1 hour)**
- Inform the patient receiving either a mydriatic or a cycloplegic that dark glasses may be needed after eye examination to prevent photophobia
- **After administering either mydriatic or cycloplegic eyedrops, minimize systemic absorption by applying pressure to the lacrimal sac at the inner canthus for 3 to 5 minutes; this prevents passage of the eyedrops via the nasolacrimal duct into areas of potential absorption, such as the nasal and pharyngeal mucosa**

OTIC DRUGS

Mechanism of action

- Anti-infectives kill or inhibit the growth of susceptible bacteria
- Anti-inflammatories reduce redness and itching
- Antihistamines and decongestants stimulate adrenergic receptors of respiratory mucosa, thereby producing vasoconstriction and reducing respiratory tissue hyperemia to open an obstructed eustachian tube
- Local anesthetics block nerve conduction at or near the application site to control pain associated with ear infections
- Ceruminolytics emulsify and loosen cerumen (earwax) deposits

Pharmacokinetics

- Absorption
  - Anti-inflammatories may be systemically absorbed with long-term use
  - Local anesthetics and ceruminolytics aren't absorbed
- Distribution: Local
- Metabolism: Unknown
- Excretion: Unknown

Drug examples

- Anti-infectives and anti-inflammatories: boric acid
- Antihistamines and decongestants: antihistamine-decongestant combinations (Actifed, Allerest, Chlor-Trimeton, Dimetane, Drixoral, Novahistine, Triaminic)
- Local anesthetics: benzocaine (Americaine-Otic, Tympagesic), antipyrine and benzocaine combination (Auralgan Otic Solution)
- Ceruminolytics: carbamide peroxide (Debrox Drops), triethanolamine polypeptide oleate-condensate (Cerumenex)

Indications

- Anti-infectives and anti-inflammatories are used to dry the ear and kill susceptible bacteria
- Antihistamines and decongestants are used as adjunctive therapy for acute otitis media, to reduce respiratory congestion, and to open an obstructed eustachian tube
- Local anesthetics are used to treat pain associated with ear infection
- Ceruminolytics remove excess cerumen (efficacy questionable)

Contraindications and precautions

- Contraindicated in patients with hypersensitivity to the drug and in those with a perforated eardrum

Adverse reactions

- May cause hypersensitivity reactions, including redness, burning, itching, stinging, urticaria, vesicular or maculopapular dermatitis, swelling, and mild irritation

Key facts about otic drugs

- Kill or inhibit the growth of susceptible bacteria
- Reduce redness and itching
- Open obstructed eustachian tube
- Block nerve conduction to control pain associated with ear infections
- Emulsify and loosen cerumen deposits
- Metabolism and excretion unknown

When to use otic drugs

- Susceptible bacterial infections
- Acute otitis media
- Respiratory congestion
- Obstructed eustachian tube
- Ear infection
- Excess cerumen

When NOT to use otic drugs

- Hypersensitivity
- Perforated eardrum

Adverse reactions to watch for

- Hypersensitivity reactions, superinfection

- Anti-infectives may cause superinfection if there is an overgrowth of non-susceptible organisms
- Local anesthetics may mask the symptoms of a middle ear infection

Interactions

- None significant

Nursing responsibilities

- Assess the patient for hearing loss, pain, and ear drainage
- **Use the correct method to instill eardrops**
  - **For a child, pull the auricle down to straighten the external canal**
  - **For an adult, pull the auricle up and back to straighten the external canal**
- Teach the patient how to administer the prescribed drug and tell him to keep his head tilted for 10 minutes to allow the drug to be absorbed; if repositioning is necessary, tell the patient to use a cottonball or earplug to keep the medication in the ear canal
- Instruct the patient to contact the physician if pain and swelling of the ear persist
- When administering a ceruminolytic
  - Moisten the cotton ball with medication before insertion
  - Avoid touching the ear with the dropper
  - Flush the ear gently with warm water, using a soft rubber bulb ear syringe within 30 minutes after instillation to remove cerumen
  - Keep the container tightly closed and away from moisture
- Tell the patient not to use ceruminolytic drops more often than prescribed (for additional teaching tips, see *Teaching about otic drugs*)
- Tell the patient to call the physician if redness, pain, or swelling persists
- Tell the patient administering a ceruminolytic not to use a swab because it may cause trauma to the inner ear
- The efficacy of ceruminolytics is questionable

Key nursing actions

- Assess patient for hearing loss, pain, and ear drainage.
- To instill eardrops in a child, pull the auricle down to straighten the external canal.
- To instill eardrops in an adult, pull the auricle up and back to straighten the external canal.

Topics for patient discussion

- Medication regimen, including proper administration
- Signs and symptoms to discuss with the physician
- Importance of notifying the physician if redness, pain, or swelling persists
- Ear care after administration
- Irrigation of ear, if indicated
- Compliance with drug therapy for full course of treatment
- Follow-up care

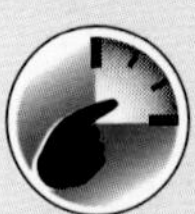

TIME-OUT FOR TEACHING

Teaching about otic drugs

Include these topics in your teaching plan for the patient receiving an otic drug.

- Medication regimen, including the drug's name, dosage, frequency, duration, and possible adverse effects
- Signs and symptoms to discuss with the physician
- Proper procedure for administering the drug
- Ear care after drug administration
- Irrigation of ear, if indicated
- Compliance with therapy for full course of treatment
- Follow-up care, including physician visits

NCLEX CHECKS

It's never too soon to begin your NCLEX preparation. Now that you've reviewed this chapter, carefully read each of the following questions and choose the best answer. Then compare your responses to the correct answers.

1. When administering eyedrops, instill the drops into which of the following locations?

- ☐ A. Conjunctival sac
- ☐ B. Inner canthus
- ☐ C. Outer canthus
- ☐ D. Vas deferens

2. Which group of ophthalmic drugs is used to prepare a patient's pupils for examination?

- ☐ A. Anti-inflammatories
- ☐ B. Cycloplegics
- ☐ C. Miotics
- ☐ D. Mydriatics

3. Your patient requires an eye examination to assess for the presence of a foreign body in his eye. To dilate a patient's pupils, which of the following drugs would you give?

- ☐ A. Carbachol (Carboptic)
- ☐ B. Cyclopentolate (Cyclogyl)
- ☐ C. Physostigmine
- ☐ D. Pilocarpine (Pilocar)

4. A physician prescribes a diuretic for a patient with glaucoma. Which class of diuretic is used to reduce intraocular pressure?

- ☐ A. Loop diuretics
- ☐ B. Osmotic diuretics
- ☐ C. Potassium-sparing diuretics
- ☐ D. Thiazide and thiazide-like diuretics

5. A 76-year-old patient is prescribed boric acid. Boric acid is an example of which type of medication?

- ☐ A. Otic anti-infective
- ☐ B. Otic anti-inflammatory
- ☐ C. Otic ceruminolytic
- ☐ D. Otic local anesthetic

6. A patient is prescribed benzocaine to reduce ear pain. You instruct her to do all of the following except:

- ☐ A. stop use of the drug if urticaria occurs.
- ☐ B. report increased ear pain to her physician.
- ☐ C. insert an ear wick before taking the agent.
- ☐ D. report hearing loss or dizziness to her physician right away.

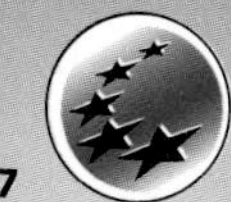

TOP 7

Items to study before your next test on drugs and the sensory system

1. Mechanisms of action of ophthalmic and otic drugs
2. Rationales for using anti-infectives, anti-inflammatories, anesthetics, lubricants, miotics, beta-adrenergic blockers, mydriatics, and cycloplegics to treat eye disorders
3. Common adverse effects of ophthalmic and otic drugs
4. Correct techniques for instilling eardrops in children and adults
5. Proper administration of different types of eye medications
6. Nursing responsibilities when administering ophthalmic and otic drugs
7. Teaching for the patient who is receiving an ophthalmic or otic drug

7. A patient was prescribed carbamide peroxide (Debrox) to treat impacted cerumen. Which instruction should you include in your teaching plan for this patient?

☐ **A.** Apply 1 drop to the affected ear canal.
☐ **B.** Flush your ears gently with warm water after using this product.
☐ **C.** Use this drug once and return to the prescriber if you don't get results.
☐ **D.** Swab the ear canal with a cotton swab after using this product.

8. The nurse is caring for a patient who underwent surgical repair of a detached retina of the right eye. Which of the following interventions should the nurse perform?

Select all that apply:

☐ **A.** Place the patient in a prone position.
☐ **B.** Approach the patient from the left side.
☐ **C.** Encourage deep breathing and coughing.
☐ **D.** Discourage bending down.
☐ **E.** Orient the patient to his environment.
☐ **F.** Administer a stool softener.

ANSWERS AND RATIONALES

1. CORRECT ANSWER: A
The conjunctival sac is the optimal site for the absorption of eye medication. You can minimize systemic absorption by pressing the inner canthus (the inner angle formed by the meeting of the upper and lower eyelids) after the drops are instilled. The outer canthus has little effect, but it's where eye ointment is applied after starting at the inner canthus. The vas deferens is part of the male reproductive system, which is nowhere near the eye.

2. CORRECT ANSWER: D
Mydriatics dilate the pupils, thereby preparing them for examination. By contrast, miotics constrict the pupils. Anti-inflammatories are often used for allergic eye conditions. Cycloplegics are used to paralyze the ciliary muscles to perform eye refraction examinations or prepare for surgery, especially in children.

3. CORRECT ANSWER: B
Cyclopentolate is an anticholinergic drug that dilates the pupils and paralyzes the ciliary muscles. All of the other options are cholinergic drugs that would have the opposite effect and constrict the pupils.

4. CORRECT ANSWER: B
Osmotic diuretics work by increasing plasma osmolarity, thereby pulling fluid into the vascular system and reducing intraocular pressure. Loop diuretics such as furosemide, potassium-sparing diuretics such as spironolactone, and thiazide and thiazide-like diuretics are best used for diuresis of edema.

5. CORRECT ANSWER: A

Boric acid makes the ear canal a less suitable environment for bacteria and infection by changing the pH. It also helps dry out the ear. It won't cure an infection when used as a sole treatment. An acid wouldn't be considered an anti-inflammatory. Boric acid doesn't have analgesic or ceruminolytic properties.

6. CORRECT ANSWER: D

Use of an ear wick isn't recommended with benzocaine. Hearing loss, dizziness, and increased pain are signs of a fulminating ear infection that should be investigated fully. Presence of urticaria denotes a hypersensitivity to the drug, and the drug should be stopped.

7. CORRECT ANSWER: B

Flushing gently with warm water is necessary with carbamide peroxide. The drug softens cerumen, and the water will gently flush out the cerumen. The correct dose is several drops to the affected ear. A swab shouldn't be used because of the risk of trauma to the inner ear.

8. CORRECT ANSWER: B, D, E, F

The nurse should approach the patient from the left side—the unaffected side—to avoid startling him. She should also discourage the patient from bending down, deep breathing, hard coughing and sneezing, and other activities that can increase intraocular pressure. The patient should be oriented to his environment to reduce the risk of injury. Stool softeners should be administered to discourage straining during defecation. The patient should lie on his back or on the unaffected side to reduce intraocular pressure on the affected eye.

18

Nutritional agents and the body

LEARNING OBJECTIVES

After studying this chapter, you should be able to:

- Discuss the purpose of each nutritional agent.
- List common adverse effects of nutritional agents.
- Identify nursing responsibilities when administering nutritional agents.
- Discuss patient teaching related to nutritional agents.

CHAPTER OVERVIEW

Nutritional agents — nutritional supplement solutions, electrolytes, vitamins, and minerals — are used to correct deficiencies in the patient's nutritional status. Enteral forms, preferred when the GI tract is functioning, are administered either orally or through a feeding tube. Parenteral forms are administered through a peripheral vein (peripheral parenteral nutrition) or a central vein (total parenteral nutrition). Nursing responsibilities include monitoring intake and output and related laboratory values, teaching proper agent administration, promoting dietary modifications, checking gastric residual (for enteral feedings), and observing for hyperglycemia (especially with total parenteral nutrition).

ANATOMY AND PHYSIOLOGY

- **Anatomy**
  - More than 50% of the average adult's body is water

- Body water contains dissolved substances (solutes) that are necessary for physiologic functioning
- Solutes include electrolytes, glucose, amino acids, and other nutrients
- Body fluid composition differs by compartment
  - The intracellular fluid (ICF) compartment consists of the fluid in the body's cells
  - The intravascular fluid compartment consists of the fluid in blood plasma and the lymphatic system
  - The interstitial fluid compartment consists of fluid distributed diffusely through the loose tissue surrounding the cells
  - Intravascular and interstitial fluids are separated by a capillary endothelium that's freely permeable to water, electrolytes, and other solutes
    - Therefore, intravascular and interstitial fluids are similar in composition
    - The intravascular and interstitial fluid compartments commonly are grouped together as a single compartment called the extracellular fluid compartment (ECF)
  - ICF composition differs from ECF composition
    - ICF has higher concentrations of protein, potassium, magnesium, phosphate, and sulfate than ECF
    - ICF has lower concentrations of sodium, calcium, chloride, and bicarbonate than ECF

Physiology

- Fluid balance
  - The body gains and loses water daily through fluid intake and output; water enters the body via the GI tract and leaves via the skin, lungs, GI tract, and urinary tract
  - Two mechanisms help maintain fluid balance
    - Thirst regulates water intake
    - Countercurrent mechanism regulates urine concentration
    - Urine excretion is the main route of water loss; output is typically 1,000 to 1,500 ml daily
- Electrolyte balance
  - Electrolytes are substances that dissociate into ions (electronically charged particles) when dissolved in water
  - Ions may be positively charged cations or negatively charged anions
    - Cations include sodium (Na^+), potassium (K^+), calcium (Ca^{++}), and magnesium (Mg^{++})
    - Anions include chloride (Cl^-), bicarbonate (HCO_3^-), and phosphate (HPO_4^-)
  - Normally, the electrical charges of the cations and anions are balanced so that body fluids are electrically neutral
  - The body uses various mechanisms to maintain electrolyte balance; the kidneys and hormones regulate most of the electrolytes
- Acid-base balance

A&P highlights

- More than 50% of the average adult's body is water, which contains dissolved substances
- Body fluid composition differs by compartment
- Three types of physiological balance: fluid balance, electrolyte balance, and acid-base balance
- Body gains and loses water daily through fluid intake and output
- Electrolytes dissociate into ions when dissolved into water
- Acid-base balance results in a stable hydrogen ion concentration in body fluids

Facts about fluid balance

- Water enters the GI tract and leaves via the skin, lungs, GI tract, and urinary tract
- Thirst regulates water intake
- Urine excretion is the main route of water loss

Facts about electrolyte balance

- Ions may be positively charged cations or negatively charged anions
- Electrical charges of cations and anions are balanced so that body fluids are electrically neutral
- Kidneys and hormones regulate most of the electrolytes

- Acid-base balance results in a stable hydrogen ion (H+) concentration in body fluids
- An acid releases hydrogen ions in water
- A base releases ions that can combine with hydrogen ions
- A hydrogen ion concentration of a fluid determines whether it's acidic or basic (alkaline)
- The body is an acid-producing organism
- Buffer systems and the lungs and kidneys maintain the blood pH within a narrow range—7.38 to 7.42—by neutralizing and eliminating acids as rapidly as they are formed, thus helping maintain the body's acid-base balance
  - Buffer systems minimize pH changes caused by excess acids or bases by reducing the effect of a sudden change in hydrogen ion concentration by converting a strong acid or base into a weak acid or base
  - The lungs affect acid-base balance by excreting carbon dioxide and regulating the carbonic acid content of the blood
  - The kidneys regulate acid-base balance by allowing tubular filtrate reabsorption of bicarbonate and by forming bicarbonate

Facts about acid-base balance

- Body is an acid-producing organism
- Hydrogen ion concentration of a fluid determines whether it's acidic or basic
- Buffer systems and lungs and kidneys maintain the blood pH within a narrow range – 7.38 to 7.42

Function

- The complex interrelationship among fluid, electrolyte, and acid-base metabolism creates the body's state of homeostasis
- Water and fluid balance is essential to physiologic functioning
- Electrolyte balance and sufficient quantities of each major electrolyte are essential to normal metabolism and function
- When acids and bases are balanced, the hydrogen ion concentration is stable and the pH is neutral (7)

ENTERAL AGENTS

Mechanism of action

- Use normal metabolic pathways and processes

Pharmacokinetics

- Absorption: Absorbed via GI tract
- Distribution: Well distributed
- Metabolism: Unknown
- Excretion: Excreted in the feces

Facts about enteral agents

- Use normal metabolic pathways and processes
- Metabolism unknown
- Excreted in feces

Drug examples

- Complete nutritional supplement feeding solutions (Amin-Aid, Arginaid, BCAD 2, Boost, Cyclinex-2, Ensure, Epulor, Glucerna, Glutarex-2, Hepatic-Aid II, Hominex-2, Immun-Aid, Isocal, I-Valex-2, Jevity, Ketonex-2, Nutrament, Osmolite, Peptamen, Peptinex, Phenex-2, Propimex-2, Pulmocare, Respalor, Suplena, Sustacal, TraumaCal, Tyrex-2, Vital, Vivonex)

Indications

- Oral intake inadequate to meet nutritional needs

Enteral feeding routes

The chart below shows various enteral feeding routes and the indications for their use.

ACCESS	INDICATIONS
Nasogastric or orogastric	• Short-term • No esophageal reflux • Gag reflex intact • Normal gastric and duodenum emptying
Nasoduodenal or nasojejunal	• Short-term • Esophageal reflux • High risk of pulmonary aspiration • Delayed gastric emptying
Esophageal or pharyngostomy	• Long-term • Head or neck tumors • Nasopharyngeal access contraindicated
Gastrostomy	• Long-term • Swallowing dysfunction • Nasoenteric access contraindicated • Normal gastric and duodenum emptying • Esophageal stricture or neoplasm
Jejunostomy	• Long-term • Esophageal reflux • High risk of pulmonary aspiration • Impaired gastric emptying • Failure to access upper GI tract • Postoperative feeding in trauma, malnourishment, or upper GI surgery

- Total or supplemental nutrition for patients who can't consume adequate calories because of physical impairments (such as dysphagia), GI tract problems (such as fistulas), psychological disturbances (dementia, depression), altered level of consciousness (delirium), or hypermetabolic states (burns, cancer, multiple trauma) (for more information, see *Enteral feeding routes*)
- Amin-Aid and Respalor are used in renal failure
- Hepatic Aid II, which contains branched-chain amino acids, is used in liver impairment
- Pulmocare (higher in fat and lower in carbohydrate, yielding less carbon dioxide) is used in pulmonary disease
- Glucerna is used for patients with glucose intolerance
- TraumaCal is used for patients in a hypermetabolic state
- Vivonex is a nutritionally complete diet that requires virtually no digestion

Contraindications and precautions

- Contraindicated in patients with bowel obstruction, vomiting, malabsorption syndrome

When to use enteral agents

- Nutritional needs
- Renal failure
- Liver impairment
- Pulmonary disease
- Glucose intolerance
- Hypermetabolic state

When NOT to use enteral agents

- Bowel obstruction
- Vomiting
- Malabsorption syndrome

Adverse reactions

- Diarrhea, nausea, aspiration

Interactions

- These agents may decrease phenytoin levels; give drug 2 hours before enteral therapy or stop enteral feeding for 2 hours before phenytoin administration

Nursing responsibilities

- Assess the patient's nutritional status; include dietary recall and anthropometric measurements; make sure that the patient has an intact digestive system
- Obtain diagnostic test results to establish baseline values, identify deficiencies, and evaluate progress after supplementation
- Weigh the patient before initiating therapy to establish a baseline; check daily weights to evaluate for changes
- Teach the patient about the nutritional agent to be used, and review any special modifications or procedures needed for administration
- Reinforce instructions on a well-balanced diet, with emphasis on food allowances and restrictions
- Know that enteral supplements may be given orally, via nasogastric tube, gastrostomy, or via needle-catheter jejunostomy
- Teach the patient how to prepare the supplement (for example, keep refrigerated, shake before using, mix powder with specified amount of water or fruit juice)
- Assist the patient with measures to enhance the taste of oral forms, such as serving the supplement cold or poured over ice
- Verify the diet and fluid order and the formula to be used before administering a tube feeding
  - Check the formula's expiration date, when it was opened, and how long it has been kept at room temperature
  - Verify whether the feeding is to be intermittent (usually given every 3 to 4 hours) or continuous (usually given over 16 to 24 hours)
  - Check for possible agent-formula interactions
- **Confirm placement and patency of the tube before an enteral feeding, flush the tube with 30 to 50 ml of water every 4 hours or according to agency policy for continuous feedings; change the feeding solution every 8 hours, and change the administration set every 24 hours**
- Check gastric residual; notify the physician if the residual is 100 ml or more (or according to agency policy)
- Position the patient upright or with the head of the bed elevated at least 45 degrees to prevent aspiration
- Provide oral care unless contraindicated
- Monitor intake and output and daily weight
- Slow the rate or reduce the concentration of the feeding if the patient complains of cramping or nausea, and notify the physician
- **Stop the feeding immediately if the patient vomits**

Adverse reactions to watch for

- Diarrhea, nausea, and aspiration

Key nursing actions

- Assess nutritional status; include dietary recall and anthropometric measurements.
- Teach about the nutritional agent to be used, and review any special modifications or procedures needed for administration.
- Verify the diet and fluid order and the formula to be used before administering a tube feeding.
- Confirm placement and patency of the tube before an enteral feeding, flush the tube with 30 to 50 ml of water every 4 hours or according to agency policy for continuous feedings.
- Change the feeding solution every 8 hours, and change the administration set every 24 hours.
- Stop the feeding immediately if the patient vomits.

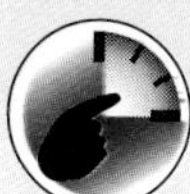

TIME-OUT FOR TEACHING

Teaching about home enteral nutrition

Include these topics in your teaching plan for the patient requiring tube feedings at home.
- Rationale for tube feeding
- Type of feeding being used
- Hand-washing and infection-control measures
- Procedure for carrying out the feeding
- Care of tube and equipment, including storage of solutions and temperatures for administration
- Assessment of tube placement
- Proper patient positioning for feeding
- Tube flushing after medication administration
- Environmental monitoring during feeding (making it as pleasant as possible)
- Signs and symptoms to discuss with the physician, including intolerance or complications
- Follow-up care, including physician visits

- Don't let feedings remain at room temperature for more than 8 hours (formulas provide an excellent media for bacterial growth)
- Don't add new formula to a feeding that has been hanging for more than 6 hours
- Provide tube insertion site care or dressing change at least daily or when the dressing is soiled
- Teach the patient and family the tube feeding procedure if they are to continue it at home (for additional teaching tips, see *Teaching about home enteral nutrition*)

Topics for patient discussion
- Tube feeding
- Care of tube and equipment
- Signs and symptoms

PARENTERAL AGENTS

Mechanism of action
- Absorb solution that's nutritionally complete except for essential fatty acids and provide the necessary calories, vitamins, electrolytes, minerals, and trace elements to the body

Pharmacokinetics
- Absorption: Administered I.V.
- Distribution: Well distributed
- Metabolism: Unknown
- Excretion: Excreted in the urine

Drug examples
- Dextrose solutions in water (D_5W, $D_{10}W$, $D_{20}W$, $D_{50}W$), amino acid solutions (Aminosyn, FreAmine), lipid emulsions (Intralipid, Liposyn II, Liposyn III), specialized amino acid formulations (Aminess, Aminosyn-

Key facts about parenteral agents
- Provide necessary calories, vitamins, electrolytes, minerals, and trace elements to the body
- Metabolism unknown
- Excreted in urine

HBC, Aminosyn-RF, FreAmine HBC, HepatAmine, NephrAmine, RenAmin)

Indications

- These agents are used for oral intake inadequate to meet nutritional needs
- Parenteral nutrition is used to achieve a zero or positive nitrogen balance when a negative balance is present; it provides enough protein to rebuild tissue
- Total parenteral nutrition (TPN) or peripheral parenteral nutrition (PPN) is used to provide carbohydrate, protein, fat, water, electrolytes, vitamins, minerals, and trace elements when the GI tract can't be used
  - PPN is used preoperatively and postoperatively to provide low-calorie nutrition supplementation and to augment enteral therapy as necessary
  - TPN is used to maintain or increase body weight, to achieve normal growth in infants and children, and to restore lean body mass and adequate tissue in emaciated patients
- D_5W and $D_{10}W$ are used for short-term nutritional support in patients who don't need more than 2,500 calories/day
- $D_{20}W$ and $D_{50}W$ (often in admixtures with amino acid solutions) provide total nutrients
- Aminess, Aminosyn, NephrAmine, and RenAmin are high-calorie, low-protein formulations used in renal failure
- HepatAmine contains branched-chain amino acids and high protein for use in liver disease
- Intralipid, Liposyn II, and Liposyn III are fat supplements that provide additional calories while sparing protein
- FreAmine HBC is a stress formula for hypermetabolic conditions

When to use parenteral agents

- Nutritional needs
- Body weight maintenance
- Normal growth in infants and children
- Lean body mass restoration
- Renal failure
- Liver disease
- Hypermetabolic conditions

Contraindications and precautions

- Contraindicated in patients with anuria, severe uncontrolled electrolyte or acid-base imbalance, or decreased circulating blood volume

When NOT to use parenteral agents

- Anuria
- Severe uncontrolled electrolyte or acid-base imbalance
- Decreasing circulating blood volume

Adverse reactions

- Pulmonary edema, fluid overload, hyperglycemia, glycosuria, electrolyte imbalances, catheter sepsis, rebound hypoglycemia, pancreatitis (lipid formulations)

Adverse reactions to watch for

- Pulmonary edema, fluid overload, hyperglycemia, glycosuria, electrolyte imbalances, catheter sepsis, rebound hypoglycemia, and pancreatitis

Interactions

- None reported; see individual manufacturer's labeling

Nursing responsibilities

- Assess the patient's nutritional status; include dietary recall and anthropometric measurements
- Obtain diagnostic test results to establish baseline values, identify deficiencies, and evaluate progress after supplementation
- Weigh the patient before initiating therapy to establish a baseline; check daily weights to evaluate for changes

- Teach the patient about the nutritional agent to be used, and review any special modifications or procedures needed for administration
- Reinforce instructions on a well-balanced diet, with emphasis on food allowances and restrictions
- **Verify the order to ensure the correct type and amount of solution to administer and the proper infusion rate**
- Follow procedures for initiating and maintaining peripheral or central vein infusion therapy
- Monitor the patient for signs and symptoms of fluid overload and electrolyte imbalance
- Monitor vital signs, intake and output, and daily weight
- Allow a solution to hang for no more than 24 hours
- Assess the patient's response to therapy as evidenced by weight gain; obtain ongoing assessment of nutritional and metabolic status as evidenced by laboratory studies
  - Monitor serum electrolyte, glucose, and blood urea nitrogen levels and hepatic function, as ordered
  - Monitor serum calcium and phosphorus levels, as ordered
- Inspect the catheter insertion site at least every 8 hours and change tubing, filters, and dressing according to agency protocol; maintain sterile technique during dressing changes
- Monitor infusion rate and administration system every hour or according to agency protocol
- Monitor the patient receiving TPN for glycosuria and ketonuria every 4 to 6 hours; perform fingerstick blood glucose levels every 4 to 6 hours or as ordered to assess for hyperglycemia
- Know that insulin may be added to the TPN solution or otherwise administered based on the patient's blood glucose level
  - Begin TPN infusion at a slow rate to allow the body to adjust to increased glucose levels; starting the TPN infusion too fast may cause hyperglycemia.
  - Infuse $D_{10}W$ if TPN solution isn't available
- **Never attempt to "catch up" a TPN solution by increasing the infusion rate**
- Discontinue TPN gradually while increasing oral or enteral feedings
- Initially infuse lipid emulsions at a rate of 0.5 to 1 ml/hour and observe for adverse effects; avoid rapid infusion, and use a pump to regulate the rate
- **Hang lipid emulsion higher than dextrose and amino acid admixture because lipids have a higher specific gravity**
- Be aware that in-line filters with pores of 1.2 microns or larger are sometimes used to remove particulate matter
- Use only the tubing supplied with the emulsion to prevent possible interaction with the material used to make the plastic more flexible
- Be aware that lipid emulsions may be mixed with amino acid solution, dextrose, electrolytes, and vitamins in the same I.V. container; check with the pharmacist for acceptable proportions and compatibility information

Key nursing actions

- Assess the patient's nutritional status; include dietary recall and anthropometric measurements.
- Verify the order to ensure the correct type and amount of solution to administer and the proper infusion rate.
- Monitor for signs and symptoms of fluid overload and electrolyte imbalance.
- Never attempt to "catch up" a TPN solution by increasing the infusion rate.
- Hang lipid emulsion higher than dextrose and amino acid admixture because lipids have a higher specific gravity.
- Be aware that lipid emulsions may be mixed with amino acid solution, dextrose, electrolytes, and vitamins in the same I.V. container; check with the pharmacist for acceptable proportions and compatibility information.
- Use lipid emulsion within 12 hours after starting the infusion; lipids support bacterial growth.

- **Use lipid emulsion within 12 hours after starting the infusion; lipids support bacterial growth**
- Lipid solutions should initially be infused slowly to observe for adverse reactions
- Monitor serum lipid levels closely; elevated lipid levels must return to normal between doses

ELECTROLYTE REPLACEMENTS

Mechanism of action

- Electrolyte agents replace and maintain electrolyte levels
- Sodium fluoride stabilizes apatite crystal of bone and teeth
- Sodium bicarbonate restores the body's buffering capacity and neutralizes excess acid
- Ammonium chloride increases free hydrogen ion concentration
- Tromethamine combines with hydrogen ions and associated acid anions with excretion of resulting salts; it also has an osmotic diuretic effect

Pharmacokinetics

- Varies with each electrolyte

Drug examples

- Ammonium chloride, calcium (see chapter 20), magnesium oxide (Mag-Ox, Maox), magnesium sulfate (see chapter 5), phosphorus, potassium chloride (Kaochlor, Kay Ciel, K-Dur, Micro K Extentabs, Slow-K), potassium phosphate (Neutra-Phos K), sodium bicarbonate, sodium fluoride (Fluoritab, Flura-Drops, Pediaflor), tromethamine (Tham)

Indications

- These agents are used for oral intake inadequate to meet nutritional needs
- Potassium is used for potassium depletion
  - Potassium chloride is used for potassium deficiency from diuretics, vomiting, diarrhea, or fistulas
  - Potassium phosphate is used to treat hypokalemia
- Sodium fluoride is indicated for supplementation to harden tooth enamel and prevent dental caries when adequate fluoride isn't provided in drinking water
- Sodium bicarbonate is indicated to correct metabolic acidosis secondary to cardiac arrest, shock, renal failure, or diabetic ketoacidosis
  - Sodium bicarbonate may be used to neutralize gastric acid but isn't recommended because of the high sodium load
  - Sodium bicarbonate may be applied topically for itching and minor burns
- Magnesium oxide may be used as a magnesium supplement during parenteral nutrition or as an antacid
- Ammonium chloride is used as a systemic acidifier in metabolic alkalosis to correct chloride depletion

Key facts about electrolyte replacements

- Replace and maintain electrolyte levels
- Sodium fluoride stabilizes apatite crystal
- Sodium bicarbonate restores the body's buffering capacity and neutralizes excess acid
- Ammonium chloride increases free hydrogen ion concentration
- Tromethamine combines with hydrogen ions and associated acid anions
- Metabolism and excretion varies

When to use electrolyte replacements

- Nutrition
- Potassium depletion
- Potassium deficiency
- Hypokalemia
- Dental caries prevention
- Metabolic acidosis correction
- Minor burns and itching
- Magnesium supplement
- Systemic acidifier in metabolic alkalosis to correct chloride depletion
- Acidosis secondary to cardiac arrest or cardiac bypass surgery
- Rapid calcium replacement is necessary
- Cardiac arrest

- Tromethamine is used to correct acidosis secondary to cardiac arrest or cardiac bypass surgery
- Calcium gluconate and calcium chloride are used when rapid calcium replacement is necessary; calcium chloride is used during cardiac arrest

Contraindications and precautions

- Sodium fluoride is contraindicated when fluoride intake from drinking water is greater than 0.7 ppm (parts per million)
- Sodium bicarbonate is contraindicated in patients with metabolic or respiratory alkalosis, in those losing chloride by vomiting or through continuous gastric suctioning, in those receiving diuretics known to produce hypochloremic alkalosis, and in those with hypocalcemia in which alkalosis may produce tetany, hypertension, seizures, or heart failure
- Ammonium chloride is contraindicated in renal or hepatic insufficiency
- Tromethamine is contraindicated in renal failure or anuria
- Potassium preparations should be used cautiously in patients with renal impairment or renal failure and in those receiving potassium-sparing diuretics
- Calcium preparations should be used with caution in patients receiving cardiac glycoside preparations and in those with ventricular fibrillation, hypercalcemia, hypophosphatemia, or renal calculi

When NOT to use electrolyte replacements

- Fluoride intake from drinking water that exceeds 0.7 ppm
- Metabolic or respiratory alkalosis
- Chloride loss by vomiting or continuous gastric suctioning
- Hypochloremic alkalosis from diuretics
- Hypocalcemia
- Renal or hepatic insufficiency
- Anuria

Adverse reactions

- Potassium preparations: phlebitis, confusion, restlessness, paralysis, cardiac arrest
- Sodium fluoride: headache, weakness, GI distress, brown discoloration of teeth (overdose)
- Sodium bicarbonate: gastric distention, renal calculi, metabolic alkalosis, hypernatremia, hyperkalemia (with overdose)
- Magnesium oxide: constipation
- Ammonium chloride: headache, confusion, twitching, tetany, bradycardia, metabolic acidosis, hyperchloremia, hypokalemia, gastric irritation
- Tromethamine: respiratory depression, hypoglycemia, hyperkalemia, I.V. thrombosis
- Calcium preparations: constipation, tingling sensation, chalky taste (after I.V. administration), hypercalcemia, vein irritation, local reactions with I.M. use

Adverse reactions to watch for

- Phlebitis, confusion, restlessness, paralysis, cardiac arrest, headache, weakness, GI distress, brown discoloration of teeth, gastric distention, renal calculi, metabolic alkalosis, hypernatremia, hyperkalemia, constipation, twitching, tetany, bradycardia, metabolic acidosis, hyperchloremia, gastric irritation, respiratory depression, hypoglycemia, I.V. thrombosis, tingling sensation, chalky taste, hypercalcemia, vein irritation, and local reactions with I.M. use

Interactions

- None significant

Nursing responsibilities

- Assess the patient's nutritional status; include dietary recall and anthropometric measurements
- Obtain diagnostic test results to establish baseline values, identify deficiencies, and evaluate progress after supplementation
- Weigh the patient before initiating therapy to establish a baseline; check daily weights to evaluate for changes

Key nursing actions

- Assess nutritional status; include dietary recall and anthropometric measurements.
- Teach about the nutritional agent to be used, and review any special modifications or procedures needed for administration.
- Administer potassium chloride orally or as an I.V. infusion
- Give oral forms of ammonium chloride after meals to minimize adverse GI effects.
- Be aware that tromethamine shouldn't be used longer than 1 day except in life-threatening situations; be prepared to adjust dosage carefully according to blood pH.
- Monitor ECG closely for changes, especially when administering potassium and calcium preparations.

Key facts about vitamins

- Act as replacements in deficiency states
- Metabolism and excretion vary with each vitamin

- Teach the patient about the nutritional agent to be used, and review any special modifications or procedures needed for administration
- Reinforce instructions on a well-balanced diet, with emphasis on food allowances and restrictions
- Evaluate the patient's serum electrolyte levels and arterial blood gases, as ordered
- Monitor serum levels closely to prevent toxicity
- Administer potassium chloride orally or as an I.V. infusion
  - Know that oral tablets should never be chewed or sucked; however, they may be crushed and added to water or fruit juice or swallowed whole
  - Administer I.V. potassium by infusion only as a dilute solution to prevent potentially fatal hyperkalemia from a too-rapid infusion
  - Never give potassium by I.V. push or I.M. injection
- Tell the patient that sodium fluoride tablets may be chewed, swallowed whole, or dissolved in liquids other than dairy products; advise him not to take fluoride within 2 hours of ingesting a dairy product
- Be aware that sodium bicarbonate isn't routinely recommended for use in cardiac arrest because it may produce a paradoxical acidosis from carbon dioxide production
- Give oral forms of ammonium chloride after meals to minimize adverse GI effects
- Be aware that tromethamine shouldn't be used longer than 1 day except in life-threatening situations; be prepared to adjust dosage carefully according to blood pH
- Give calcium chloride by I.V. only, using an in-line filter; watch for possible precipitate if added to parenteral solutions containing other additives, such as phosphorus and phosphates
- Monitor the patient's ECG closely for changes, especially when administering potassium and calcium preparations
- Know that calcium gluconate is the antidote for magnesium sulfate toxicity; it should be immediately available at all times during magnesium sulfate administration

VITAMINS

Mechanism of action

- Act as replacements in deficiency states

Pharmacokinetics

- Varies with each vitamin

Drug examples

- Water-soluble vitamins: thiamine (B_1), riboflavin (B_2), nicotinic acid (niacin [B_3]), pyridoxine (B_6), folic acid (B_9 [Folvite]), cyanocobalamin (B_{12}), vitamin C (ascorbic acid), calcium pantothenate (B_5)
- Fat-soluble vitamins: vitamin A (Aquasol A), ergocalciferol (D_2 [Calciferol]), vitamin E (tocopherol [Aquasol E, Vita-Plus E]), phytonadione (K_1)

Indications

- Vitamins are used for oral intake inadequate to meet nutritional needs
- Thiamine is a coenzyme used in carbohydrate metabolism, beriberi, and treatment of neuritis in pregnancy and alcoholism
- Riboflavin is used as a supplement to combat pellagra and beriberi
- Pyridoxine is used with isoniazid in alcoholic polyneuritis
- Folic acid is used to treat megaloblastic anemia
- Cyanocobalamin is used to treat pernicious anemia
- Ascorbic acid is used to maintain collagen, blood vessels, and skin cartilage; in wound healing; and to provide resistance to infection (such as the common cold)
- Calcium pantothenate is used as a calcium supplement, although calcium is plentiful in most diets
- Vitamin A is used in pregnancy, breast-feeding, gastrectomy, and psoriasis and to promote bone growth and development, mucosal integrity, and night vision
- Vitamin K is indicated in the treatment of hypoprothrombinemia secondary to vitamin K deficiency or hepatic failure; it's also used prophylactically for neonatal hemorrhagic disease

Contraindications and precautions

- All vitamins are contraindicated in patients with hypersensitivity
- Vitamin A is contraindicated in patients with malabsorption syndrome or hypervitaminosis A

Adverse reactions

- Riboflavin: yellow discoloration of urine
- Vitamin A: hypervitaminosis manifested by malaise, lethargy, abdominal pain, anorexia, nausea
- Thiamine: hypotension (after rapid I.V. administration), angioedema
- Vitamin C: epigastric distress, renal failure

Interactions

- Vary with each vitamin

Nursing responsibilities

- Assess the patient's nutritional status; include dietary recall and anthropometric measurements
- Obtain diagnostic test results to establish baseline values, identify deficiencies, and evaluate progress after supplementation
- Weigh the patient before initiating therapy to establish a baseline; check daily weights to evaluate for changes
- Teach the patient about the vitamin to be used, and review any special modifications or procedures needed for administration
- Reinforce instructions on a well-balanced diet, with emphasis on food allowances and restrictions
- Know that oral, I.V., and I.M. preparations of thiamine are available
- **Administer I.V. thiamine carefully because cardiovascular collapse and anaphylaxis have been reported**

When to use vitamins

- Nutrition
- Carbohydrate metabolism
- Neuritis in pregnancy and alcoholism
- Pellagra and beriberi
- Alcoholic polyneuritis
- Megaloblastic anemia
- Pernicious anemia
- Collagen, blood vessels, and skin cartilage maintenance
- Wound healing
- Infection resistance
- Pregnancy
- Breast-feeding
- Gastrectomy
- Psoriasis
- Bone growth and development
- Mucosal integrity
- Night vision
- Hypoprothrombinemia
- Neonatal hemorrhagic disease

When NOT to use vitamins

- Hypersensitivity
- Malabsorption syndrome
- Hypervitaminosis A

Adverse reactions to watch for

- Yellow discoloration of urine, hypervitaminosis, hypotension, angioedema, epigastric distress, and renal failure

Key nursing actions

- Assess nutritional status; include dietary recall and anthropometric measurements.
- Administer I.V. thiamine carefully because cardiovascular collapse and anaphylaxis have been reported.

Key facts about minerals

- Act as the component of many enzyme actions
- Chromium potentiates the action of insulin and regulation of lipoprotein metabolism
- Iron is an essential mineral that's a component of hemoglobin, myoglobin, and other enzymes
- Metabolism and excretion varies

When to use minerals

- Nutrition
- Long-term TPN
- Goiter
- Hypothyroidism
- Iron deficiency anemia
- Zinc deficiencies

When NOT to use minerals

- Shellfish or iodine allergies

Adverse reactions to watch for

- Nausea, vomiting, gastric ulceration, rash, joint swelling, bronchospasms, convulsion, coma, kidney or liver damage, diarrhea, lethargy, altered behavior, diminished reflexes, photophobia, metallic taste, skin lesions, eyelid swelling, increased saliva production, goiter, bloody diarrhea, fever, depression, mouth tenderness, GI irritation, constipation, and darkened or blackened stools, stained teeth, anorexia, headache, Parkinson disease–like symptoms, gout-like symptoms, alopecia, garlic breath odor, gastric ulceration, elevated serum amylase level, hypothermia, hypotension

- To avoid toxicity, advise the patient against self-dosing with megadoses of vitamins without specific indications
- Instruct the patient in food sources of vitamins
- Monitor prothrombin time of a patient receiving vitamin K to determine effectiveness

MINERALS

Mechanism of action

- Act as the component of many enzyme actions
- Chromium potentiates the action of insulin and regulation of lipoprotein metabolism
- Iron is an essential mineral that's a component of hemoglobin, myoglobin, and other enzymes and is a major factor in oxygen transport

Pharmacokinetics

- Varies with each mineral

Drug examples

- Chromium (Chroma-Pak), copper (Coppertrace), iodine (SSKI solution), iron sulfate (ferrous sulfate [Feosol]), manganese (Manganese Gluconate), molybdenum (Molypen), selenium (Sele-Pak), zinc (Orazinc)

Indications

- Minerals are used for oral intake inadequate to meet nutritional needs
- Chromium and molybdenum are used primarily in patients receiving long-term TPN
- Copper and selenium are used as supplements in TPN
- Iodine is used to treat goiter and hypothyroidism caused by iodine deficiency
- Iron is used to correct iron deficiency anemia or as iron supplementation
- Manganese is used as a dietary supplement
- Zinc is used to treat zinc deficiencies

Contraindications and precautions

- Don't give preparations containing iodine to patients allergic to shellfish or iodine
- Take seizure precautions in patients receiving large doses of chromium

Adverse reactions

- Chromium: nausea, vomiting, gastric ulceration, rash, joint swelling, bronchospasms, convulsion, coma, kidney or liver damage
- Copper: diarrhea, lethargy, altered behavior, diminished reflexes, photophobia
- Iodine: metallic taste, skin lesions, eyelid swelling, increased saliva production, goiter, bloody diarrhea, fever, depression, and mouth, gum, and salivary gland tenderness
- Iron: may cause nausea, vomiting, GI irritation, constipation, diarrhea, and darkened or blackened stools, and may stain teeth (liquid form)

- Manganese: anorexia, diarrhea, headache, Parkinson disease–like symptoms
- Molybdenum: gout-like symptoms
- Selenium: alopecia, skin lesions, GI irritation, garlic breath odor
- Zinc: stomach irritation, gastric ulceration, diarrhea, vomiting, elevated serum amylase level, hypothermia, hypotension

Interactions

- None significant

Nursing responsibilities

- Assess the patient's nutritional status; include dietary recall and anthropometric measurements
- Obtain diagnostic test results to establish baseline values, identify deficiencies, and evaluate progress after supplementation
- Weigh the patient before initiating therapy to establish a baseline; check daily weights to evaluate for changes
- Teach the patient about the mineral to be used, and review any special modifications or procedures needed for administration
- Reinforce instructions on a well-balanced diet, with emphasis on food allowances and restrictions
- Dilute liquid preparations well before administration
- Monitor hydration if the patient experiences vomiting or diarrhea
- Dilute parenteral solution well and administer via a central venous line
- Monitor the patient closely for signs and symptoms of toxicity
- Institute seizure precautions for patients receiving large doses of chromium
- **Assess the patient for allergies to iodine or shellfish before administering an iodine preparation**
- Consider the mineral content of a patient's diet in addition to mineral supplements to prevent possible toxicity
- Give iron on an empty stomach; however, if GI upset occurs, give after meals or with food
- Don't give iron within 2 hours of antacids, tetracyclines, or fluoroquinolones
- **Give iron liquid preparations in water or juice and through a straw to prevent tooth stains**
- **When giving iron parenterally, use the Z-track method to prevent staining the skin**

Key nursing actions

- Assess nutritional status; include dietary recall and anthropometric measurements.
- Teach about the mineral to be used, and review any special modifications or procedures needed for administration.
- Monitor closely for signs and symptoms of toxicity.
- Assess for allergies to iodine or shellfish before administering an iodine preparation.
- Give iron liquid preparations in water or juice and through a straw to prevent tooth stains.
- When giving iron parenterally, use the Z-track method to prevent staining the skin.

NCLEX CHECKS

It's never too soon to begin your NCLEX preparation. Now that you've reviewed this chapter, carefully read each of the following questions and choose the best answer. Then compare your responses to the correct answers.

1. A 78-year-old woman who weighs 94 lb (42.6 kg) is to receive Sustacal, 240 ml, between meals as a nutritional supplement. The most important factor to consider before giving this product is that:

- [ ] A. it provides 20 cal/ml.
- [ ] B. it's a low-carbohydrate, high-protein supplement.
- [ ] C. the patient must have an intact digestive system.
- [ ] D. when given by itself, it's nutritionally incomplete.

2. A patient with intestinal cancer is started on total parenteral nutrition (TPN) at 25 ml/hour for the first 12 hours. This rate was selected because it:

- [ ] A. helps prevent catheter-site infections.
- [ ] B. reverses fluid volume deficit from low oral intake of fluids.
- [ ] C. allows the body to adjust to the increased glucose levels.
- [ ] D. reverses the negative nitrogen balance caused by the patient's cancer.

3. Magnesium sulfate is prescribed to a patient diagnosed with preeclampsia (pregnancy-induced hypertension). Which statement about magnesium sulfate is correct?

- [ ] A. Calcium gluconate is the antidote for magnesium toxicity.
- [ ] B. Magnesium sulfate is incompatible with normal saline solution.
- [ ] C. Magnesium sulfate increases acetylcholine released by nerve impulses.
- [ ] D. Enhanced knee jerk and patellar reflexes are signs of impending magnesium toxicity.

4. A patient is diagnosed with pernicious anemia. Which drug is used in the treatment of pernicious anemia?

- [ ] A. Ferrous sulfate (Feosol)
- [ ] B. Iron dextran (INFeD)
- [ ] C. Thiamine (Biamine)
- [ ] D. Cyanocobalamin (Vitamin B_{12})

5. You're teaching a patient taking ferrous sulfate (Feosol). Which of the following statements by the patient indicates that your teaching was successful?

- [ ] A. "If I miss a dose, I need to double the next dose."
- [ ] B. "I should eat extra fiber and whole-grain cereals."
- [ ] C. "I only need to take it when my stomach hurts bad."
- [ ] D. "Smoking won't harm the drug's effectiveness. It might even help."

6. The physician orders an I.V. infusion of dextrose 5% in quarter-normal saline solution to be infused at 7 ml/kg/hour for a 10-month-old infant. The infant weighs 22 lb. How many ml/hr should the nurse infuse of the ordered solution?

____

TOP 4

Items to study before your next test on nutritional agents and the body

1. Purpose of each nutritional agent
2. Common adverse effects of nutritional agents
3. Nursing responsibilities when administering nutritional agents
4. Patient teaching related to nutritional agents

ANSWERS AND RATIONALES

1. CORRECT ANSWER: C

Sustacal, like many other supplements, is a milk-based product that requires an intact digestive system for breakdown and absorption of the supplement. Sustacal provides 1 cal/ml and is a nutritionally complete product. It's high in carbohydrates and fats, but lower in proteins.

2. CORRECT ANSWER: C
The high glucose content of TPN can cause hyperglycemia if TPN is started at too fast a rate, so TPN is started at a slow rate to allow the body to adjust to increased glucose levels. 25 ml/hour is considered a slow rate for TPN and would be appropriate to infuse the TPN for the first 12 hours. Catheter-site infections are best prevented by good aseptic technique. The rate would need to be faster to affect fluid volume deficit. The negative nitrogen balance would be reversed with faster rates of TPN.

3. CORRECT ANSWER: A
Calcium gluconate reverses magnesium toxicity. Because magnesium toxicity is a danger with magnesium sulfate therapy, this antidote should be immediately available at all times during magnesium sulfate therapy. Magnesium sulfate is compatible with normal saline solution. Magnesium sulfate decreases (not increases) acetylcholine released by nerve impulses. The absence (not the presence) of knee-jerk and patellar reflexes is a sign of impending magnesium toxicity.

4. CORRECT ANSWER: D
Pernicious anemia results from the lack of intrinsic factor, which is essential for vitamin B_{12} absorption. Lifelong vitamin B_{12} therapy is given to patients lacking intrinsic factor. Ferrous sulfate and iron dextran are indicated for treatment of iron deficiency anemia. Thiamine is indicated for anemia that results from thiamine deficiency.

5. CORRECT ANSWER: B
Constipation is a common adverse reaction to ferrous sulfate therapy. Eating extra fiber and whole-grain cereals will help decrease the risk of constipation. Missed doses of ferrous sulfate should be taken as soon as possible, but doses should never be doubled. Ferrous sulfate should be taken on a scheduled basis, not in response to symptoms, for the full term of therapy. Smoking should always be avoided.

6. CORRECT ANSWER: 70
To perform this dosage calculation, the nurse should first convert the infant's weight to kilograms:

$$2.2 \text{ lb/kg} = 22 \text{ lb/X kg}$$

$$X = 22 \div 2.2$$

$$X = 10 \text{ kg}$$

Next, she should multiply the infant's weight by the ordered rate:

$$10 \text{ kg} \times 7 \text{ ml/kg/hr} = 70 \text{ ml/hr}$$

Herbal drugs

HERBAL MEDICINE	COMMON USES	SPECIAL CONSIDERATIONS
Aloe	*Oral* • Constipation • Bowel evacuation *Topical* • Minor burns • Skin irritation	• The laxative actions of aloe may take up to 10 hours after ingestion to be effective. • Monitor the patient for signs of dehydration; geriatric patients are particularly at risk.
Chamomile	*Oral* • Anxiety or restlessness • Diarrhea • Motion sickness • Indigestion *Topical* • Inflammation • Wound healing • Cutaneous burns *Teas* • Sedation • Relaxation	• People sensitive to ragweed and chrysanthemums or others in the *Compositae* family may be more susceptible to contact allergies and anaphylaxis. • Patients with hay fever or bronchial asthma caused by pollens are more susceptible to anaphylactic reactions. • Pregnant women should not use chamomile. • Chamomile may enhance anticoagulant's effect.
Cranberry	• Prophylaxis for UTI • Treatment of UTI • Prevention of renal calculi	• Only the unsweetened form of cranberry prevents bacteria from adhering to the bladder wall and preventing or treating UTIs
Echinacea	• Supportive therapy to prevent and treat common cold and acute and chronic infections of the upper respiratory tract	• Echinacea is considered supportive therapy and should not be used in place of antibiotic therapy.
Feverfew	• Prevention and treatment of migraines and headaches • Hot flashes • Rheumatoid arthritis • Asthma • Menstrual problems	• Avoid using in pregnant patients because feverfew is also an abortifacient. • Feverfew may increase the risk of abnormal bleeding when combined with an anticoagulant or antiplatelet. • Abruptly stopping feverfew may cause "postfeverfew syndrome" involving tension headaches, insomnia, joint stiffness and pain, and lethargy.
Garlic	• Decrease cholesterol and triglyceride levels • Prevent atherosclerosis • Age-related vascular changes • Prevent GI cancer • Coughs, colds, fevers, and sore throats	• Odor of garlic may be apparent on breath and skin. • Garlic may prolong bleeding time in patients receiving anticoagulants. • Excess raw garlic intake may increase the risk of adverse reactions. • Garlic should not be used in patients with diabetes, insomnia, pemphigus, organ transplants, or rheumatoid arthritis or in those who have recently undergone surgery.
Ginger	• Nausea (antiemetic) • Motion sickness • Morning sickness • GI upset (colic, flatulence, indigestion) • Hypercholesteremia • Liver toxicity	• Ginger may increase the risk of bleeding, bruising, or nosebleeds. • Pregnant women should obtain medical advice before using ginger medicinally. • Ginger may interfere with the intended therapeutic effects of certain conventional drugs.

HERBAL MEDICINE	COMMON USES	SPECIAL CONSIDERATIONS
Ginger *(continued)*	• Burns • Ulcers • Depression	
Ginkgo biloba	• "Memory" agent • Alzheimer's disease • Multi-infarct dementia • Cerebral insufficiency • Intermittent claudication • Tinnitus • Headache	• Adverse effects occur in less than 1% of patients; the most common is GI upset. • Ginkgo biloba may potentiate anticoagulants and increase the risk of bleeding. • Ginkgo extracts are considered standardized if they contain 24% flavonoid glycosides and 6% terpene lactones. • Seizures have been reported in children after ingestion of more then 50 seeds. • Treatment should continue for 6 to 8 weeks but for no more than 3 months.
Ginseng	• Fatigue • Improve concentration • Treat atherosclerosis • Also believed to strengthen the body and increase resistance to disease after sickness or weakness	• Ginseng may cause severe adverse reactions when taken in large doses (> 3 g per day for 2 years), such as increased motor and cognitive activity with significant diarrhea, nervousness, insomnia, hypertension, edema, and skin eruptions. • Ginseng may potentiate anticoagulants and increase the risk of bleeding.
Green tea	• Prevent cancer • Hyperlipidemia • Atherosclerosis • Dental caries • Headaches • CNS stimulant • Mild diuretic	• Green tea contains caffeine. • Avoid prolonged and high caffeine intake, which may cause restlessness, irritability, insomnia, palpitations, vertigo, headache, and adverse GI effects. • Adding milk may decrease adverse GI effects of green tea. • Green tea may potentiate anticoagulants and increase the risk of bleeding.
Kava	• Anti-anxiety • Stress • Restlessness • Sedation • Promote wound healing • Headache • Seizure disorders • Common cold • Respiratory infections	• Kava is contraindicated in pregnancy and lactation. • Kava should not be used in combination with St. John's wort. • Kava should not be taken with other CNS depressants, MAO inhibitors, levodopa, antiplatelets, alcohol, or anxiolytics. • Kava can cause drowsiness and may impair motor reflexes and mental acuity; advise the patient to avoid hazardous activities. • Effects should appear within 2 days of initiation of therapy.
St. John's wort	• Mild to moderate depression • Anxiety • Psychovegetative disorders • Sciatica • Viral infections	• Effects may take several weeks; however, if no improvement occurs after 4 to 6 weeks, consider alternative therapy. • St. John's wort interacts with many different types of drugs. • St. John's wort should not be used in combination with prescription antidepressants or anti-anxiety medications.
Vitex	• Premenstrual syndrome	• Vitex should be taken in the morning with water. • Vitex is a very slow acting substance; it may take several cycles to see an effect.
Yohimbine	• Impotence (works as an aphrodisiac)	• Yohimbine may cause CNS excitation, including tremor, sleeplessness, anxiety, increased blood pressure, and tachycardia. • Don't use in patients with renal or hepatic insufficiency.

Commonly abused substances

SUBSTANCE	IMMEDIATE EFFECTS	WITHDRAWAL SYMPTOMS	ROUTE
Tobacco/nicotine	• Stimulant • Increased heart rate	Intense craving, tension, irritability, difficulty concentrating, drowsiness, weight gain, headache	• Chewing, smoking
Caffeine	• Stimulant • Increased alertness, sleep delay • May increase heart rate in sufficient quantities	Severe throbbing headaches, drowsiness or decreased sociability and anxiety, muscle stiffness, nausea and waves of hot or cold sensations sweeping the body	• Oral via drinks or OTC products
Amphetamine ("Speed")	• Stimulant • Excitement, increased activity, decreased appetite, may delay sleep	Anxiety, agitation, fatigue, extended sleep increased appetite, psychosis, suicidal thoughts	• Snorting • Injecting • Oral • Rectally
Cocaine	• Feeling of self-confidence and power • Increased energy • Decreased appetite	Agitation, depression, intense craving for the drug, extreme fatigue, anxiety, angry outbursts, lack of motivation, nausea and vomiting, shaking, irritability, muscle pain, disturbed sleep	• Snorting • Injecting • Oral • Smoking • Rectally
MDMA ("Ecstasy")	• Increased confidence • Feeling of closeness with others • Sensation of floating, anxiety, nausea, paranoia	Depression, anxiety, sleeplessness, depersonalization, de-realization, paranoid delusions	• Oral • Injecting • Rectally
Alcohol	• Slurring of speech • Loss of inhibitions, relaxation, feeling of happiness and well-being • Large amounts can lead to unconsciousness	Tremors, nausea, anxiety, sweats, sleep disturbances, visual or tactile hallucinations, seizure, vomiting, diarrhea	• Oral
Benzodiazepines (Ativan, Valium, Xanax, Serax)	• Calmness, relief of tension, drowsiness, muscle relaxation, blurred vision	Anxiety, sleep disturbances, hypersensitivity to light, noise, touch, perceptual disturbances, feelings of unreality, memory impairment, headache, depression, suicidal thoughts, agoraphobia, seizure	• Oral • Injecting • Rectally
Opioids (heroin, morphine, Dillaudid, oxycodone, methadone)	• Pain relief and anxiety • Feeling of well-being • Diminished awareness of outside world • Drowsiness • Large doses may lead to unconsciousness and death	Lacrimination, rhinorrhea, perspiration, restlessness, insomnia, dilated pupils, anorexia, nausea, weakness, muscle aches, abdominal cramps, diarrhea, fatigue	• Oral • Injecting • Rectal • Smoking • Snorting
Marijuana	• Relaxation, increased appetite, slowing down of time • Poor coordination, blood shot eyes • May be hallucinogenic	Irritability, anxiety, physical tension, decreases in appetite and mood	• Oral • Smoking

SUBSTANCE	IMMEDIATE EFFECTS	WITHDRAWAL SYMPTOMS	ROUTE
Hydrocarbon (petrol, glue, aerosol cans, butane gas)	• Feeling of happiness, relaxation, drowsiness	Sweating, rapid pulse, hand tremors, insomnia, nausea or vomiting, hallucinations, and, in severe cases, grand mal seizures	• Inhalation
LSD ("Magic mushroom," "Trip")	• Hallucinations • Anxious feelings, panic • Nausea	Minimal physical withdrawal	• Oral
GHB (gamma hydroxybutyrate) ("Fantasy")	• Euphoria, happy, sociable; with high doses, dizziness, sleepiness, vomiting, muscle spasms, loss of consciousness	Early symptoms: insomnia, tremor, anxiety, confusion, nausea and vomiting Later symptoms: agitation, vivid hallucinations, combative behavior, disorientation	• Oral
2CB ("Nexus," "Venus," "Brom")	• Hallucinogen, heightened visual imagery, acute awareness of body, increased sensitivity to smells and tastes, sexual stimulation	Depression, anxiety, sleeplessness, depersonalization, de-realization, paranoid delusions	• Primarily oral, but can be snorted or smoked
Rohypnol ("Date rape drug," "Rib," "Roofies," "R2," "Roachies")	• Tranquilization for brief period	Headache, muscle pain, confusion, hallucinations, seizures	• Oral

Glossary

accommodation: adjustment of the eye by contraction of ciliary muscles and a change in the lens curvature that allows focusing at various distances; inhibited by cycloplegic drugs, which paralyze ciliary muscles

acetylcholinesterase inhibitors: drugs that increase parasympathetic activity and block the action of acetylcholinesterase, an enzyme that inhibits the action of acetylcholine

action potential: electrical impulse across nerve or muscle fibers that have been stimulated

adrenergic agonists: drugs that mimic the effects of the sympathetic nervous system

adrenergic blocking drugs: drugs that interfere with transmission of nerve impulses to adrenergic receptors, allowing a parasympathetic response

adrenocortical: pertaining to the adrenal cortex (the largest portion of the adrenal gland), which produces androgens, glucocorticoids, mineralocorticoids, and other hormones

afterload: pressure in the arteries leading from the left ventricle that must be overcome by the left ventricle during systole to open the semilunar valves and eject blood

agranulocytosis: severe and acute decrease in granulocytes (basophils, eosinophils, and neutrophils) as an adverse reaction to a drug or radiation therapy resulting in high fever, exhaustion, and bleeding ulcers of the throat, mucus membranes, and GI tract

akinesia: complete or partial loss of movement

alopecia: loss of hair

angioedema: life-threatening reaction causing sudden swelling of tissues around the face, neck, lips, tongue, throat, hands, feed, genitals, or intestines

angiotensin: polypeptide in the blood that causes vasoconstriction (angiotensin I, which is physiologically inactive, is the precursor of angiotensin II)

anticoagulant drugs: drugs that prevent clot formation or extension but do not speed dissolution of preexisting clots (which occurs naturally in 7 days)

antilipemic drugs: drugs used to prevent or treat increased accumulation of fatty substances (lipids) in the blood

antipyretic: pertaining to a substance or procedure that reduces fever

aphakic: without a lens

aplastic anemia: anemia characterized by a decrease in erythrocytes and hemoglobin, usually caused by bone marrow failure from neoplastic bone marrow disease or by destruction of the bone marrow by exposure to toxic chemicals, radiation, or certain medications; usually associated with granulocytopenia and thrombocytopenia; also known as *pancytopenia*

arthralgia: any joint pain

ataxia: incoordination of voluntary muscle action, particularly during such activities as walking and reaching for objects

atrial fibrillation: extremely rapid atrial contraction (200 to 400 contractions per minute) with a variable ventricular contraction response

atrioventricular block: slowed conduction or cessation of the excitatory impulse of the heart, occurring at the atrioventricular node or the bundle of His or its branches

attention deficit hyperactivity disorder: syndrome that may include decreased attention span, increased impulsiveness and emotional lability, and impairment in such areas as perception, language, memory, and motor skills; usually also includes hyperactivity

azotemia: toxic renal condition caused by insufficient kidney function and subsequent retention of urea in the blood; also known as *uremia*

bacteriocidal: causing death of bacteria

bacteriostatic: inhibiting or retarding bacterial growth

bioavailability: rate and extent to which a drug enters the circulation, thereby gaining access to target tissue

bipolar affective disorders: affective disorders characterized by mania and overactivity, depression and decreased activity, or a combination or alternation of the two

blood-brain barrier: barrier separating the parenchyma of the central nervous system from the circulating blood, preventing certain substances from reaching the brain or cerebrospinal fluid

blood dyscrasias: diseases of the blood

bone age: determination of the stage of development of the ossification centers of long bones, where cartilage is replaced with true bone during development

bone marrow depression: hematologic toxicity causing a decrease in blood cell production that may lead to thrombocytopenia, leukopenia, and anemia

bradykinesia: abnormally slow body movements

bronchospasm: narrowing of the bronchioles resulting from an increase in smooth muscle tone; causes wheezing

cardioacceleration: increase in heart muscle action

cell-mediated immunity: immunity mediated by T lymphocytes; involved in such responses as delayed hypersensitivity reactions, graft rejection, and defense against certain bacterial, viral, and fungal pathogens

cholinergic crisis: situation caused by overdose of an antimyasthenic drug, resulting in muscle weakness, dyspnea, and dysphagia (usually within 1 hour of drug administration); other symptoms may include increased respiratory secretions and saliva, nausea, vomiting, cramping, diarrhea, and diaphoresis

Chvostek's sign: abnormal spasm of facial muscles elicited by light taps on the facial nerve; indicates hypocalcemic tetany

controlled substances: depressant and stimulant drugs and drugs of abuse or potential abuse whose distribution and use are controlled under the Comprehensive Drug Abuse Prevention Act of 1970

corneal reflex: closing of the eyelids on direct touch or irritation of the eye; disappears with application of corneal anesthetics

cross-sensitivity: hypersensitivity or allergy to one anti-infective drug in a particular class (for example, penicillins) that may cause an allergic reaction to another anti-infective drug in the same class

crystalluria: presence of crystals in urine

Cushing's syndrome: metabolic disorder caused by an increased production of corticotropin from a tumor of the adrenal cortex or of the anterior lobe of the pituitary gland or by excessive intake of glucocorticoids; characterized by central obesity, "moon face," glucose intolerance, growth suppression in children, and muscle weakness

cyclic adenosine monophosphate: nucleotide produced by stimulation of $beta_2$ receptors in the lungs; causes bronchodilation when released

debriding drugs: those used to remove foreign material and dead or damaged tissue from a wound or burn

depolarizing neuromuscular blocking drugs: drugs (such as succinylcholine) that disrupt nerve impulse transmissions at the motor end plate, resulting in skeletal muscle relaxation

digitalization: administration of a larger-than-maintenance dose (loading dose) of cardiac glycosides to attain a therapeutic serum level rapidly; necessitates close patient observation to detect toxicity

disseminated intravascular coagulation: life-threatening coagulopathy caused by overstimulation of the body's clotting and anti-clotting processes in response to disease, septicemia, neoplasms, obstetric emergencies, severe trauma, prolonged surgery, and hemorrhage

distal tubule: portion of the renal tubule located after the loop of Henle that regulates water and acid-base balance

dysphoria: feelings of unrest, restlessness, and anxiety

emesis: vomiting

endometriosis: abnormal condition characterized by ectopic growth and function of the endometrium

enuresis: urinary incontinence, especially in bed at night (called *nocturnal enuresis*)

eosinophilia: increase number of eosinophils in the blood accompanying many inflammatory conditions; substantial increases are usually from an allergic reaction

epiphyses: ends of a long bone that are separated from the shaft by a cartilaginous disk (epiphyseal plate) until growth stops

erythema: redness of the skin caused by dilatation and congestion of the capillaries; often signifies an inflammation or infection

erythropoiesis: formation of red blood cells

extrapyramidal symptoms: symptoms caused by an imbalance in the extrapyramidal portion of the nervous system; typically include pill-rolling motions, drooling, tremors, rigidity, and shuffling gait

extravasation: infiltration of intravenous fluid

gingival hyperplasia: overgrowth of gum tissue

glomerular filtrate: fluid remaining in the renal tubule after filtration of blood in the glomerulus

glucocorticoids: steroid hormones secreted by the adrenal cortex that promote formation of carbohydrates from noncarbohydrate molecules and exert an anti-inflammatory effect (among their many functions); may be administered exogenously as replacement therapy for adrenocortical insufficiency

goiter: enlarged thyroid gland, usually manifested as a swelling in the neck

gonadal suppression: condition characterized by a decrease in the number or function of reproductive cells

gout: disorder of purine metabolism causing high serum uric acid levels; leads to joint pain and inflammation, usually begins in the knee or foot

gram-negative: having the pink color of the counterstain used in Gram's method of staining microorganisms

gram-positive: retaining the violet color of stain used in Gram's method of staining microorganisms

gray baby syndrome: life-threatening condition in neonates (especially premature babies) who are given chloramphenicol for a bacterial infection, like meningitis; symptoms usually appear 2 to 9 days after therapy has started and include vomiting, loose green stools, refusal to suck, hypotension, cyanosis or gray coloring, low body temperature, and cardiovascular collapse

hemochromatosis: rare disorder of iron storage characterized by excessive accumulation of iron

hemolytic anemia: anemia resulting from hemolysis, or premature destruction of red blood cells

hepatic encephalopathy: condition usually caused by severe liver impairment, characterized by changes in level of consciousness, personality changes, memory loss, flapping tremor of the hand, hyperreflexia, and hyperventilation

hepatotoxicity: quality of being toxic to or capable of destroying liver cells

herpes keratitis: infection of the cornea by the herpes simplex virus, leading to chronic inflammation, scarring, and possible vision loss

herpetic encephalitis: acute brain disease caused by herpes simplex virus, characterized by early repeated seizures and signs indicating temporal or frontal lobe involvement

hirsutism: excessive growth of dark and course body hair in a masculine distribution

histamine-2 receptors: cells in the gastric mucosa that respond to histamine release by increasing gastric acid secretion

host cells: cells in which a parasitic organism is nourished and harbored

hypercalcemia: excessive amounts of calcium in the blood, causing confusion, anorexia, abdominal pain, muscle pain, and weakness

hyperglycemia: abnormally high blood glucose level, usually associated with diabetes mellitus; typically results in frequent urination, fatigue, excessive thirst, weight loss, blurred vision, poor wound healing, flushed dry skin, and fruity breath odor

hyperkalemia: excessive potassium in the blood causing nausea, vomiting, fatigue, weakness, palpitations, and irregular heartbeat

hyperlipoproteinemia: abnormally high levels of serum lipoproteins

hypermagnesemia: excessive magnesium in the blood; toxic levels may cause cardiac arrhythmias, respiratory depression, and deep tendon reflex depression

hypernatremia: excessive sodium levels in the blood, causing confusion, seizures, coma, dysrhythmic muscle twitching, lethargy, tachycardia, and irritability

hyperplasia: increase number of cells

hypertensive crisis: medical emergency characterized by a sudden, severe increase in diastolic blood pressure to a level exceeding 120 mm Hg

hyperthyroidism: disorder caused by oversecretion of the thyroid gland, characterized by increased metabolism and goiter

hypocalcemia: decreased serum calcium levels that may cause cardiac arrhythmias, muscle twitching or cramping, and numbness and tingling of the hands, feet, lips, and tongue

hypoglycemia: abnormally low serum glucose level, usually caused by administration of too much insulin, excessive insulin secretion by pancreatic islet cells, or dietary deficiency; typically leads to anxiety, chills, cold sweats, confusion, cool pale skin, difficulty concentrating, drowsiness, excessive hunger, nausea, irritability, nervousness, rapid pulse, unusual fatigue, and weakness

hypokalemia: abnormally low serum potassium level, typically resulting in muscular weakness, tetany, and orthostatic hypotension

hypomagnesemia: abnormally low serum magnesium level, causing nausea, vomiting, muscle weakness, tremors, tetany, and lethargy

hyponatremia: low sodium level that may cause anorexia, headache, muscle cramps, obtundation, coma, or seizures

hypothyroidism: disorder caused by undersecretion of the thyroid gland, characterized by decreased metabolism, fatigue, and cold sensitivity

idiopathic: of unknown cause

keratin: protein that is the main constituent of the epidermis, hair, and nails

leukocytosis: abnormal increase in circulating WBCs

leukopenia: abnormal decrease in WBCs to fewer than 5,000 cells/μl

lipid pneumonia: pneumonia resulting from aspiration of oil, such as oily nose drops or mineral oil

lipodystrophy: thickening of tissues and accumulation of fat at an injection site; results from too-frequent injection of insulin in the same site

loop of Henle: U-shaped portion of a renal tubule, consisting of a thin descending limb and a thick ascending limb; changes in its permeability to water and sodium alter urine osmolality

malaise: general overall feeling or discomfort, uneasiness, or fatigue; often the first indication of an infection or other disease

malignant hyperthermia: potentially fatal reaction to an inhalation anesthetic characterized by a marked increase in the rate of muscle metabolism, a rapid temperature rise, and muscular rigidity

mineralocorticoids: steroid hormones secreted by the adrenal cortex that maintain normal blood volume and promote sodium retention and urinary excretion of potassium; may be administered exogenously as replacement therapy for adrenocortical insufficiency

mitosis: division of a parent cell into two daughter cells

monoamine oxidase: enzyme that catalyzes the oxidation of amines (including dopamine)

muscarinic receptors: receptors in effector cells that are stimulated by acetylcholine, muscarine, or a similar substance

myalgia: diffuse muscle pain, usually associated with malaise

myasthenia gravis: disease characterized by muscle weakness that may involve all skeletal muscle groups, including muscles responsible for swallowing and breathing

myasthenic crisis: situation caused by underdose of or resistance to an antimyasthenic drug; signs and symptoms, such as muscle weakness, dyspnea, and dysphagia usually occur 3 or more hours after drug administration

mydriasis: dilation of the pupil

myocardial oxygen consumption: amount of oxygen the heart uses during each beat; increases as the work of the heart increases (such as from increased preload and afterload)

myopia: vision defect in which objects can be seen distinctly only when held close to the eyes (also called *nearsightedness*)

narcolepsy: chronic ailment characterized by recurrent attacks of drowsiness and sleep; the patient cannot control the spells but is easily awakened

National Formulary: official source of detailed drug information used in the United States

necrotic: pertaining to localized tissue death

nephrotic syndrome: abnormal kidney condition characterized by marked proteinuria, hypoalbuminemia, and edema

nephrotoxicity: quality of being toxic to or capable of destruction of kidney cells

neuroleptic malignant syndrome: life-threatening, rare syndrome caused by antipsychotic drugs, characterized by extreme diaphoresis, muscle rigidity, tachycardia, fever, and renal failure

neurotransmitter: substance (such as acetylcholine, dopamine, or norepinephrine) that is released when an axon terminal of a presynaptic neuron is excited; the substance then travels across the synapse to the target cell to inhibit or excite it

neutropenia: abnormal decrease in circulating neutrophils

nicotinic receptors: receptors in effector cells that are stimulated by acetylcholine and nicotine

nondepolarizing neuromuscular blocking drugs: drugs that block nicotinic receptors, ultimately blocking acetylcholine's transmission and preventing muscle membrane depolarization

nonproductive cough: dry, hacking cough that does not produce sputum

nonpyogenic: without pus production

norepinephrine: neurotransmitter that increases blood pressure by vasoconstriction without affecting cardiac output

nystagmus: constant involuntary eye movement

occult bleeding: bleeding that is not visible by gross inspection and can be detected only by chemical methods (guaiac) or with a microscope

opioid agonist-antagonists: drugs that possess partial antagonist properties (they block further narcotic binding at the opiate receptor sites they occupy) and may cause withdrawal symptoms in patients with physical dependence on opioids

optic neuritis: inflammation, and usually degeneration, of the optic nerve

orthostatic hypotension: abnormally low blood pressure that occurs when a person stands; also known as *postural hypotension*

osmotic pressure: pressure that develops between two solutions of different concentrations separated by a semipermeable membrane

otitis externa: infection or inflammation of the external ear canal or auricle

otitis media: infection or inflammation of the middle ear

ototoxicity: potentially irreversible damage to the auditory and vestibular branches of the eighth cranial nerve; may cause hearing or balance loss

Paget's disease: chronic progressive bone disorder characterized by excessive bone destruction and unorganized bone repair

pancytopenia: abnormal decrease in erythrocytes, WBCs and platelets; also known as *aplastic anemia*

parasympatholytic drugs: drugs that block the effects of the parasympathetic nervous system, allowing a sympathetic response

parasympathomimetic drugs: drugs that mimic the effects of the parasympathetic nervous system

paresthesia: abnormal sensations (including numbness, prickling, and tingling) with no known cause

Parkinson's disease: idiopathic form of parkinsonism caused by degeneration of dopamine-containing neurons in the basal ganglia of the brain

parkinsonism: neurologic disorder characterized by tremors, muscle rigidity and weakness, and hypokinesia

partial thromboplastin time: diagnostic test for coagulation defects of the intrinsic system (except factors VII and XIII)

peak and trough drug concentration levels: serum drug concentration levels measured to determine whether the dosing regimen is therapeutic or toxic; blood for peak concentration level is drawn immediately after the dose is administered; blood for trough concentration level is drawn just before the next dose is administered

peptic ulcer: lesion of the mucous membrane of the stomach, duodenum, or other part of the GI system that is exposed to acid and pepsin gastric juices

peripheral neuropathy: inflammation and degeneration of peripheral nerves; usually associated with numbness, tingling, burning, or pain in extremities

pernicious anemia: chronic anemia caused by failure of the stomach to secrete enough intrinsic factor to ensure intestinal absorption of vitamin B_{12}

phlebitis: inflammation of a vein

photosensitivity reaction: increased reaction of the skin to sunlight; may result in edema, papules, urticaria, or acute burns

pituitary dwarfism: form of dwarfism (underdevelopment of the body) caused by deficient production of growth hormone by the anterior pituitary gland

potentiate: to increase the action of another drug so that the combined effect of both drugs is greater than the effect of either drug alone

preload: volume of blood in the ventricles at the end of diastole

priapism: abnormal, painful, prolonged, or constant penile erection, usually without sexual desire

proteinuria: presence of an abnormally large amount of protein (usually albumin) in the urine

prothrombin time: diagnostic test for coagulation defects caused by deficiency of factor V, VII, or X

pruritus: itching

pseudomembranous colitis: complication of prolonged antibiotic therapy that causes severe inflammation of the colon, usually from *Clostridium difficile*; causes watery diarrhea, abdominal pain and cramping, and fevers

pseudotumor cerebri: benign intracranial hypertension, most common in women ages 20 to 50, caused by increased pressure in the brain, causing headache, dizziness, nausea, vomiting, and ringing or rushing in the ears

psychosis: major mental illness characterized by personality disintegration and loss of touch with reality; may include auditory and visual hallucinations and delusions

rhabdomyolysis: acute and potentially fatal skeletal muscle disease

Raynaud's disease: vasospastic disorder characterized by bilaterally symmetrical pallor and cyanosis of the fingers and precipitated by cold or emotional upset

refractory period: period of relaxation after muscle excitement

Reye syndrome: encephalopathy affecting children linked to use of aspirin and other salicylate-containing medications, as well as other causes; syndrome may follow an upper respiratory infection or chicken pox; its onset is rapid, usually starting with irritable, combative behavior, and vomiting and progressing to unconsciousness, coma, seizures and, possibly, death

sedative-hypnotic drugs: drugs that exert a soothing or tranquilizing effect while dulling the senses or inducing sleep

serotonin: neurotransmitter that acts as a powerful vasoconstrictor and is thought to be involved in sleep and sensory perception

serotonin syndrome: adverse reaction causing confusion, agitation, restlessness, tachycardia, muscle rigidity or twitching, tremors, and nausea, most often reported in patients taking two or more medications that increase CNS serotonin levels; most common drug combinations are MAO inhibitors, SSRIs, and TCAs

serum drug level: amount of a drug present in the blood at a given moment

sick sinus syndrome: degeneration of the conductive tissue that maintains heart rhythm

Somogyi effect: rebound hyperglycemia caused by an excessive insulin dosage

spasticity: continuous resistance to muscle stretching that results from increased tension and muscle tone, usually caused by an upper motor neuron lesion; results in stiff, awkward movements

status epilepticus: rapid succession of seizures without intervals of consciousness; constitutes a medical emergency

stomatitis: inflammation and possible ulceration of the mucous membranes of the mouth

superinfections: new infections caused by an organism that is usually resistant to the anti-infective prescribed to treat the initial infection; causes such signs and symptoms as furry overgrowth on the tongue, loose or foul-smelling stools, and vaginal itching or discharge

sympatholytic drugs: drugs that inhibit sympathetic activity; may block receptors or prevent release of norepinephrine

sympathomimetic drugs: drugs that mimic the effects of the sympathetic nervous system

syncope: brief loss of consciousness caused by lack of oxygen to the brain

tardive dyskinesia: disorder characterized by involuntary repetitious movements of the muscles of the face, limbs, and trunk; most commonly results from extended periods of treatment with phenothiazine drugs

teratogenic: pertaining to the production of physical defects in an embryo or a fetus

thrombocytopenia: abnormal decrease in platelets, predisposing the patient to bleeding

thrombocytopenic purpura: bleeding disorder characterized by marked decrease in platelets, causing multiple bruises, petechiae, and tissue hemorrhage

thrombolytic drugs: drugs that dissolve a thrombus by activating plasminogen and converting it to plasmin

thyrotoxicosis: toxic condition resulting from thyroid hyperactivity; causes thyroid enlargement, a rapid heart rate, tremors, increased basal metabolism, exophthalmos, nervousness, and weight loss

tinnitus: ringing, buzzing, or whistling in one or both ears occurring without external stimuli; may be caused by an ear infection, drugs, head trauma, or blocked ear canal

T lymphocytes: lymphocytic cells that develop in the thymus and initiate the cell-mediated immune response

Tourette syndrome: neurologic disorder characterized by multiple tics (such as blinking, grimacing, and shrugging) that progresses to grunting, shouting, barking, and in some cases compulsive swearing

transplant rejection: destruction of transplanted material at the cellular level by the immune response of the host

triglyceride: chief lipid in the blood; a fatty acid-glycerol compound that constitutes most animal and vegetable fats

Trousseau's sign: carpal spasm elicited by applying pressure to the upper arm (for example, with a blood pressure cuff); usually indicates hypocalcemic tetany

United States Pharmacopeia (USP): compendium of drugs and their preparation that is issued annually by a national committee of experts; adopted in 1906 as the official standard for drug information in the United States

uric acid: product of protein metabolism that is present in the blood and excreted in the urine

urticaria: itchy skin inflammation characterized by pale wheals with well-defined red edges; usually an allergic response to insect bits, food, or certain drugs

vasospastic angina: uncommon form of angina in which attacks occur during rest rather than activity (also called *Prinzmetal's angina*)

virustatic: quality of slowing the growth of a virus

von Willebrand's disease: inherited coagulation disorder caused by deficiency of factor VIII and characterized by prolonged bleeding time, spontaneous nosebleeds, and gingival bleeding; affects equal numbers of males and females

widening pulse pressure: increase in the differential between systolic and diastolic blood pressures

withdrawal symptoms: unpleasant and sometimes life-threatening physiologic changes occurring when certain drugs are withdrawn after prolonged, regular use; with barbiturates, withdrawal symptoms include anxiety, restlessness, tremors, weakness, dizziness, nausea, vomiting, nightmares, hallucinations, and seizures

Selected references

American Hospital Formulary Service. *Drug Information 2003*. Bethesda, Md.: American Society of Hospital Pharmacists, 2003.

Aschenbrenner, D.S., et al. *Drug Therapy in Nursing.* Philadelphia: Lippincott Williams & Wilkins, 2002.

Drug Information for the Health Care Provider-USPDI, 22nd ed. Rockville, Md.: United States Pharmacopeial Convention, 2002.

Facts and Comparisons. St. Louis: C.V. Mosby Co., 2003.

Illustrated Manual of Nursing Practice, 3rd ed. Springhouse, Pa.: Lippincott Williams & Wilkins, 2002.

Nursing2004 Drug Handbook. Springhouse, Pa.: Lippincott Williams & Wilkins, 2004.

Physician's Drug Reference, 57th ed. Montvale, Md.: Thomson PDR, 2003.

Roach, S., and Scherer, J.C. *Introductory Clinical Pharmacology,* 6th ed. Philadelphia: Lippincott Williams & Wilkins, 2000.

Springhouse Nurse's Drug Guide 2004, 5th ed. Springhouse, Pa.: Lippincott Williams & Wilkins, 2004.

Index

t refers to a table.

ABOUT THE CD-ROM

The enclosed CD-ROM is just one more reason why the *Straight A's* series is at the head of its class. The more than 250 additional NCLEX-style questions contained on the CD provide you with another opportunity to review the material and gauge your knowledge. The program allows you to:

- take tests of varying lengths on subject areas of your choice
- learn the rationales for correct and incorrect answers
- print the results of your tests to measure progress over time.

Minimum system requirements

To operate the *Straight A's* CD-ROM, we recommend that you have the following computer equipment:

- Windows 98 or higher
- Pentium 166 or higher
- 64 MB RAM or more
- 8 MB of free hard-disk space
- SVGA monitor with High Color (16-bit)
- CD-ROM drive
- mouse.

Installation

Before installing the CD-ROM, make sure that your monitor is set to High Color (16-bit) and your display area is set to 800 × 600. If it isn't, consult your monitor's user's manual for instructions about changing the display settings. (The display settings are typically found in Start/Settings/Control Panel/Display/Settings tab.)

To run this program, you must install it onto the hard drive of your computer, following these three steps:

1. Start Windows 98 or higher.
2. Place the CD in your CD-ROM drive. After a few moments, the install process will automatically begin. *Note:* If the install process doesn't automatically begin, click the Start menu and select Run. Type *D:\setup.exe* (where *D:* is the letter of your CD-ROM drive) and then click OK.
3. Follow the on-screen instructions for installation.

Technical support

For technical support, call toll-free 1-800-638-3030, Monday through Friday, 8:30 a.m. to 5 p.m. Eastern Time. You may also write to Lippincott Williams & Wilkins Technical Support, 351 W. Camden Street, Baltimore, MD 21201-2436, or e-mail us at techsupp@lww.com.

This work is protected by copyright. No part of this work may be reproduced in any form or by any means, including photocopying, or utilized by any information storage and retrieval system without written permission from the copyright owner.